Psychiatric Interview of Children and Adolescents

Psychiatric Interview of Children and Adolescents

Claudio Cepeda, M.D.

Adjunct Clinical Professor, Department of Psychiatry,
University of Texas Health Science Center at San Antonio

Lucille Gotanco, M.D.

Assistant Medical Director of Inpatient Services,
Clarity Child Guidance Center, San Antonio, Texas;
Adjunct Assistant Professor, Child and Adolescent
Psychiatry Division, University of Texas Health Science
Center at San Antonio

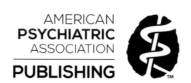

AMERICAN
PSYCHIATRIC
ASSOCIATION
PUBLISHING

If you wish to buy 50 or more copies of the same title, please go to www.appi.org/specialdiscounts for more information.

Copyright © 2017 American Psychiatric Association Publishing

ALL RIGHTS RESERVED

First Edition

Manufactured in the United States of America on acid-free paper

26   25   24   23   5   4   3

American Psychiatric Association Publishing
800 Maine Avenue SW, Suite 900
Washington, DC 20024-2812
www.appi.org

Library of Congress Cataloging-in-Publication Data
Names: Cepeda, Claudio, author. | Gotanco, Lucille, author. | American Psychiatric Association Publishing, publisher.
Title: Psychiatric interview of children and adolescents / Claudio Cepeda, Lucille Gotanco.
Description: First edition. | Arlington, Virginia : American Psychiatric Association Publishing, [2017] | Includes bibliographical references and index.
Identifiers: LCCN 2016039069 (print) | LCCN 2016039706 (ebook) | ISBN 9781615370481 (pbk. : alk. paper) | ISBN 9781615371174 (ebook)
Subjects: | MESH: Interview, Psychological—methods | Child | Mental Disorders—diagnosis | Adolescent | Child Psychiatry—methods | Adolescent Psychiatry—methods
Classification: LCC RJ499.3 (print) | LCC RJ499.3 (ebook) | NLM WS 105 | DDC 618.92/89—dc23
LC record available at https://lccn.loc.gov/2016039069

British Library Cataloguing in Publication Data
A CIP record is available from the British Library.

To my wife, Rosalba,

and to my children,
Claudio Rene and Mary, Adrian and Michelle,
and Joe and Chante

C.C.

Contents

Preface

This book has its roots in the late 1990s, when I was preparing to teach a class on child and adolescent interviewing to fellows in the Child and Adolescent Psychiatry Division at the University of Texas Health Science Center at San Antonio (UTHSCSA). As I began to think about my upcoming course, I sketched out some ideas in writing, which would later serve as the preliminary work for my first book. When I was a medical student, I was highly inspired by one of my internal medicine professors, Professor Rios, whom I grew to admire greatly. He was very detailed in his physical examinations, and he seemed able "to read" the patient's body, listening to the signs and determining organ impairment, by thoroughly inspecting the physical body. This mystified me and my fellow medical student peers. As I began to sketch out the initial version of my book, I wondered whether something similar could be achieved in psychiatry.

This book is the result of an evolution that started with *Concise Guide to the Psychiatric Interview of Children and Adolescents,* published in 2000 by American Psychiatric Press. That book was translated into Japanese, Spanish, and Slovak. A revised and augmented version became *Clinical Manual for the Psychiatric Interview of Children and Adolescents,* published in 2010 by American Psychiatric Publishing. (It was an honor to have Doody Enterprises Inc. review this book and award it five stars and 100 points, the maximum score given by these reviewers.) That text was translated into Polish. I am extraordinarily pleased by the reception of these prior two versions of the present book. The acceptance of these books in the United States and in the international market has been beyond this author's wildest dreams!

The present publication is an updated and revised version of the clinical manual. The chapter on interviewing preschoolers is new, as is the first subsection on bullying in the chapter on the evaluation of abuse and other symptoms.

I asked my colleague and former pupil Lucille Gotanco, M.D., to join me in the project of updating and revising the manual for the present publication. Lucille is a superb practitioner and a dedicated and methodical clinician. Lucille wrote the chapter on the assessment of preschoolers and the subsection on bullying. My thanks go out to her for her contribution.

I would also like to extend my gratitude to Frederick ("Fred") Hines, President of Clarity Child Guidance Center (Clarity CGC),[1] in San Antonio, Texas, for his support of the new publication. Fred gave all the administrative, IT, and secretarial support needed to carry out this project, and he gave his permission to publish the most recent assessment protocol for the written documentation of all the psychiatric evaluations done at Clarity CGC. Under Mr. Hines's leadership, the association of the Division of Child and Adolescent Psychiatry at UTHSCSA with Clarity CGC became closer. Clarity is now the principal clinical site for the training of Child and Adolescent Psychiatry residents in the San Antonio area.

Geoff Gentry, Ph.D., Clarity CGC Senior Vice President of Clinical Services, merits recognition for his unswerving commitment to improving the quality standards at Clarity CGC. The protocol for documentation of the psychiatric evaluations reflects how his efforts have evolved and crystallized.

I also want to express my appreciation to Katrina Hallmark, Psy.D., neuropsychologist and Chief of Psychological Services at Clarity CGC, for reading the draft of the chapter on the neuropsychiatric interview and examination and for the feedback she gave on that chapter. My thanks also go out to Mr. Rick Edwards, Chief of Clinical Services at Clarity CGC, for the case example involving Phillip in the chapter on the comprensive psychiatric formulation.

I have worked at Clarity CGC for 30 years in various clinical roles, including as the Medical Director for a number of years. Currently I am Medical Director of the Urgent Care Clinic and Partial Hospital Services at the Westover Hills Clinic in San Antonio, Texas. It has been a pleasure to work with such a wonderful group of caring professionals.

I would like to express a special appreciation to Ms. Leticia O. Leal, LPC, for the excellent work she did in formatting the draft for the final review and for digitizing the family organigrams/genograms.

---

[1]Clarity Child Guidance Clinic, in San Antonio, Texas, is a nonprofit, comprehensive mental health organization for children and adolescents. This organization started services to the Southwest Texas community in the late 1800s and has been associated with the Department of Psychiatry, University of Texas Health Science Center at San Antonio (UTHSCSA) since the inception of the medical school in 1968. Clarity CGC is a major Clinical Site for the training of child and adolescent psychiatry residents from the Department of Psychiatry, UTHSCSA, and is also a training site for advanced psychology candidates, and for psychiatric nursing and occupational therapy students.

Gratitude also goes out to the staff at American Psychiatric Association Publishing for the thoroughness of the manuscript review and assistance in improving the readability and clarity of the text.

Lastly, I want to reiterate my gratitude to the excellent teachers I had at the University of Michigan in the late 1970's and early 1980's: Humberto Nagera, Jose Carrera, Morton Chethik, Mary Lou Kemme, to name only a few. I carry perpetual memories of their inspiration and teachings.

Claudio Cepeda, M.D.

CHAPTER 1

Diagnostic and Therapeutic Engagement

The diagnostic engagement relates to the rational and emotional involvement of the child or adolescent and his or her family with the examiner for the purpose of establishing a psychiatric diagnosis and developing a therapeutic plan. This process entails the creation of a therapeutic alliance—that is, the building of a collaborative relationship with the objective of obtaining pertinent and accurate data to ascertain diagnoses and define treatment options. *Engagement* relates to the active efforts by the examiner to bring the patient and family within the expert influence of the examiner, surmounting apprehensions and concerns, with the goal of promoting a cooperative and effective diagnostic and therapeutic relationship.

The quality of the relationship between the examiner and the patient and family has an important bearing on the accuracy of the diagnosis and on the patient's compliance with treatment recommendations. A good interview achieves its objectives when the examiner promotes optimal participation from the patient and family in providing accurate and thorough information; this is achieved when wariness, defensiveness, and self-consciousness are stimulated to a minimum.

The interviewing process, by its very nature, is a stressful event for all involved, including the examiner. The art of interviewing rests on the examiner's ability to minimize discomfort and to foster a natural and easy interaction.

1

When the interview is done in a tactful and sensitive way, the patient's and family's apprehension of being "in the hot seat" is diminished.

Truthfulness relates to the veracity with which the family and child inform the examiner about the main issues, or the facts, related to the patient's dysfunction at home, at school, or in other milieus. Truthfulness also relates to the quality of disclosure—that is, the reporting of the presence of the predominant dysfunctions and their degree of severity as well and their impact in adaptation and development. Frequently, during the process of obtaining diagnostic data, the examiner receives partial truths, distorted facts, and sometimes outright lies from both the patient and the family; he or she also may receive selectively biased data or even deliberate omission of relevant information. The examiner will always be looking for coherence of the data, for the transparency of the information provided, and for a causal chain in the construction of an evidence-based factual diagnosis.

Pertinence and *relevance* relate to what is important to the family and the patient. What the family or the patient considers important is not necessarily in accord with what the examiner believes to be the major issues in a particular case. The examiner needs to heed how the child and/or family construes the nature of the problem and will try to align his or her scientific explanation with the family or patient's believes. Parents' perceptions and their priority of issues that need to be attended to should be considered and included when treatment recommendations are being implemented.

We believe that failures in the process of engagement are at the root of misdiagnoses in medicine in general, and in psychiatry in particular. This view is in agreement with Groopman (2007), who asserted, "While modern medicine is aided by a dazzling array of technologies, like high-resolution MRI [magnetic resonance imaging] scans and pinpoint DNA analysis, language is still the bedrock of clinical practice [the interview process]" (p. 8).

We also believe that failures of engagement are related to failures of compliance in medicine. The progress that has been made in medicine and psychiatry and the potential benefits of the contemporary technologies and treatments options offered to patients are irrelevant if treatment recommendations are not followed through. Quite often, physicians fail to engage patients in the process of cure. Modern technical medicine has neglected the importance and power of the process of treatment engagement.

Rapport has been referred to as the emotional climate between the child and the examiner that evolves throughout the interview. *Engagement* relates to the quality of relatedness and the technical measures used by the examiner to facilitate the child's participation during the interview. In other words, engagement relates to the means by which the examiner increases rapport. When a positive emotional bond is created between the examiner and the child and family, engagement is achieved.

The psychiatrist or mental health experts are responsible for creating the diagnostic and treatment ambiance, in line with the expression "creating rapport" that was in vogue some years back. With this interpretation, one can easily understand that rapport could be created in dealing with a depressed, hostile, or psychotic child, or with an aggravated or irrational family. Because of the ambiguous meanings that the concept of rapport has evolved, we prefer the concept of engagement because it has a connotation of deliverance of the process of winning over the child and the family trust.

Engagement entails warmth, acceptance, playfulness, humor, compassion, helpfulness, and empathic attunement on the part of the examiner. Furthermore, the examiner must have an accepting and tolerant attitude toward human vicissitudes and must be sensitive to emotional developmental levels. (Table 1–1 lists the ingredients of engagement.) Engagement is also fostered when the examiner uses positive and encouraging comments and demonstrates sensitivity to cultural norms and to religious practices. Engagement is achieved when the examiner conveys to the child and family that he or she understands their circumstances and when the examiner expresses compassion related to the child's and family's problematic situation.

To build rapport with children and adolescents, the examiner should be flexible and patient, should possess an in-depth understanding of child and adolescent development, and should be conversant with topics and areas that children and adolescents find familiar and interesting (Schulenberg et al. 2008). What are the consequences of not building rapport? As Schulenberg et al. (2008) note, "Absence of rapport [engagement] can negatively influence the evaluation to the extent that the results are invalid; it is necessary to prepare [interest] individuals and encourage [stimulate] them to do their best on measures of ability [disclosure] and to respond frankly [openly] in personality instruments [probing examination]" (pp. 522–523). These ideas are certainly a corollary to ideas presented in this chapter.

Diagnostic and treatment engagement is not only a caring, deliberate intervention but also a subtle and sophisticated clinical skill. Table 1–2 summarizes factors that facilitate engagement of the child, whereas Table 1–3 lists techniques that are not helpful in the engagement process.

The engagement of the child is facilitated when the examiner involves the patient in the diagnostic assessment and in the development of the treatment plan. Therefore, the psychiatric evaluations should be initiated with the child or adolescent and family together. In some cases, the examination needs to be conducted separately with child and family, and making separate examinations and evaluations (see Benny's case [Case Example 1] below). The need for separate evaluations is rare, even in the most severe psychiatric conditions. Occasionally, an angry and alienated adolescent demands a separate assessment, or a parent or parents request a meeting without the child. The

Table 1–1.   Ingredients of engagement

Warmth	Helpfulness
Compassion	Responsiveness
Benevolence	Immersion
Interest	Humanness
Caring	Equanimity
Active listening	Wholesomeness
Empathy	Calm demeanor
Sympathy	Humor
Sensitivity	Developmental knowledge
Acceptance	Positive and encouraging comments
Playfulness	Awareness and sensitivity to cultural norms
Understanding	Sensitivity to spiritual and religious beliefs

Source.   Modified from Cepeda 2010, p. 4.

exceptions typically represent situations in which the child feels very alienated from the family or in which the parents feel powerless in the face of the child's aggression or defiant behaviors. A number of parents want to meet with the examiner separately to prime the doctor regarding issues they do not feel comfortable confronting the adolescent about (e.g., drugs, sex, conduct problems, aggressive and intimidating behaviors). Our position about the importance of the conjoint evaluation is in accord with Pruett's (2007) philosophical stance: "It also struck me as extremely shortsighted to dissect out the child—even intellectually—from the family for diagnostic studies, economies of time, convenience of intervention, or cost containment. Such a myopia was like a celestial navigator trying to identify a constellation by fixating on but one star with his sextant; then as now, a really good way to get good and lost" (p. 2).

In the conjoint meeting, the examiner starts by asking the child for his or her name and for help with the appropriate spelling, questions the child about the day of the week and the date, and then asks the child to explain his or her understanding about why they are meeting. Depending on the child's openness, defensiveness, or guardedness, the examiner proceeds to gather information from the child or calls on a parent to assist with the provision of the data.

In our experience, even the most personal issues can be explored and discussed in conjoined meetings. Details and particulars about acting-out behaviors (e.g., drug use, sexual activity, delinquent behavior) may be deferred

Table 1–2. Factors that facilitate engagement of the child and family

Courteous and sensitive demeanor

Attention to voice tone and melody

Attention to and focus on patient's presenting problem

Attentive listening

Use of appropriately attuned language

Parallel nonverbal behavior

Balanced focus on problems and strengths

Sensitive use of humor

Praise of prosocial and adaptive behaviors

Praise of problem-solving behaviors

Positive and encouraging comments

Awareness of and sensitivity to cultural norms

Sensitivity to religious practices

Expression of interest in the patient's interests and preferences

Respect for family ethos and cultural norms

Source. Modified from Cepeda 2010, p. 5.

for further elaboration in follow-up individual interviews. In this regard, any specific denial (about drugs, sex, and so forth) during the conjoint interview ought to be corroborated in the individual interviews with either the child or the family. The same is true regarding probing on some family practices or discipline styles, marriage life, marital conflicts, and other family matters.

At the beginning of the first psychiatric examination of the child, the examiner should start with a warm greeting and a mutual introduction. The examiner may start by asking simple questions such as "What is your name?" "How old are you?" "Where do you go to school?" The examiner may ask if the child knows where he or she is, what kind of doctor the examiner is, why the child is at the doctor's office now, and/or why the child needs to see a psychiatrist. After these preliminary questions, the specific interviewing process begins.

Engagement is fostered when the examiner promotes a positive bond with the child and family; this process is boosted when the examiner expresses empathy for the child's or family's circumstances and when the examiner identifies with the child's or family's perspectives. Engagement is facilitated when the examiner gives the child positive feedback for behaving adaptively

Table 1–3. Techniques not considered helpful for fostering engagement

Writing excessively during interview, and paying undue attention to the electronic medical record

Conveying disinterest, not listening

Lacking warmth

Lacking empathy for patient's symptoms or circumstances

Relying excessively on surveys or questionnaires

Patronizing

Criticizing

Presenting alternatives, preferences, or recommendations to the family or patients without prior development of a therapeutic alliance

Source. Modified from Cepeda 2010, p. 5.

or in a developmentally appropriate manner or when the examiner praises the parent for opportune and sensitive redirection during the interview. For example, when evaluating a 5-year-old boy who has a prolonged history of hyperactivity and destructiveness, the examiner could praise the child for responding to structuring, not going into certain areas of the office, not playing with the telephone or the computer, and so forth, or praise the parents when they provide sensitive redirection and when they demonstrate attunement with the child's needs. The child may be praised for displaying behavioral organization (see section "Using AMSIT" in Chapter 8, "Documenting the Examination"), responding to the limits established, respecting the examiner's structure, or putting away toys at the end of the session on hearing that the interview is about to end. Engagement is also facilitated when the examiner supports the child's adaptive efforts. This point is illustrated in the following case example.

Case Example 1

Benny, a 16-year-old Caucasian male, was brought by his paternal grandmother to a psychiatric evaluation for aggressive and oppositional behaviors at home and at school. The grandmother had had custody of Benny and his 12-year-old sister for many years, because of the children's parents' addiction issues and their not being able to care for their son and daughter.

Benny had an extensive psychiatric history, including acute psychiatric hospitalizations and residential treatment for anger dyscontrol, conduct difficulties, unstable mood, and drug abuse. Benny had spent some time at a juvenile detention center and had received drug treatment at a residential drug program. At the time of the psychiatric examination, he was on probation.

Benny's grandmother had previously brought her granddaughter for a psychiatric evaluation secondary to aggressive and extreme oppositional behaviors. At that time, the examiner learned that both children hated their grandmother and that both were abusive to her. From the moment the grandmother and Benny entered the examination room, an atmosphere of tension and hostility permeated the interview. Benny stated at the outset, "Either she leaves and I stay, or I go and she stays." When the examiner attempted to elicit information regarding the grandmother's concerns, Benny issued a new warning: "I am not going to stay in the same room with her." When the examiner asked a general question to both of them, Benny stood up and left the room. The examiner asked the grandmother a number of questions regarding her concerns about Benny. The grandmother was concerned about Benny's aggressive and unruly behaviors and suspected that he was using drugs again. After spending some time with the grandmother, the examiner escorted her out and invited Benny to rejoin him.

Benny was a robust and rough-looking adolescent. His hair was shaved close to the scalp, and he had several scars on his face. He was dressed seasonally in a short-sleeve shirt. An inch-round cigarette burn was conspicuous on his left forearm. With overt hostility, Benny repeated defiantly that he did not need to be examined and that he came to the interview only "to get my grandmother off my back." Benny displayed a defensive and reserved posture and conveyed through nonverbal behavior that he wanted the evaluation to be over as soon as possible.

When the examiner asked Benny about school, he said, "My grades are getting better this semester." He said that he liked school and that he had not been skipping school during the current semester. The examiner praised him for that. When the examiner asked Benny about his drug use, Benny proudly responded, "I haven't touched the stuff for 50 days; today is the 50th day I've been without drugs. I've been going to PDAP [a juvenile drug abuse outpatient program] regularly." Upon hearing this, the examiner stood up, walked over to Benny, and shook his hand, congratulating him. The examiner praised Benny for his effort to stay away from drugs and said that he hoped Benny would remain abstinent.

Benny smiled with appreciation, and his demeanor toward the examiner changed demonstrably. He apologized for his previous rude behavior, saying, "I'm tired of psychiatrists and of taking medicines. They don't help." Because Benny seemed open to further exploration, the examiner proceeded to inquire about Benny's self-abusive behavior. The examiner invited Benny to discuss the cigarette burn on his arm. Benny said that he enjoyed pain and that he did not see it as a problem. He denied suicidal ideation. He said he was looking forward to turning 17 because he expected to leave his grandmother's custody at that time. He said, "That would be a relief!"

The examiner asked Benny how he controlled his anger. Benny said that he tried to control it all the time. He mentioned a couple of fights at school, explaining that he had been provoked and that he would not allow "those punks to run over me." The examiner said that Benny seemed very angry at his grandmother. Benny said, "I can't stand her." The examiner asked Benny if he thought about killing her. Benny reported that he thought about it all the time. He attempted to reassure himself by saying, "I am not stupid. I know

that if I were to kill her, I'd be the first suspect. If I knew a way, I would do it."
He added, "I don't want to have a [legal] record because I'm planning to join the
Marines." The examiner praised Benny again for thinking about his future and
for avoiding things that would stand in his way of achieving his goals. Benny
confessed that when his anger became too intense, he would burn himself
because "it helps me to get back in control."

Benny was able to review other difficult and sensitive topics (e.g., his relationships with his parents and sister). Benny said that he would like to have
more contact with his father. He was very negative and critical of his mother.
Benny was happy that his mother was in trouble and intimated that she was
going to jail: "She's responsible for what she's doing, and she should pay for
it." He didn't care about her at all. Benny did not seem to like his sister, either;
she was in a residential placement at the time of the interview.

To close the interview, the examiner asked Benny if there was any way a
psychiatrist could help him. Benny said that he did not need any help right now.
The examiner gave Benny his business card and offered his services any time
Benny felt in need of help. Benny shook the examiner's hand warmly and appeared appreciative when he departed.

In the preceding case, the patient arrived at the evaluation with a very angry
and antagonistic demeanor. He came prepared to battle with the examiner.
However, a clear, if not dramatic, change in his attitude toward the interview
occurred after the examiner praised him for his efforts to control himself and
for staying off drugs.

Engagement is also fostered when the examiner initiates the examination
by picking up on themes or preoccupations the child brings to the evaluation,
as in the following case example.

Case Example 2

Rudy, a 14-year-old Caucasian male, was evaluated for paranoia. He brought
to the examination two large dragon drawings. The examiner demonstrated
interest in the drawings, which showed dragons puffing fire with no other
figures or beings present. The examiner asked Rudy what the dragons were
doing. Rudy said, "The dragons are puffing fire." The examiner commented,
"The dragons seem very lonely; there is nobody else around them." Rudy responded, "The dragons don't like to be around other people." He added, "Others don't like dragons because they are very angry." The examiner added that
the dragons puffed a lot of fire and that they were very angry. To this, Rudy
said, "Although one of the dragons puffs fire, the other puffs only smoke." The
child added, "I don't need anybody. I don't need to be loved." The examiner
interjected, "Love is essential for life. Without it we can't live." Rudy said, "I am
trying very hard not to need love." After this exchange, Rudy began to talk about
the problems he had with his parents, and the interview continued in a productive manner.

By supporting this conflicted adolescent's efforts at adaptive behavior with the
use of displacement (see Chapter 3, "Special Interviewing Techniques"), his

guardedness decreased and rapport with the examiner increased, and the interviewee became more open and revealing.

The child may open the interview by talking about sports, a movie star, a television show, or some other issue that at first glance may seem banal or immaterial to the main concerns of the examination. By joining the child's prevailing fantasy or immediate interest, the examiner gains a number of benefits: 1) the examiner gets access to what is uppermost in the child's mind; 2) the examiner learns about important aspects of the child's psychological world; and 3) by paying close attention to the content and the process of the child's communication, the examiner gains significant insights into the child's cognitive capacities, language functions, manner of relating, reality testing, and other psychological and adaptive functions.

The engagement phase needs to be as unstructured as possible. During this phase, the child should be allowed to speak about anything he or she wants and to discuss whatever is uppermost in his or her mind. While listening, the examiner develops a sense or understanding of the sources of the patient's anxieties. This approach parallels an open-ended exploration. The examiner pays particular attention to the child's emotional expression and to the manner in which the child articulates the difficulties (thought processes). This allows the examiner to appreciate the child's prevailing mood, cognitive organization, and adaptive resources.

Observations made during the engagement phase stimulate a number of clinical hunches or incipient hypotheses. These impressions may serve as bases for exploring further or for probing a number of diagnostic areas. Also, by listening attentively and by demonstrating interest and empathy, the examiner conveys to the child that his or her concerns are considered seriously and that whatever the child has in mind is of interest to the psychiatrist. In this manner, the child perceives that the examiner is caring, attentive, and interested in what he or she has to say.

An important early goal of the examiner is to facilitate the child's and the family's participation in defining the problems and in finding ways to solve them. If everything proceeds well, later, during the interpretive phase of the evaluation (see Chapter 5, "Providing Post-evaluation Feedback to Families"), the child's, parents', and examiner's views regarding what the problems are and what needs to done about them will converge.

Factors That Facilitate Engagement of Family

The examiner increases engagement of the family by demonstrating respect for each family member and by listening attentively to what each member, even the smallest, has to say. If a baby were in the session, the examiner might raise the question, "If the baby could talk, what would the baby say about what is going on?" The examiner also gains engagement by respecting the family's culture, customs, and traditions. For example, addressing the father first is important in Hispanic and Asian families.

The examiner should welcome all the members the family has brought in and invite all of them to the diagnostic interview: the presence of family members gives the examiner a broader view of the family's circumstances, provides new perspectives on the nature of the presenting problems, and acquaints the examiner with untapped resources to deal with the problems. Many family members may have been on the sidelines waiting for an opportunity to assist in the ongoing family difficulties or to help in the resolution of the problems.

An unsound practice during initial evaluations is for the examiner to interject personal views or to challenge the family's philosophy, religion, political views, lifestyle, or composition, be that recombined, interracial, gay, or otherwise. The examiner needs to avoid criticizing or patronizing the members, or entering into power struggles with the families regarding authority or discipline within the family, unless such family practices are questionable or abusive. The same should be said about the family's theory of illness or the therapeutic interventions that the family believes are indicated.

By paying attention to the larger picture of the family, the examiner is able to observe lines of authority, family coalitions, family subsystems, generation boundaries, and so forth. Furthermore, attending to the whole family gives the examiner the opportunity to find major foci of dysfunction and to attend to forces that undermine parental authority or interfere with the resolution of the problems. On the other hand, the examiner may encounter resources or areas of strength in different family members or subsystems. These resources may be instrumental in solving major conflicts within the family or in solving problems of the family transacting with other systems (see Chapter 4, "Family Assessment").

A priority of the examiner is to focus on establishing alliances with both parents, or at least with the parent who is the family gatekeeper. The examiner needs to make this effort even if the parent looks ostensibly unconventional or is physically or mentally impaired—that is, the examiner should keep in mind that "a parent is a parent."

Other Factors That Facilitate Engagement With Child and Family

The examiner needs to create a sensitive and empathic environment for the child and family. The interview environment needs to be inviting and to communicate genuine warmth and receptivity. The child needs to feel respected and understood at all times. Except with preschoolers, with whom there is a universal tendency to use "baby talk," the examiner should use his or her natural voice and inflection. Children sense when they are being patronized or manipulated by adults or when they are being addressed in an artificial manner.

To engage families, the examiner must show equanimity, compassion, and tolerance to human frailty. Broad personal experience is also important. The process of engaging the child and the family is facilitated by the examiner's equidistant relationship with various family members. Traditionally, the child psychiatrist has been cast in the role of the child's advocate. This special role should not be exercised at the expense of alienating other family members or at the risk of being unduly partial to the child.

Obstacles to Development of Engagement

During the psychiatric assessment, the mind of the examining psychiatrist is occupied and preoccupied with two professional tasks: the need to document and the need to determine a diagnosis. This attentional split interferes with listening attentively to what the child and family need to express.

Nobody would disagree that documentation is necessary and that good record keeping is a standard of solid and good medical practice; however, some patients and families get put off by the examiner's incessant writing, attention to the electronic medical record, lack of eye contact, or lack of attention to their verbal and nonverbal communications. In the same vein, the examiner needs to limit the use of electronic devices during the examination. Nowadays, it is not unusual for the parents or caretaker to bring smart phones or tablets to the examination and to review emails or even to carry on texting during the interview. The examiner needs to reorient the adults to the matters at hand.

Some patients and families leave the office believing that the physician has not listened to them or that the examiner does not care about their problems. Interviewers need to accomplish documentation without sacrificing therapeutic engagement during the interview. In other words, the physician needs to make an effort to maintain engagement at all times.

The goal of diagnostic and therapeutic engagement is to ensure that the patient's and family's feel that they are understood. The examiner's lack of attention to the patient's and family's subjectivity—that is, to what they want or need to say—leaves them with a sense of psychological "dis-ease," and particularly with the feeling of not being understood. Building a diagnostic and therapeutic alliance is impossible under those conditions. Unfortunately, in some contemporary psychiatric circles, the notion of therapeutic alliance is a dated objective.

In an effort to achieve expediency in clinical practice, many practitioners rely a great deal on the use of symptom checklists and related symptom surveys. Although checklists have a place in clinical practice and may assist in the diagnostic process and treatment evaluations, depending on them exclusively for assessment purposes hinders opportunities to enrich the diagnostic process and to foster a treatment alliance.

Reverse Engagement

The engagement process is the responsibility of the examiner. When the child initiates the engagement or attempts to befriend the examiner, the situation is called *reverse engagement*. Two groups of children commonly attempt reverse engagement.

The first group, children with disinhibited social engagement disorder (American Psychiatric Association 2013, pp. 268–270), may try to befriend and/or ingratiate themselves to the examiner. These children initiate the engagement from the very beginning. They do not consider anyone a stranger, and they believe that everybody or anybody can be a friend. With these patients, the examiner needs to be attentive to setting prompt limits (see Chapter 2, "General Principles of Interviewing," and Chapter 3, "Special Interviewing Techniques") and should immediately respond to violations of personal boundaries.

The second group, children with conduct disorder traits, attempt to befriend the examiner with ulterior motives. The ingratiation and befriending behaviors are manipulative. Seductive behavior is common in adolescents with borderline or histrionic personality disorders. Occasionally, children with a background of trauma, particularly sexual abuse, may try to reenact the traumatic experiences with the examiner. Some of these children may display overt sexualized behavior during the interview.

To reveal the primacy and importance of a child's emotional bonding, the examiner can ask, "Tell me, who is the most important person in the whole world?" A child who is securely attached and feels loved immediately responds, "My mom" (or other primary attachment figure). The examiner then asks, "Who is the second most important?" Commonly, the patient replies that this person is the father or an equivalent. The examiner proceeds, "Who is the next one?" A grandparent or other significant person such as a sibling is often mentioned third. The answers to this line of inquiry are illuminating as to who is really important in the child's psychological life. Many children reveal their conflictive attachments in this short list or hint at the degree of disconnection with their immediate family. For some adolescents, a girlfriend or boyfriend is high on the list. A special friend may also occupy a place of importance; for others a pet may be the source of trust and affection. Some patients feel baffled and confused by the question and strain to indicate any person to whom they feel close. The most disconnected and detached patients respond, "Me," and depressed adolescents who feel unloved may respond, "No one." Adolescents in active conflicts with parents commonly say, "A friend"; in these circumstances, parents are usually at the bottom of the list.

Key Points

- Engagement is a fundamental and indispensable component of the diagnostic examination.
- Engagement relates to a positive and benevolent bond between the child and family and the examiner.
- The examiner is responsible for the creation and maintenance of the process of engagement.
- Success in the establishment of engagement is correlated with success in the diagnostic process and with compliance with treatment.

CHAPTER 2

General Principles of Interviewing

Diagnostic interviewing of a child or adolescent is a collaborative process that involves the psychiatric examiner, the identified patient, and the patient's family, among others. Its purpose is to reach a comprehensive diagnostic formulation (see Chapter 13, "Comprehensive Psychiatric Formulation") that will serve as the foundation of a comprehensive treatment plan. Conducting the family assessment is discussed in Chapter 4, "Family Assessment." In this chapter, we focus on general principles of interviewing.

The Interview Setting

The diagnostic interview is usually conducted in a professional setting, ideally in an appropriately suited office space; however, a productive diagnostic interview may take place in other locations, such as a classroom, a hospital at the child's bedside, a playground, and other settings. The setting is determined by the spirit, purpose, and objectives of the interview rather than by the nature of the space or the environment surrounding the patient and the examiner. The most important element of the interview setting is the climate of respect, receptivity, warmth, and cooperative interest that the examiner creates. No matter where the interview is carried out, the child and the child's family need to feel welcome, respected, and understood. An attitude of hope and helpfulness should permeate all transactions with the child and the family, regardless of the clinical condition.

Safety—the child's and the examiner's—is a basic consideration for all evaluations. In professional settings, any objects located in the examiner's office (e.g., decorative items) may be transformed by the child into playing objects or may become weapons in moments of dyscontrol. The examiner should keep this risk in mind when making decisions regarding the examination space and the office decor. A child, especially a preschooler, should not be left in the reception area without adult supervision. This recommendation applies particularly to children with a history of impulsive or destructive behavior.

Preparation for the Psychiatric Examination

Ideally, children and adolescents should be prepared for the psychiatric examination ahead of time. The examiner should provide guidance to the parents regarding what to tell the child about the examination. The type of guidance depends on the nature of the problem and the relationship between the parents and the child. If open hostility exists between the two, the child may not be amenable to adequate preparation.

In general, parents need to address the distressing symptoms that disturb the child or the problematic behaviors that put the child in conflict with others. If the child feels depressed, for instance, parents could explain that the child will be taken to a child psychiatrist to find out why he or she feels that way and to get help. In some cases, parents may want to tell the child that the psychiatrist will help the child discover, for example, why he or she is getting into trouble at school or at home. Occasionally, parents are not forthright with a child regarding the need for the psychiatric evaluation. When parents feel intimidated or when they fear the child's response, they are likely to be less than candid with the child about the evaluation. In these circumstances, parents often cajole or deceive the child by saying that he or she will be taken to a medical doctor, a counselor, a special school, or somewhere else. In crisis or emergency situations, the preparatory aspects of the interview are usually dispensed with.

Children rarely express explicit concerns about their symptoms, but this does not mean they are happy with their problems. Children with psychiatric symptoms are unhappy to a greater or lesser extent; some prefer to save face rather than acknowledge responsibility for maladaptive behaviors. Others may be unwilling to discuss their problems and to seek change until the right person and the right circumstances present themselves. If the child is given this opportunity, the chances for involving him or her in the examination and in the treatment process may increase.

For some children, the interview may become a turning point in their lives and may have a longlasting, positive effect. The interview, therefore, needs to be considered in a broader perspective rather than with narrow and immediate objectives. If the examiner is unsuccessful, or worse, becomes aversive or psychologically negative to the child, the end result may be detrimental for future evaluations or psychiatric interventions.

The Interview Process

Before a face-to-face interview with the parents and the child, the examiner needs to clarify the nature of the problem(s) that prompted the evaluation. Contact with the referral agent (e.g., medical professional, school, other agency) helps the examiner sort out issues that need to be addressed during the assessment. The referral agent may be able to provide useful information or clarify the questions at hand. This preliminary review of the situation will stimulate broad hypotheses that will give initial organization to the psychiatric examination.

An important consideration is who or what has prompted the need for the assessment. Does the concern originate within the family or from an external source (e.g., school, court)? It makes a big difference if the concerns come from within the immediate family rather than from external sources. An evaluation that is initiated by someone outside the family typically is fraught with greater difficulties and overt obstacles (in the form of open resistances) from the start (see Chapter 15, "Diagnostic Obstacles [Resistances]").

Caveats of the Interviewing Process

The examiner needs to avoid premature closures. In particular, the examiner needs to consider that observations gathered during the consultation may not be typical of the child's or family's behaviors. There are other caveats the examiner needs to consider, as described by Charman et al. (2015):

> A good-quality clinical assessment of children and adolescents and their families is time consuming and requires expertise, but a few-hour assessment provides only a limit snap-shot of the child's functioning. Moreover, children's behavior in the clinic [office] may not be representative of their behavior elsewhere. For example, a child who is polite, quiet and compliant may be highly disruptive in familiar settings. Parental reports may misrepresent the child's difficulties because of biases related to parents' background or problems. The father of a child with autism, for example, may underplay the difficulties noting "I was just like that at his age and I don't have any problems now." School reports, too, can be biased. A well-behaved child with learning problems may be described as not having discernible difficulties, while a disruptive child of average IQ may be reported as failing academically as well as socially. Despite standardization of questionnaires, these, too, are not bias-free, and if respondents have intellectual or language problems they may not necessarily interpret questions correctly. In such circumstances, the only way to obtain more reliable information on the child and the factors that contribute to his or her difficulties is to supplement the clinical assessment with direct observations. (p. 438)

Maintaining Dependency Ties During the Interview

Many evaluations are marred from the very beginning because the examiner inadvertently or prematurely threatens to sever strong dependency ties between the child and the parents. This risk is greater during the examination of adolescents when the examiner assumes more individuation and autonomy than the child has achieved or more independence than the parents are able or willing to grant. The following case example illustrates this point.

Case Example 1

Nick, a 17-year-old Caucasian male, had just been withdrawn by his mother from an acute psychiatric hospital, where he had been admitted 48 hours earlier for an acute psychotic episode. The mother alleged that the former psychiatrist "had been insensitive" and that the doctor "had rushed into judgment regarding the diagnosis" (she was told that her son had schizophrenia and that he needed acute psychiatric hospitalization). She complained that the psychiatrist had spoken to Nick "alone for only 10 minutes." She objected to having been separated from her son and was upset that she could not be around to comfort him. She said that she was going to start a national campaign "to ensure that parents of hospitalized adolescents could stay in the hospital with them." According to the former psychiatrist, Nick arrived at the hospital in a state of incoherence and displayed florid psychosis. Nick's mother claimed that prior to the referral to the psychiatric hospital, she had taken him to a local emergency room, where "he had an episode of respiratory arrest." The acute psychotic break coincided with Nick's father's recent departure for a consulting job in another state.

Nick, a valedictorian of his high school class, had been markedly driven to excel, had been an honor student, and was seeking entrance into an Ivy League college. He got up at 4:30 A.M. to study on a regular basis and was involved in multiple extracurricular activities. According to Nick's mother, most of the family members, including Nick's father, were shy. His father had a severe stuttering disorder, and Nick's mother used to speak for him in social situations. There was a strong history of bipolar disorder in the mother's extended family.

Nick was born a few weeks prematurely and weighed about 5 lbs. He was born with respiratory distress syndrome. His parents were told to make funeral arrangements for him. Nick survived but required an incubator and oxygen for the first 3 months of his life. At age 3 months, he had spinal meningitis but never had seizures. His development was delayed: he first sat at age 11 months and walked at 18 months. Nick's mother could not tell if there had been any delay in Nick's speech production. Nick had always been of smaller stature than his peers, and this had been a source of difficulty with his classmates. His superior intelligence was recognized when he entered school.

During the diagnostic evaluation, Nick's mother responded when the examiner asked Nick questions. She was very anxious and intrusive. She minimized the nature of the recent psychotic episode and did not lose any opportunity to extol the virtues and accomplishments of her "special child." The examiner recognized and accepted the dependent relationship of this adolescent with his mother and made no attempt to disrupt the symbiotic bond.

Nick was guarded and suspicious and maintained limited eye contact. He was thin and small and had a frail appearance. He was mildly depressed and very constricted in the affective sphere and had problems developing rapport with the examiner. He was coherent, but his speech was moderately pressured and uninterrupted (he did not punctuate his sentences). His associations were loose and tended to be very circumstantial. Nick was overtly paranoid. A number of times he asked his mother to bring a lawyer because he feared the examiner might "tamper" with his mind. His mother appropriately reassured him at those times.

Nick denied he was experiencing auditory or visual hallucinations but acknowledged that he had experienced them recently. He denied any suicidal or homicidal ideation. He also denied there was anything wrong with him. He wanted to go back home right away, "to catch up with my studies and to continue the college search."

Nick's mother was told that Nick still needed intense psychiatric monitoring in an acute psychiatric hospital. She persuaded Nick to follow the examiner's recommendation. Nick recovered promptly and completely from the psychotic episode. Shortly afterward, his mother informed the examiner that Nick had been awarded the president's scholarship to attend a prominent university in New England.

Despite multiple risk factors, Nick demonstrated an exceptional cognitive and academic outcome. His mother's fear for his life and Nick's behavioral inhibition had contributed to his strong dependency needs. Nick's long-term psychiatric outcome was uncertain.

The preceding case illustrates the importance of beginning the evaluation with a family interview and alerts the examiner to the risks of prematurely separating the child from the family for the individual interview.

Conducting the Individual Interview

Once the family assessment has been completed (see Chapter 4, "Family Assessment"), the child can be interviewed alone. An important goal for the examiner during the individual interview is to facilitate the child's verbalization of his or her problems so that the child may put into his or her own words the nature of the difficulties or the manner in which the child perceives them. Without the child's understanding, the quality of diagnostic data will be compromised and incomplete. The examiner's facilitation of the child's verbalizations also helps in building a diagnostic and therapeutic alliance.

Creating Engagement

As described in Chapter 1 ("Diagnostic and Therapeutic Engagement"), one of the first goals of the examiner is to create engagement. Toward this goal, experienced clinicians display an automatic behavioral repertoire (adaptive professional demeanor) and make instantaneous adjustments when they interview children. For example, they change body posture, vocabulary, tone of voice, and even their affective display. These adjustments of verbal and nonverbal communication put the clinicians in immediate contact with the child's developmental level. The following case example illustrates the process of engagement in an impaired and defensive early adolescent.

Case Example 2

George, a 12-year-old Asian American male, was a very defensive and uncooperative child. He was clever and liked to outsmart adults and his peers. He had a history of chronic affective psychosis and had an extensive psychiatric history, including prolonged hospitalizations for suicidal and aggressive behaviors. He was intelligent but had a history of chronic school problems, including aggression toward his teachers. For many years, George had received neuroleptic medications to control the psychotic symptoms, and he had developed a severe case of tardive dyskinesia. As a result, all antipsychotic medication had been stopped.

When George was interviewed for the first time, he fidgeted a great deal in his chair; at times, he rocked and tilted the chair in such a way that the examiner feared for George's safety. The examiner said to George, "That makes me uneasy." George reassured the examiner that he would not get hurt and continued tilting the chair back and forth. When asked why he was brought to the hospital, George said, "Drugs." The examiner asked, "Which ones?" George answered, "Marijuana." He said that he had used marijuana for a long time, adding that his parents did not know anything about his drug use. To this the examiner said, "It takes a lot of cleverness to hide this from the family." George responded with an enthusiastic, "Yes!" George then proceeded to talk about the buzz he got from gasoline: it made him feel like he was floating, as if he could fly. The examiner then asked George whether he had ever attempted to fly. George said that from time to time he felt like Superman and had tried to fly from the roof of his home. On one occasion, George "tried and fell on my belly and it got hurt pretty bad." He denied he had broken any bones while trying to fly.

Later in the interview, when the examiner and George discussed his suicidal behavior and prior suicide attempts, George said he had a secret plan to kill himself and stressed that he was not going to share the plan with anybody. He stated that he frequently daydreamed about flying over a highway bridge and being killed by a car. He said he believed he would go straight to heaven, adding that he was not meant to be in this life, because "I can't make it in life." George then described how bad he felt about himself. For example, when he looked at himself in the mirror, he used to see a monster with horns. This monster talked to him and told him to do bad things. On one occasion, the monster told him to hurt somebody, but George shouted, "No!"

The preceding case example illustrates successful engagement of a resistant child. By joining the child's grandiosity, the examiner facilitated the development of rapport. The child provided meaningful information after the examiner achieved an emotional connection with him.

The Psychiatric Examination

First and foremost, during the psychiatric examination, the clinician should use language appropriate for the child's developmental level. Special attention is required to avoid the use of sophisticated or professional language. Furthermore, the examiner should understand that when the child or the family uses common words such as "depression," the meaning they give to such words is not necessarily the same as the meaning the examiner gives to them. Currently, with the heightened awareness of bipolar disorders, laypersons commonly use the expressions "chemical imbalance" and "mood swings" without a common basis for use of the terms.

The examiner must ascertain whether the child understands the initial verbal transactions; if the child does not understand, the clinician should suspect an auditory sensory defect, delirium, or a receptive language disorder (see Chapter 12, "Neuropsychiatric Interview and Examination"). When working with children who have receptive language difficulties, the examiner needs to modify the communication approach. The clinician must speak slowly and in a deliberate manner to make contact with the child, striving toward attentive eye contact and face-to-face communication. The examiner could also use alternative media (e.g., play, drawing) to interact and communicate with the child. If delirium is suspected, a detailed examination of the sensorium is mandatory. If the child does not seem to respond to the examiner's utterances, the examiner should determine whether the child's auditory functions are intact or whether autistic features are present. If the child has a hearing impairment and the psychiatrist is not fluent in sign language, arrangements should be made in advance to procure the assistance of a qualified interpreter.

Sensitive comments to the child about signs of illness or injury (e.g., limping, a crutch, a sling, a cast) help the examiner to build rapport and increase the diagnostic alliance with the patient. For example, the examiner can convey to the child that he or she has noticed that the child is sick or may have been injured in some way.

Phases of the Psychiatric Examination

As listed in Table 2–1, the psychiatric examination has seven phases. The first four are discussed in this section.

Beginning the Interview (Engagement)

The beginning or engagement phase of the psychiatric examination involves the initial contact between the examiner and the child, and possibly his or her family. Leon's (1982) comments regarding the first meeting between the adult patient and the doctor are applicable to child psychiatry (in which case

Table 2–1.   Phases of the psychiatric examination

Beginning the interview (engagement)

Elaborating the presenting problem

Extending the exploration

Completing the mental status examination

Closing the interview

Interpreting the results

Presenting treatment recommendations

Source.   Modified from Cepeda 2010, p. 25.

"physician" represents the child psychiatrist and "patient" refers to the child and family):

> Although the physician may already have seen many patients that day, this is the first meeting of this patient and doctor. For the patient, it is important. The patient has been anticipating this meeting with a mixture of fear and hope. The patient's fear comes from many sources. What will the doctor be like? Will the patient be judged adversely? What will be found? Will the doctor want to help? The hope is that the doctor can relieve the stress. (p. 15)

In a similar fashion, Katz's (1990) description of the adolescent's anxiety preceding the initial interview with a therapist could be aptly applied to the first meeting between the child and the psychiatrist:

> While the first few minutes of an interview are significant with all patients, they are particularly significant with adolescents, as many of them are struggling for independence, trying to establish an identity, and choosing their place in the world. They are particularly sensitive to any signals from the therapist [examiner] that their power of decision, their intelligence, and their perceptions will be ignored. (p. 70)

Depending on how the preliminary contact goes and what impressions are made, a warm-up stage or engagement phase takes precedence in the initial encounter (see Chapter 1, "Diagnostic and Therapeutic Engagement"). The goal is to help the patient and family feel at ease and as comfortable as possible, thereby promoting cooperation and a decrease in anxiety and wariness. In general, this phase is more prolonged with preadolescents and with younger, immature, and regressed children. With adolescents, the engagement phase may not take long. The extent and duration of the engagement phase depend on the degree of psychopathology, the degree of dystonicity (discomfort) or reaction against the symptoms, and the patient's awareness of a need to change.

The engagement phase allows the examiner to determine the patient's and family's openness and their likely degree of participation in the diagnostic process. It also provides an incipient sense of the patient's and family's relatedness (i.e., the quality of interpersonal relations within the family and with the child). These preliminary perceptions guide the examiner in judging the degree of overt psychopathology, the level of cooperation and rapport, and the amount of structuring (i.e., direction) that will be necessary to ensure success in the diagnostic process.

Once the family's concerns have been explored and the family members have been given the opportunity to express their views on the problem(s), the family may be asked to leave, and the child's examination continues.

Elaborating the Presenting Problem

The major purpose of the elaboration phase is to explore the presenting problem as fully as possible. This phase parallels what Brown and Rutter (1996) called the "systematic exploratory style" of interviewing, which involves a fact-oriented style and feeling-oriented techniques. Systematic questioning and specific probing have definite advantages in eliciting factual information. This approach seems to be successful in eliciting the "detailed, relevant data needed for an adequate diagnostic formulation" (Cox et al. 1981a, p. 289):

> The structured and systematic exploratory styles are far superior in providing evidence on the definitive absence of problems....The implication is clear: if psychiatrists are to obtain sufficient detail about family problems and child symptoms for them to make an adequate formulation on which to base treatment plans, systematic and detailed probing and questioning must occur. (Cox et al. 1981b, pp. 31–32)

The approach parallels Shea's (1998) Chronological Assessment of Suicide Events (CASE) approach, described later in this section. Table 2–2 lists the goals involved in this phase. The priority during this phase is to obtain a clear and detailed account of the presenting problem. The examiner asks what, how, when, and where questions to delve into the facts, events, and circumstances related to the presenting problem. Questions regarding "how much"— frequency, intensity, and other factors that bring on the problem—are of major relevance. After this exploration is completed, the examination of the psychological factors that may contribute to the problem—that is, the "why" questions—may be in order. The why questions relate to opinions, psychological explanations, rationalizations, and belief systems that are subjective by nature. For instance, if the presenting problem is anger dyscontrol, the examiner needs to consider the following questions: What does the patient do when he or she loses control? Does the patient become aggressive? How? Does the patient become destructive? Does the patient become self-abusive? In what ways does the patient become self-destructive? Has the patient ever tried to hurt himself or herself, or to hurt others? (Note that the examiner is conducting a mental status examination while exploring the presenting problem.) How often does the patient lose control? Where does the patient lose control? How long does it take for the patient to regain control? What factors make the patient lose control? What happens after the patient loses control? Has the patient ever received any treatment? Has the patient complied with therapeutic or medical recommendations? How does the patient see his or her loss of control? Does the patient see dyscontrol as a problem? Note that the most introspective questions come last. The same format may be followed with other symptoms (e.g., depression, suicidal behavior, drug abuse, running away).

When the issue at hand is suicidality or homicidality, standard questions are, in the case of suicidality, "How close have you been to killing yourself?" and "Do you have a plan to kill yourself?"; or, in the case of homicidality, "How close have you been to killing someone?" "Whom have you thought of killing?" and "Do you have a plan to kill that person now?" The examiner must assess the patient's potential risk to harm others and must remember his or her duty to warn potential victims, a result of the 1976 *Tarasoff vs. Regents of the University of California* decision (Nurcombe 1996).

Systematic interviewing parallels Shea's (1998) approach for the evaluation of suicidal ideation. In this approach, the examiner uses a number of questioning techniques, including 1) behavioral incidents, 2) gentle assumptions, and 3) denial of the specific. *Behavioral incidents* questions probe for specific facts, details, or trains of thought (e.g., "Describe what happened. How did you try to kill yourself?"). This approach is similar to asking what, how, when, and where questions. *Gentle assumptions* questions focus on areas or topics that the patient hesitates to talk about (e.g., "How often do you think about suicide? How do you intend to kill yourself?"). These open-ended and leading questions explore areas the patient rarely discusses spontaneously. *Denial of the specific* questions include specific probes to rule out symptoms or a variety of problems (e.g., "Have you had thoughts of shooting yourself?" "Have you tried to hang yourself?").

In Shea's approach, the examiner explores the four following chronological areas: 1) present ideation and suicidal behaviors, 2) recent ideation and behaviors over the last 6–8 weeks, 3) past suicidal ideation and behaviors, 4) immediate ideations and plans for the future. Shea warned that many times patients will erect a façade for the mental health professional or the primary care physician while describing the suicide event that led them to seek help. This barrier may sometimes arise out of a sense of embarrassment or perhaps because the patient is genuinely feeling a little better since sharing his pain at the time of the presentation. Such a reassuring interplay can lull the clinician into a false sense of security. Any time the patient displays any hint

Table 2–2. Elaborating the presenting problem

Clarifying major concerns regarding the evaluation or consultation

Listening attentively to verbal and nonverbal behaviors

Making efforts to understand the presenting symptoms

Exploring the multiple dimensions of the presenting symptoms

Keeping focus in the presenting problem before exploring other areas

Connecting the presenting problem with major dimensions in the child's life:

Family

School

Girlfriends/boyfriends

Friends

Developmental concerns

Hygiene and personal care

Issues of abuse

Ongoing history of abuse

Past history of abuse

Source.   Modified from Cepeda 2010, p. 27.

of ambivalence about suicide (or being alive), the subject should be explored at once. Suicide usually requires considerable forethought and internal debate arising from many days of intense pain. The degree to which this pain has taken the patient to the edge of suicide in the recent past may serve as one of the best indicators of whether the patient will cross that line in the near future (Shea 1998, pp. 472–495).

In the evaluation of suicidal behavior in children and adolescents, the examiner needs to determine the factor of intentionality. The intention to commit suicide is the core from which all suicidal behavior and a great deal of self-destructive behaviors originate. Simply exploring whether the patient has suicidal ideation is not enough. The examiner must explore all the possible means the patient has in mind. This point is illustrated in the following case example.

Case Example 3

Matthew, a 6-year-old Caucasian male, was referred by a social worker for a psychiatric evaluation because of concerns regarding the child's depressive state and possible suicidal behavior. One year earlier, Matthew had undergone a psychiatric evaluation for aggressive behaviors at home and at school.

His disturbance seemed to have started 1 year before the previous evaluation, when his father moved out and his older brother was hospitalized. Shortly afterward, Matthew began to kill small animals, to trip and hit his peers, and to hit his teenage sister. Matthew threw things around and was quite angry at his mother. Earlier, Matthew's preschool teacher had described him as very disruptive and withdrawn; he also was said to be careless and destructive with his schoolwork. Matthew displayed a prominent fear of fires; this had begun after a fire drill. Matthew had not been abused but had witnessed his father's abusive behavior toward his mother. Matthew's developmental milestones and history prior to his father's leaving home were unremarkable. Both parents had depression and anxiety, and Matthew's older brother had been diagnosed with oppositional defiant disorder and a behavioral disturbance associated with a brain disorder, possibly secondary to marijuana exposure in utero.

At the time of the current evaluation, Matthew's mental status examination revealed a handsome, bright, and articulate child who appeared his stated age. He looked unhappy and depressed and exhibited marked retardation in psychomotor activity. His affect was markedly constricted, and he appeared anhedonic and hopeless. When questioned about suicidal ideation, Matthew confirmed it readily. When asked how he thought he would kill himself, he said he had thought of using a knife. The examiner asked Matthew if he had considered other means of hurting himself. Matthew said that he had wanted to jump from the roof of the house. He had also thought about using a gun, lying down in the road so that he could be run over by a car, or crushing his brain somehow. He said that he had stood on his head many times, hoping to "drown" his brain with blood. Matthew missed his father a great deal and hated living with his mother. He was very unhappy with his mother's recent remarriage. Also, he hated school and had difficulties concentrating. No psychotic features were evident. Matthew was given the diagnosis of a major depressive episode and was placed on an antidepressant.

The preceding case example illustrates a severe affective disorder in an early latency child and also demonstrates the variety of self-destructive means a child had devised. This case illustrates full melancholic symptomatology in early preadolescence. The same comprehensive and thorough exploratory approach is mandatory with adolescents, and if necessary with the parents.

Issues related to the child's psychiatric history and ongoing treatments are also explored during the elaboration phase of the interview. Data related to the presenting problem become the core organizer of the interview process. All data gathering will have the presenting problem as its reference point and as its integrative core.

Extending the Exploration

The third phase of the psychiatric examination is equivalent to the review of systems conducted when a physician is completing the history and examination in the field of physical medicine. During this phase, the examiner extends the exploration to other areas and attempts to find threads connecting to the presenting problem. For example, the parents of a 12-year-old girl with anger dyscontrol may tell the examiner that their daughter is aggressive at home. The examiner explores other areas: Does the child also lose control at school or in the neighborhood? Has she ever had any other problems at school? If so, what kind of problems has she had? How does this child do academically? How are her peer relationships? The examiner pursues any leads pertinent to the evolving hypothesis. For example, the exploration may branch into questions related to oppositional behavior, conduct problems, gang affiliation, or drug use.

Examiners should approach sensitive areas (e.g., suicidal or homicidal behaviors, drug abuse) from many different angles. They should never be satisfied with a single denial to a question related to a sensitive issue. Sometimes, rephrasing a question or using different language brings about productive diagnostic information. Some children who have denied having suicidal thoughts respond differently when asked, "Have you had thoughts of killing yourself?" The use of vernacular language may be quite appropriate in this regard.

Sometimes, despite careful exploration, the examiner does not find corroboration for some clinical impressions (intuitions or "hunches"). In cases of suicidality, homicidality, psychosis, substance abuse, and other areas, the clinician must remain cautious and avoid making premature closures, because his clinical impressions may be correct, despite a lack of explicit clinical proof. When the examiner has an uneasy feeling about a concerning issue, despite the patient's denials regarding suicidal or homicidal thoughts, drug abuse, or another issue, the examiner should heed his clinical sense and background experience.

The examiner should attempt further clarification of the clinical incongruencies because they may indicate that the patient is withholding (voluntarily or involuntarily) relevant information or that other lines of inquiry may need to be pursued to achieve full clarity. Some children tenaciously withhold sensitive information. Children are adept at keeping certain secrets (e.g., suicidal intentions, homicidal plans, psychotic experiences, drug abuse, physical or sexual abuse, and sexual activity). The examiner also needs to be aware of countertransference responses, because tactful utilization of these responses may be helpful in the diagnostic process (see Chapter 16, "Countertransference").

A number of areas need to be explored in every child or adolescent interview (Table 2–3). These areas include the child's relationships with family members, the kind of discipline the child receives, the child's history of physical or sexual abuse, his or her school life (e.g., academic performance, school difficulties), and his or her friendships. The child's drug use, conduct difficulties, and sexual behavior should also be explored.

Table 2–3.   Extending the exploration

Sleep

   Sleep habits; difficulties falling or staying sleep

   Issues at night time: worrying feelings at bedtime; being scared at night and other issues at night

   Insomnias, nightmares

   Psychotic features at night

Awakening at morning

   Mood at morning, behavioral organization

   Issues related to getting ready to go to school

   Transportation issues

School

   Academic performance

   Behavioral issues at school; issues related to school discipline

   Bullying

   Tardiness and absences

   Alternative placement

   Issues with special education and remedial services

Behaviors after returning home

   Use of electronics and social media

   Visitation of inappropriate places in the Internet (pornography, violence, terrorism, chatrooms)

Hygiene

   Showering, dental hygiene

   Hygiene during menstrual cycles

   Personal care, hair care; clothing

   Perforations, tattoos

Friendships

Gender issues

   Gender preference: do you prefer boy or girls?

   Family reaction to gender preference, to sexual choice?

   Quality of friends

Table 2–3.   Extending the exploration *(continued)*

Respect for home rules

    Leaving home without permission; sneaking out of the house at night

    Letting people into the room at night

    Running away

    Conduct Problems

    Sexual behavior; birth control

    Delinquent behavior; gang participation

Substance abuse must be evaluated privately, because adolescents do not want their parents to know about this aspect of their lives. The examiner should not merely ask an adolescent, "Have you used drugs?" This type of question gives the adolescent an easy way out; he may respond with a fast denial. Instead, the examiner needs to conduct a detailed inquiry, using gentle assumption questions, such as the following: "What drugs have you tried?" "Do you drink wine coolers, beer, or liquor?" "How many times a week do you drink?" "How often do you get drunk?" "What kinds of problems have you gotten into because of alcohol?" "Do you drive after drinking?" "Have you received any citations for driving while intoxicated?" "What other drugs do you use when you drink?" "Have you been sexually involved when you've been drinking?"

The examiner should inquire individually about the following substances of abuse: marijuana, amphetamines, cocaine, crack, LSD (lysergic acid diethylamide), sedatives (benzodiazepines and others), steroids, inhalants, and other hallucinogenic and mind-altering substances. The examiner should systematically ask the patient these questions: "When did your use of [drug] start?" "How much do you use it, and how often do you use it?" "When was the last time you used [the drug]?" This methodical inquiry needs to be repeated with each drug the patient admits to using (Senay 1997).

The examiner also must attempt to ascertain whether the child has ever experienced any withdrawal symptoms or has ever been delirious or psychotic under the influence of drugs. Furthermore, the examiner should explore impairment and lapses of judgment during drug use. For example, the examiner may ask questions such as these: "When you use [the drug], do you fight?" "Do you get sexually involved?" The examiner must explore whether the adolescent has used intravenous drugs and whether the adolescent has been sexually involved with individuals who have HIV (human immunodeficiency virus) or hepatitis. If the examiner has not inquired about sexually transmitted diseases, this is the opportune time to approach the topic. (For more information about evaluating alcohol and substance abuse in adolescence, see Chapter 10, "Evaluation of Externalizing Symptoms.")

The patient's sexual behavior should be explored systematically. The examiner should not simply ask the patient, "Have you ever had sex?" It is better to assume that adolescents are sexually active. The patient needs to be asked about issues related to unprotected sex and history of pregnancy. Sexually active adolescent females must be asked, "Have you ever been pregnant?" Similarly, sexually active adolescent males should be asked, "Have you ever impregnated a girl?" Asking the patient whether he or she likes girls or boys opens the door to explore the patient's sexual orientation and his or her sense of gender. The adolescent may start a conversation about gender dysphoria.

Because children tend to be protective of their caregivers, denials to direct questions such as "Have you been physically abused?" need to be considered carefully. A more tactful question could be, "When you do something wrong, how are you disciplined?" More specific questions about abuse should follow.

During the exploratory phase, the patient's medical history is also investigated. A history of head trauma, seizures, congenital problems, cardiovascular issues, or neurological problems may be relevant in the diagnostic process. A selected family and developmental history also may be illuminating (see Chapter 4, "Family Assessment").

Completing the Mental Status Examination

During the fourth phase of the psychiatric examination, completing the mental status examination, the examiner finishes exploring areas of the patient's mental status that were not covered earlier. In the process of exploring the presenting problem, the examiner has the opportunity to assess a number of areas typically covered on a mental status examination. These findings may not need to be formally explored again if the examiner has a solid understanding about areas already covered. For example, if during the interview, the examiner has noticed that the child or adolescent gives accurate details about his or her own history, including dates and precise locations, the examiner can safely assume that the patient's recent memory is probably intact. If the child is in advanced math classes (e.g., calculus) at school, the child's calculation ability may not need to be tested, unless there are good reasons for doing so. In the same vein, if the examiner previously determined that the child had hallucinatory experiences and the examiner ascertained the nature of those perceptions, the examiner may not need to inquire about them again.

When beginning to explore the patient's sensorium and intellectual capacities, the examiner should mark the transition to a different kind of questioning by telling the patient that the next series of questions will test his memory, orientation, and so on. The examiner might say, for instance, "These are questions that are asked of all children." Children who have neuropsychological deficits may be sensitive to this examination. If, despite reassurances, the patient remains apprehensive or exhibits narcissistic mortification, this line of exploration should be interrupted or postponed. Once the mental status examination is complete, the examiner should ask the patient and family if they have any additional important information to share. After any additional data gathering is complete, the psychiatrist will move into the interpretive phase of the interview.

Modalities of the Psychiatric Examination

The psychiatric examination is comprehensive when most of the possible areas of psychopathology are reviewed; it is considered focal or selective if only selected areas of the patient's psychopathology or of the mental status examination are explored. The interview is also classified as unstructured or structured.

Unstructured Interviews

The psychiatric interview is unstructured if the examiner does not follow a predetermined scheme to conduct the interview process. In this modality, the examiner does not follow a prearranged path in exploring the relevant issues or completing the mental status examination. This modality gives the examiner a great deal of flexibility; he or she can adapt the examination to the relevant issues or to the most salient aspects that emerge during the examination. The examiner attempts to follow a coherent thread in the flow of emerging data and takes advantage of the patient's emotional abreactions to understand the nature of the patient's internal conflicts.

In unstructured interviewing, the examiner emphasizes the process and the vicissitudes of affect and attempts to help the patient to see and make connections between the content of the interview and troublesome emotional factors that the patient is experiencing. In this modality, the empathic and emotional processes are emphasized, and building rapport and establishing a solid therapeutic alliance are the examination's major objectives. The patient's relatedness to the examiner becomes more important than the data and the thoroughness of the examination. The unstructured modality does not cover all the relevant areas of a psychiatric examination in a consistent and systematic fashion and frequently leaves important areas unexplored. Furthermore, unstructured interviewing leaves significant room for subjective inferences regarding observations and diagnoses.

Structured Interviews

The structured interview is used when consistent and systematic data gathering and high levels of reliability are desired in the psychiatric examination and diagnostic process. In the most structured form of interview, the examiner uses a standardized set of questions. The examiner stays with the predetermined format of the examination, without deviating, until the interview is completed. Structured interviewing has a unique role in research (i.e., to ascertain change in any given diagnostic category resulting from, or secondary to, a given intervention), in epidemiological studies (i.e., to establish incidence and prevalence of psychiatric disorders), and in developmental studies (i.e., to compare contemporary examination data to baseline assessments with the purpose of ascertaining developmental change). In structured interviewing, the degree of the examiner's inferences is decreased to a minimum. (For more information about structured and unstructured interviews, see Note 1 at the end of this chapter.)

In clinical practice, behavioral rating scales, checklists, and symptom inventories are commonly used. Parents, teachers, patients themselves, clinicians, child care workers, and others can administer them. Table 2–4 lists the advantages and limitations of behavioral rating scales (Achenbach 1995).

Strategies for Evaluation of Preadolescents

The interviewing space needs to be inviting to children and spacious enough to allow small children to play comfortably on the floor. It should contain a medium-size table and appropriate chairs for playing and other diagnostic and therapeutic activities. For a small child or a preadolescent, sitting at a table feels more natural than sitting in a chair, face to face with the examiner. A variety of materials and toys should be readily available to the child. Table 2–5 outlines the basic toys necessary for the psychiatric assessment of preadolescents.

The examiner can foster engagement with the preadolescent by addressing the child warmly and engagingly and making the child an active participant of the diagnostic process from the very beginning. A common strategy is for the examiner to begin by asking simple questions to the preadolescent during the family meeting. For example, while taking notes, the examiner could ask the preadolescent how his or her name is spelled, what the current day or date is, and so on. The child's demeanor and responses provide important information about the child's alertness and intelligence.

The examiner may also reach an agreement with the child regarding the family member to whom questions should be addressed. The patient may be told that he or she is going to be asked the questions and that if a question becomes too difficult to answer or if the patient does not want to answer the question, the parents will be asked for an answer. This strategy gives the child a prominent role in the interview and helps to create a positive working and diagnostic alliance; usually, the family agrees with this arrangement. This ap-

Table 2–4. Advantages and limitations of behavioral rating scales

Advantages

Behavioral rating scales are convenient and economical.

The basic instrument is usually printed.

Relevant observations can usually be made under a variety of conditions without rigid standardization of the observational interval, setting, or inputs to subjects and raters.

Behavioral rating scales can be completed quickly.

They can be completed by diverse informants without specialized training.

They can cover a wide range of data, from specific behaviors to inferential judgments.

They provide scores that are easy to analyze.

High test-retest and inter-observer reliability are obtainable.

Limitations

Exclusive reliance on predetermined items may cause important characteristics to be overlooked.

Rating scales compare individuals in terms of item and scale scores but may not provide ideographic (individualized) descriptions of persons apart from their specific pattern of scores.

Rating scales are affected by the cooperation, knowledgeability, and candor of the rater, although gross distortions are clinically informative and can usually be detected by comparisons with other data.

Rating scales are subject to misuse by being over-interpreted or interpreted too literally in isolation from other data about the case. Ratings from different informants should therefore be compared with each other and with other types of data about the case.

Source. Adapted from Achenbach 1995, pp. 3–4. Modified from Cepeda 2010, p. 36.

proach gives centrality to the child's problems and concerns. When a mental status examination outline exists, the child may be "invited" to help the clinician fill in the requested information. Often, the child takes an interest in this cooperative enterprise.

A face-to-face interaction in an adult-like setting is an awkward situation for the preadolescent. The examiner should be sensitive to the patient's anxiety about the new situation and environment. Even with the best of preparation, the child will arrive with fears and negative expectations about the

Table 2–5.   Toys required for a diagnostic examination

Playhouse with furniture and a toilet

Doll family, with a dad, a mom, and children

Dolls with different ethnic features (e.g., white, black, Hispanic, Asian)

Wood and plastic building blocks, building bricks (e.g., Legos), disposable activity dough (e.g., Play-Doh)

Paper and pencils for drawing and writing

Crayons for coloring

Play telephones

Action figures representing men with associated weaponery

Table games and other structures games (e.g., checkers, Parcheesi)

Source.   Modified from Cepeda 2010, p. 37.

interview. A format in which the child and the examiner sit at a table gives the child a sense of comfort. The child is more likely to feel at ease if the interview is conducted in a specially furnished playroom. The younger the child, the greater the need is for nonverbal approaches such as play or the use of nonverbal media (e.g., drawing, puppetry, games; see Chapter 3, "Special Interviewing Techniques"). The nature of the media depends on the child's developmental level, as well as the examiner's style, preference, and technical experience.

After the child is properly situated in the office, the examiner attempts to engage the child. After some engagement is achieved, the examiner tells the child what he or she already knows about the presenting problems and then discusses with the child the known concerns. Most children start a verbal engagement when they are invited to discuss what is already known; more often than not, they express their thoughts about the problems without major difficulties. The exploration then proceeds. Instead of asking the child questions about issues the examiner already knows about, the examiner should disclose to the child what has already been learned about the problem and encourage the child to present his or her point of view.

Technical Issues of the Diagnostic Inquiry

Open and Leading Questioning

Open questions give children the opportunity to express themselves and allow the examiner to observe a spontaneous flow of thought processes and the emergence of preconscious affect and of emotional conflicts. When patients elaborate on some issues, the examiner observes the nature of the thought process, the integrity of reality testing, the degree of relatedness, the status of receptive and expressive language, the quality of cognitive abilities and social and adaptive skills, and so forth. The following are examples of open questions: "How are you feeling today?" "How is your day going?" "How did you sleep last night?"

Leading questions constrain the patient's answers, often result in monosyllabic (usually yes or no) answers, and stifle the communication and engagement between the examiner and the patient and family. Worse, leading questions frequently include or suggest the answer to the question. The following examples are counterparts of the open questions: "Are you feeling OK?" "Is your day going well today?" "Did you sleep well last night?"

The clinician needs to develop the discipline to avoid leading questions consistently. Leading questions may be dangerously reassuring. Care must be taken not to ask leading questions when exploring sensitive areas (e.g., "You didn't want to kill yourself, did you?") or to ask questions that would result in yes or no answers (e.g., "Do you sleep well every night?"). Leading questions (e.g., "Did you really intend to kill yourself?") are inappropriate in a couple of ways: 1) the questioner is deferring the assessment of such a serious behavior onto the patient, and 2) the question gives the patient an easy way out (by responding "no"). The examiner, not the patient, is responsible for assessing the nature of this and related serious matters. Therefore, the examiner should ask open-ended questions (e.g., "What did you intend when you overdosed?" "How is your sleep?") and must pay close attention to the patient's responses, including the associations generated and the patient's flow and change of affect. We believe that the use of leading questions is the source of many misdiagnoses and medical errors.

Some situations obligate the examiner to ask leading questions. These include instances when engaging the patient is difficult, when the child's verbal productivity is limited, or when the child's comprehension capacity is poor. Even in these circumstances, leading questions should be structured in a way to offer the patient choices. For example, if the examiner were to ask the child, "How are you feeling today?" and the patient does not respond, the examiner could ask, "Are you feeling the same, worse, or better than yesterday?" Based on the response, the examiner continues attempting to clarify the nature of the answer.

In general, open-ended questions are more productive than closed ones: "Closed questions...may inhibit emotional expression not only because they suggest a very brief factual reply but also because they suggest that the examiner has already decided what is important and relevant" (Hopkinson et al. 1981, p. 413).

Interpretive and Declaratory Comments

During diagnostic inquiry, the examiner may find interpretations and declaratory comments to be productive. Interpretations and expressions of sympathy explicitly indicate the examiner's interest and attention in the emotions, feelings, and attitudes of patients and families. Expressions of sympathy are also likely to be reinforcing because they indicate that the examiner cares. When such caring responses follow the expression of emotions or feelings, the informant is likely to be encouraged to continue showing feelings. Interpretations might draw the informant's attention to feelings that had been below the surface (Hopkinson et al. 1981), such as when the child or the family discloses the death of a significant other, a serious illness of a family member or close friend, the departure of a dear one, and so on.

Declaratory statements often elicit more information and create less resistance than do questions, particularly if the questions explore issues the patient is not yet ready to broach. For instance, when a patient is displaying a particular emotional state, making a gentle assumption (see subsection "Phases of the Psychiatric Examination" earlier in this chapter) such as "You look angry [or scared or nervous,]" is likely to be more productive than asking, "Are you angry [or scared or nervous]?" A statement such as "I understand you have problems at home" is a far better opener than the question "Do you have problems at home?" Asking a question like "Do you have any problems?" will certainly start the interview on the wrong foot.

If the examiner knows that the child has a particular problem, the examiner should state the problem up front, thereby presenting the issues directly and getting to the heart of the matter from the very start. For example, the examiner could start by saying, "I understand you have problems controlling yourself" or "It seems that you do not want to live anymore."

Use of Developmentally Attuned Language With Preadolescents

In communicating with a preadolescent, the examiner needs to use vocabulary calibrated to the child's developmental and cognitive level. Although smart and verbally advanced children may have sophisticated language skills and a rich vocabulary, this is not true of most children, even those from well-educated families. The examiner should avoid using technical jargon. For example, simple terms such as *sad* and *feel bad* are better than *depressed* and *guilty*. In contrast, most children are familiar with the term *suicide*. In fact, inquiring about the meaning of this term is a smooth way to explore suicidal intentions or suicidal behavior in young children. Table 2–6 lists some terms often used in adult psychiatric evaluations and the less complex equivalents appropriate for use with preschoolers and early latency children. When exam-

Table 2-6. **Developmentally appropriate terms and phrases for communicating with young children**

Adult diction	Terms for use with children
frightened	scared
frightful	scary
cruel or malicious	mean
anxious	nervous, antsy
angry or frustrated	upset, mad
of a sexual nature	nasty
irritable	grouchy or cranky
feel guilty about…	feel bad about…
compulsion	urges
depressed	feel down or feel sad
self-concept	feeling good or feel bad about oneself
feel hopeless	feel like not caring anymore
improve	feel better
learning problems	have trouble learning or hard to learn

Source. Modified from Cepeda 2010, p. 41.

ined carefully, the words *upset, scary, nasty, sad, bad,* and *good* seem to carry more affect than do their more sophisticated synonyms; the latter are most frequently used at the service of defense intellectualization or isolation of affect. The word *progress* is seldom understood by preadolescents; instead, they will readily understand when an examiner asks, "Do you feel any better or any worse?"

The examiner needs to pay equal attention to the use of idioms; even the most common idioms may be beyond a child's comprehension. Preadolescents and even early adolescents tend to be concrete thinkers and often interpret idioms literally. No subject is taboo in any diagnostic interview. Any topic can be discussed with children if appropriate language and judicious timing are used.

Dealing With Nonverbal Behavior During Diagnostic Assessment

During a diagnostic examination, preadolescents and early adolescents sometimes resort to responding with nonverbal behavior rather than verbal answers. For example, a preadolescent might respond to a question with a facial gesture, shrugging of the shoulders, or a penetrating stare. This covert and guarded nonverbal communicative language needs to be transformed into a declarative language.

When the patient responds with a stare during the diagnostic inquiry, the examiner could tell the patient, "Your eyes said a lot; now is the time for your mouth to speak, for your mouth to tell me what your eyes said." For patients who shrug their shoulders, the examiner can approach the issue in a rather humorous manner by saying, "My ears can't hear what your shoulders are trying to tell me." A similar approach may be used with other nonverbal behaviors, such as bowel sounds, knuckle cracking, and changes of body position. The examiner must make a deliberate effort to translate or transform the nonverbal language into a verbal narrative. A related issue, nonverbal enactments, is described in the section "Enactments During the Psychiatric Examination" later in this chapter.

Process Interviewing

In the process interview, the examiner notices how things are said and presented. The *content* of a communication refers to the explicit aspects of the communication. The *process* refers to the implicit aspects of the communication—to the way the communication is presented. To assess the communication process, the examiner pays special attention to the way the patient communicates. The way things are conveyed may be more important than what is said. For example, the patient may be saying one thing with words and a very different thing with his or her voice or body language. The examiner should inform the patient about any discrepancy between verbal and nonverbal behaviors and make the patient aware of atypical nonverbal communications. Any incongruity between verbal and nonverbal behaviors requires elucidation. Every time an abreaction of affect occurs, the examiner should ask the patient about the thoughts or memories that brought on those emotions. When the patient interrupts his or her own narrative or when unexpected transitions occur in the patient's train of thought, the examiner should ask about these interruptions or transitions. It is meaningful to know whether the patient has noticed these events. The following case example illustrates process interviewing.

Case Example 4

Donna, a 16-year-old Caucasian female, was being evaluated for protracted depression and suicidal behavior. According to Donna, her depression went back to when she was 7 or 8 years old, and she revealed that she had felt suicidal for a long time. Donna's mother and maternal grandmother had received a diagnoses of schizophrenia. A maternal aunt had raised Donna since early childhood. Donna had received both inpatient and prolonged outpatient treatments, with limited success.

At the time of the evaluation, Donna's aunt was in the process of giving up custody rights to the state because she could not handle Donna and could no longer afford to pay for Donna's psychiatric services. Donna had been involved in a lesbian relationship with a female 3 years her senior and had displayed significant behavioral problems at school and at home. Donna also had problems with substance abuse: she had abused marijuana, cocaine, LSD, and other mind-altering drugs. Donna had been a bright and articulate child who had excelled in school. Her academic performance had suffered during the previous year. She was described as a gifted and creative adolescent. Donna was fairly well kept and groomed, but she was a rather unattractive adolescent; she was withdrawn and maintained poor eye contact. Her psychomotor activity was low. She appeared distant and was not spontaneous; there was an air of apprehension and fear about her. Her mood was very depressed, and she exhibited marked constriction of affect, both in range and in intensity. She rarely smiled. Donna used sophisticated language, and her responses were filled with intellectualization and isolation of affect.

When the examiner asked questions, Donna took a long time to answer and noticeably hesitated while responding. When the examiner asked Donna how she felt about her aunt (whom Donna called "mother") giving up her guardianship rights to the state, Donna gave a bland and unemotional response. The examiner gave Donna feedback about the way she communicated and presented her thoughts. She expressed surprise and claimed that in all the time she had been in treatment, nobody had given her feedback about how she came across. She said, "My thoughts are in a different channel from other people. I always feel empty." When the examiner asked Donna why her thoughts were in a different channel from others, she said, "I need to build a barrier around people." Donna was able to discuss her apprehension and paranoid feelings and her difficulties with trusting and feeling close to people.

The content of Donna's delusional depression is presented as a case example (Case Example 11) in Chapter 8, "Documenting the Examination." The process interview is illustrated further in Chapter 9, "Evaluation of Internalizing Symptoms" (see Kurt's case [Case Example 11] example).

Technical Issues in the Evaluation of Adolescents

The adolescent evaluation should begin with the adolescent and the family together. The benefits of such a meeting are multiple: the examiner hears the parents' concerns directly, and the examiner has the opportunity to observe how the adolescent relates to the parents and how the parents or family members relate to one another. During the family meeting, the examiner completes most of the preliminary exploration and overall assessment of the presenting problem and the adolescent's level of functioning. The examiner explores the adolescent's school and family functioning; the parents' knowledge of their child's behaviors, such as drug use; and other serious concerns.

As these issues are addressed, the examiner invites and encourages the adolescent's participation. How the parents and adolescent handle conflicts gives the examiner a sense of the nature and intensity of the conflicts between them and of the problem-solving capacities within the adolescent and within the family.

After the parents express their concerns, the examiner asks them to leave. The adolescent is then given the opportunity to expand on or to present his or her side regarding the parents' concerns. The adolescent is asked to talk about issues the parents may not have any knowledge about, such as suicidal thoughts, school truancy, alcohol or drug use, illicit activities, sexual life, gang participation, cults, or other issues related to the presenting problem. Even if during the conjoined interview the adolescent made a number of denials about specific probes (e.g., suicide, homicide), those denials should not be taken as the definitive response. They need to be corroborated during the individual interview. Also, during the individual interview with the adolescent, a comprehensive mental status examination must be completed.

If the adolescent is not cooperative and displays hostility or resistance from the very beginning of the interview, the examiner may need to consider a different approach. Katz (1990, pp. 74–79) proposed four basic strategies to deal with an adolescent's immediate resistances. These strategies plus two others are presented in Table 2–7 and are discussed more fully in Chapter 15, "Diagnostic Obstacles (Resistances)."

Physical Contact

No rigid rules exist regarding physical contact with young children. Each clinical situation requires consideration of the child's developmental level, but the clinician may wish to keep some key points in mind when making decisions regarding appropriate physical contact. In general, the examiner should exercise restraint in initiating physical contact with a child except when the child is a toddler or a preschooler in need of guidance toward the office. Such guidance is achieved by holding the child's hand or making ongoing contact with the child's shoulder in a comforting and reassuring manner. The examiner may respond to any physical contact related to social courtesies (e.g., handshaking). The examiner needs to be sensitive to cultural norms. Rejecting the family's cultural norms may be interpreted as a sign of rejection and rudeness. A family from Mexico City came to the author's office to request an evaluation for their youngest child, a 9-year-old preadolescent boy who had neurodevelopmental problems. On the day of the appointment, as soon as the examiner came in to the waiting area, the mother advanced toward the examiner and kissed him on the cheek. Following this, the mother ordered her two daughters, a 13-year-old and a 15-year-old to greet the doctor. The ad-

Table 2–7. Strategies used in the psychiatric examination of adolescents

1. **Clarify the examiner's role as a stranger.** When the examiner detects an immediate distrust, he or she should respond with the ready acceptance of the distrust, pointing out to the patient that the examiner is a stranger and that the patient has no reason to trust the examiner.

2. **Analyze the situation to the patient.** When the examiner finds himself herself in trouble with a patient, the examiner should analyze the situation to the patient and enlist the patient's assistance. Often the patient revels information that can be helpful.

3. **Seek opportunities to empathize with the patient.** The examiner should demonstrate as quickly as possible his or her powers as a therapist—the power to see things from the patient's point of view—and the power to understand what is going on in the patient.

4. **Offer immediate help to the patient.** Each adolescent who comes to the office unwillingly is faced with the evidence of his or her own helplessness. The examiner offers power in the form of knowledge, and offers help, if appropriate, by intervening on the patient's situation.

5. **Reverse role with the patient.** The examiner asks the patient to take the examiner's role, while the examiner takes the patient's role. Acting as the adolescent, the examiner presents his or her concerns and seeks help from the adolescent (see Chapter 3, "Special Interviewing Techniques").

6. **Support adaptive behavior.** The examiner validates, praises, and promotes normative and adaptive behavior.

Source. Modified from Cepeda 2010, p. 45.

olescents readily came in and kissed the physician on the cheek. The greeting occurred in the presence of their consenting father. Although this manner of greeting is certainly not condoned in the United States, the examiner needs to be open to cultural differences in manners of greeting; he or she is right to respect differences in social/cultural norms.

With older adolescents, the examiner may initiate handshaking upon greeting the patient. Younger children sometimes initiate affectionate contact and may seek comfort by bodily proximity or by holding the examiner's hand. Children may want to show appreciation and make affectionate physical contact. If the contact is genuine and appropriate, the clinician may indicate that it is accepted and appreciated. However, the examiner should remind the child that he or she can express emotions with words and that words of appreciation are as good as hugs or other physical expressions of affection. Spontaneous embracing to express gratitude or to say good-bye is uncommon in children who are loved and well cared for. For small children in need of re-assurance and support, a tap on the shoulder or a delicate tapping on the head may be sufficient. Table 2–8 lists principles of physical contact with children.

With children older than mid-latency age, the examiner should exercise clinical judgment as to when it is appropriate to receive or accept physical con-tact, when it should be avoided, and when limits need to be imposed. Caution should be exercised when the examiner and the patient are of the opposite sex and when allegations of sexual abuse have been made; in such a case, no matter how young the child, physical contact should be discouraged, if not avoided.

When the child is female and a male examiner detects promiscuous relat-ing or inappropriate sexualization, he needs to exercise caution and set lim-its on boundary violations. The examiner should be particularly alert to any kind of physical contact with an overtly seductive female child or adolescent. The same caution applies to situations in which the examiner is female and the patient is male. Examiners of either gender may also be the focus of homo-sexual behavior by children or adolescents who have been abused or by pa-tients who are struggling with consolidation of their sexual identities.

With children who have not been sexually abused, an examiner may oc-casionally want to convey affirmation, approval, or reassurance by a gentle touch or when the doctor and patient converge in emotional rapport. In this case, sensitive contact could be appropriate and developmentally fitting.

Physical contact is obligatory in some situations. For example, the examiner must hold a small child who is beginning to harm himself or herself or to dis-play aggressive behavior toward the examiner; a firm hold may be necessary in these circumstances. The examiner should emphasize that the child will not be allowed to harm himself or herself or hurt the doctor. If the patient is an adolescent who gets out of control, the examiner should warn the patient that if the aggressive or intimidating behavior persists, the evaluation will be terminated immediately. If the patient persists, the examination should end at once. If the adolescent gives signs of being on the verge of losing control and asks to leave, the examiner should give this opportunity without objections by asking, "Do you need time to chill out?" or "Would you like time to get a hold of yourself?" and letting the patient leave. The examiner should inform the parents that the adolescent has left the evaluation in a state of dyscontrol. The examiner should establish procedures to follow in the event that he or she is at risk or in danger. The examiner must take precautionary actions if a patient is out of control and is at risk of self-harm or of harming others.

Physician contact with preadolescent and adolescent patients during the physical and neurological examination merits special comment. Contact is obligatory during this process. Some child and adolescent psychiatrists del-

Table 2–8. Principles of physical contact

Tenderness is the legitimate foundation for contact with the child.

The examiner should be judicious when contemplating physical contact.

In general, it is better to respond to than to initiate physical contact.

Physical contact is more appropriate and fitting with preadolescents than with adolescents.

Preschoolers and early preadolescents often seek physical contact.

Physical contacts are legitimate and fitting when related to affirmation or praise for achievements or good deeds (e.g., the child passed a test, gained an award, or is celebrating a birthday).

Supportive contact is indicated when the child is emoting pain or sadness or when the child breaks down under the influence of strong emotions or traumatic memories.

Caution is needed when responding to or initiating contact with abused children.

Physically abused children rarely seek or accept physical contact.

Neglected children are promiscuous in the search for body contact. The examiner should enforce body boundaries and provide consistent limit setting.

The examiner should beware of physical contact with sexually abused children; these children either are apprehensive about retraumatization and misperceive body contact or may attempt to recreate a sexual abuse experience.

The examiner needs to respect social manners and be attuned to cultural norms.

Source.   Modified from Cepeda 2010, p. 46.

egate all aspects of physical examination and medical care to pediatrician colleagues or other physicians, but multiple reasons exist for the evaluating and treating psychiatrist to conduct the physical examination.

The observations gathered during the physical and neurological examination are invaluable for achieving a comprehensive and integrative view of the patient. Findings frequently shed light on the diagnosis (e.g., evidence of a neurocutaneous disorder), aid in the examiner's understanding of the problem's etiology (e.g., evidence of self-inflicted injuries), or demonstrate the extent of a given identified problem (e.g., marked gynecomastia in an adolescent who has doubts about his sexual identity). In other cases, the physical examination redirects the process of assessment and treatment (e.g., when the physician observes ample evidence of physical abuse or drug addiction, even though the patient has denied such abuse or addiction throughout the interview). The examiner should explore methodically the history of every traumatic or surgical scar. These are only a few examples of the usefulness of conducting the physical examination during a comprehensive psychiatric examination. Neurological examination findings are equally valuable in patients with neuropsychiatric disorders.

The benefits of having the evaluating psychiatrist perform both the physical examination and the psychiatric examination far outweigh the risks (see Table 2–8). This is in agreement with Towbin's (2015) assertion that "[t]he physical examination in child psychiatry is part of the doctor's relationship with the patient, the patient's family, and in many cases, other health providers in the patient's life" (p. 449). Some basic precautions minimize the potential negative risks. "The physician must also be aware of and protect the patient's modesty and anxiety (Towbin 2015, p. 452). The physician should always conduct the examination in the presence of a nurse, or better yet, in the presence of one of the patient's parents. When evaluating female adolescents, the examiner should always invite the mother to be present during the examination. The physician should always tell the patient what is about to happen during the examination (e.g., "Now I'm going to examine your ears and your eyes," "Now I'm going to examine your belly"). The physician should remember that boys with a background of sexual abuse are as anxious about the physical examination as are girls with the same history. Some patients may object adamantly to a physical examination. Except in cases of medical emergency, a patient's refusal should be respected, and the examination should be deferred to the child's pediatrician or family doctor.

Special sensitivity needs to be demonstrated when examining the female thorax: that is, when listening to heart sounds and when exploring the hypogastric and inguinal areas. Pelvic examination, when indicated, should be referred to a gynecologist. If the examiner is a male and a female patient asks for a female physician to conduct the physical examination, this request must be granted.

In our experience, after thousands of physical examinations on preadolescents and adolescents, on only two occasions have patients misperceived the physical examination experience. In one case, a 12-year-old early adolescent girl with schizophrenia said, "I know you have the 'hots' for me. I know that because of the way you touched my breasts." Reality testing addressed her misperceptions. In the other case, a 9-year-old overanxious girl felt very anxious during the physical examination and complained about it afterward. For most female patients and for children in general, the physical examination is an uneventful experience with no detrimental psychological consequences. These indispensable procedures pose no significant risk in the building of a therapeutic patient-doctor alliance.

Activity, Structuring, and Support During the Psychiatric Examination

The examiner strives to create the optimal level of activity—that is, prompting and questioning—needed to elicit from the patient and the family information relevant to the diagnostic assessment. Excessive prompting tends to stifle the patient's spontaneity and may render the interview mechanical and emotionally sterile. When the interview has been too structured, the patient or the family may leave the office feeling dissatisfied, intruded upon, or even baffled, and with the sense that they could have said more if they had been given the opportunity. In contrast, in unstructured interviews, the data may be partial, incomplete, or irrelevant to the diagnostic goals if the patient is not given enough guidance and structure. The goal is to achieve a balance between activity and passivity (see subsection "Modalities of the Psychiatric Examination" earlier in this chapter).

Structuring is the process by which the examiner establishes conditions, contingencies, or limits during the psychiatric examination; these measures are necessary to ensure the integrity of the interviewing process, the integrity of the interviewing environment, and the safety of the child, the family, and the examiner. Simply, the examiner sets the structure to contain the child's or the family's acting out.

Structuring entails the control of a number of variables during the interview. The examiner has control of factors such as the interview space (e.g., limiting the child's actions or movements to a restricted area), the type of play and the toys used, the nature of the probing (e.g., using open-ended questioning or structured interviewing), and the degree and quality of nonverbal behavior (e.g., physical contact with the examiner). With verbal children, the examiner may direct the content and the process of the communication. Active structuring and limit setting are needed with hyperactive, impulsive, aggressive, self-abusive, seductive, or disorganized children.

The quality and degree of structure needed varies in each interview, depending on the child's developmental level, quality and intensity of psychopathology, dystonicity of symptoms, willingness to participate in the interview, and interest in working on his or her problems. Without appropriate structuring, a safe, effective, and productive interview cannot be achieved.

The examiner must convey to the child and family that the interview will be conducted in a safe atmosphere in which all verbalizations will be permitted and encouraged. Any personal or physical aggression will not be tolerated. The child needs to know that if he or she loses control, the examiner will help the child to regain it. If the child expresses aggression or self-abusive behaviors, the examiner will note the context in which these behaviors originated. The examiner's priority is to help the child regain control and to return the interview to its exploratory mode. The examiner must actively monitor safety conditions throughout the psychiatric examination.

The child needs to be supported or confronted as needed. There is no contradiction if the examiner is supportive and empathic during some parts of the interview, yet challenging and confrontational during other parts. The examiner should demonstrate empathy toward the child's emotional pain and circumstances but must confront the child's maladaptive behaviors. The examiner should help the patient assert self-control when an impulsive action is about to be carried out and should appeal to the child's adaptive functioning when the child entertains any impulsive or destructive action.

Balancing empathy and confrontation is an important skill for dealing with children and adolescents. For children with certain clinical presentations (e.g., acting-out behaviors, externalizing disorders), sensitive confrontations are always required (see Chapter 3, "Special Interviewing Techniques"); in contrast, for children with internalizing disorders (e.g., anxiety, depression), empathic interventions are the most helpful and productive.

The child psychiatrist will likely be asked to evaluate potentially dangerous adolescents. In these cases, the examiner needs to be alert to identifying (and anticipating) moments of potential danger during the examination. Limit setting needs to be enforced when the patient displays inappropriate familiarity with the examiner or when the patient behaves in a physically or sexually inappropriate manner toward the examiner.

Carrying the Psychiatric Examination

In a psychiatric examination, the concept of *carrying* relates to the process of assisting a patient to enhance verbal communication and to maintain a smooth verbalization flow throughout the interview. Carrying requires a number of therapeutic skills—including engagement, appropriate management of silences, and use of humor—and a good balance of exploratory and supportive approaches. This active assistance is of particular importance when interviewing patients who are developmentally arrested, resistant, or neuropsychologically impaired.

When the patient has cognitive or neuropsychological limitations, major challenges for the examiner include aiding the patient in the initiation of verbalization, helping the patient with a sensitive management of silences, and prompting the patient to be introspective. The more impaired a child is, the greater the need for communication assistance and the greater the examiner's responsibility to actively assist the child via the function of carrying the interview.

In general, small children do not tolerate silence; the tension created by silence is too much for them to bear. Prolonged silence is intimidating and erodes the engagement effort because the child may interpret silence as withholding or an expression of aggression on the part of the psychiatrist. For very small children, silences should last no longer than 10 seconds; for early preadolescents, no more than 15 seconds; and for adolescents, no more than 20–25 seconds. If the patient becomes silent following a question, the examiner needs to break the silence and move onto something else.

Enactments During the Psychiatric Examination

Enactments are nonverbal dramatizations of internal emotional conflicts that may occur when the patient is either unaware of the problems or has difficulties communicating them in verbal language. Enactments represent conflictive dramatizations that need assistance for verbal representation. The examiner needs to transform nonverbal communication (e.g., gestures, actions, motor displays) into an explicitly verbalized problem. The following are some case examples:

Members of a gang had raped a 12-year-old Hispanic female. When interviewed 2 years later, the girl was sitting by a metallic table that had multiple holes. As she discussed the rape, she stuck her fingers in and out of the holes in an obvious copulatory gesture. This adolescent felt terrible about herself and had attempted to kill herself a number of times because she felt like "damaged goods" after the rape. The girl exhibited active symptoms of posttraumatic stress disorder. The enactment indicated how active and disorganizing the gang rape incident still was for her.

A 14-year-old Caucasian male with a history of neuropsychological deficits, low intellectual functioning, and significant language difficulties was seen in consultation for persistent regressive behavior and enuresis. The examiner had been informed that the child seemed to enjoy urinating on himself. During the interview, the boy repeatedly twisted and compulsively tightened the edge of his shirt around his fingers. This behavior appeared to be an enactment of the child's effort and conflict surrounding his enuresis.

A 13-year-old Asian American male with a history of bipolar disorder was evaluated for depressive features after the manic state began to recede. When the patient was actively manic, he was busy all day long, lifting weights without feeling tired or experiencing muscle pain. He had an inordinate amount of energy. At the time of the interview, while talking about how much better he was feeling, he began to display his muscles and began contracting his biceps in both arms, touching the bulk of each bicep in a clearly exhibitionistic manner. The examiner reminded the patient about the feelings he had while in the manic state and pointed out to him that he might be missing the abundant energy he had before. This helped the patient understand some of his depressive feelings.

A 13-year-old Caucasian male with a history of marked impulsivity and overt manic features was evaluated for issues regarding sexual identity: he had conspicuous gynecomastia and clearly effeminate traits. During the assessment, the boy placed his hands under his sweatshirt and formed with his fists two prominences on his upper chest, simulating female breasts. When the examiner asked, "What are you doing?" the boy responded, "Mountains." The examiner understood the patient was enacting, in a seductive and histrionic fashion, his concerns about his sexual identity in general and his gynecomastia (i.e., the "mountains") in particular.

Qualities of the Diagnostic Interview

During the diagnostic interview, the examiner's goal is to achieve the best quality interview possible. The important qualities of the interview are described in more detail below and are summarized in Table 2–9.

Sensitivity

Sensitivity relates to the examiner's ability to empathize with the child (and family) and to adjust his or her approach to the child's developmental level, to the family's circumstances, and to the nature of the presenting problem. Sensitivity also implies that the examiner is attentive to the child's level of anxiety and attempts to carry out the evaluation process with the least amount of stress possible. An optimal level of engagement and empathic attunement to the child's emotions and anxiety level are good markers of sensitivity.

Fluidity

The examiner strives to maintain a natural and smooth flow of the child's verbal and nonverbal communication. A sense of fluidity and cohesion is created when the examiner facilitates smooth transitions from one topic to the next and closely follows the thread of the child's communications and emotional expressions.

Depth

The examiner seeks to clarify and explore the main issues at hand, including their ramifications and meanings, before moving on to other areas. He or she gives special attention to the child's verbal and nonverbal manifestations of affect. Every time an emotional abreaction occurs, the examiner asks the child to verbalize what made him or her feel in that particular way. In the same vein, when the child narrates events that by their nature are filled with emotion and the child does not display the corresponding affect, the examiner queries the child regarding the reason for the discrepancy. In the latter case, the examiner attempts to draw out the child's suppressed emotions and to give the child an understanding of the abreacted emotional states. The interview gains a sense of depth when the examiner connects the child's affects with ongoing events at home or school, or with concerns regarding the child's presenting problem.

Table 2-9.   Qualities of the diagnostic interview

Sensitivity	Comprehensiveness
Fluidity	Meaningfulness
Depth	Versatility
Coherence	Efficiency
Specificity	

Source.   Reprinted from Cepeda 2010, p. 53.

Coherence

As the examiner strives to connect and to integrate the information gathered during the interview, he or she gives to the process a sense of connection or coherence. Inexperienced examiners often give the interview process a quality of discontinuity or fragmentation. An observer is left with the impression that the communication is unclear or disjointed, that certain areas were inadequately explored, or that certain topics were missed altogether. When coherence is not achieved, the patient feels irritated and misunderstood.

Specificity

Specificity of the psychiatric interview refers to the examiner's understanding and identification of the presenting complaints and clarification of the context in which the symptoms appear. A complementary idea is the concept of functional assessment. Because psychopathology and problems of adaptation go hand in hand, the examiner needs to clarify how psychopathology interferes with the patient's adaptive capacity.

Comprehensiveness

The examiner strives to be thorough. Comprehensiveness is achieved by exploring all the possible ramifications of a given problem in the context of the child's developmental history and current family and school circumstances (i.e., other relevant medical or psychiatric history).

Meaningfulness

The interview should make overall integrative sense to achieve meaningfulness. By following through with a topic until full understanding is achieved, the examiner gains depth and breadth of meaning.

Versatility

Versatility relates to the examiner's skill in meeting and engaging diverse presentations of child and family dysfunctions. The diagnostic interview needs to be tailored to each child's and family's needs. To build a bridge of trust and to create an atmosphere of understanding, the examiner needs to address the specific issues related to the child and family's presenting problem. A monotonous or ritualistic survey of symptoms will not fulfill this need.

Efficiency

The examiner needs to keep up a diligent pace in the process of diagnostic data gathering. He or she must be efficient with time. To achieve efficiency, the examiner needs to have a flexible but clear plan in mind. The goals of the interview need to be pursued, even in the presence of intrinsic or extrinsic pressures. The experienced examiner knows how to differentiate the essential from the unimportant. He or she learns to obtain the fundamental data in the least possible time and to use the obstacles discovered in data gathering as vehicles to increase his or her understanding of the child and the child's circumstances. An efficient and experienced examiner is able to complete a comprehensive assessment of a child and family in 1.5–2 hours. Although a solid diagnostic interview may be accomplished in one sitting, circumstances may dictate additional diagnostic sessions. We agree with Strakowski (2016, p. 1), who observes, "Some psychiatrists feel the need to nail down a diagnosis after a single session, which is often unrealistic, especially with bipolar disorder." The same may be said in evaluating multiple complex psychiatric conditions in children and adolescents.

Validity of the Psychiatric Examination

Establishing validity of the psychiatric diagnoses based on diagnostic interviews is frequently problematic because no gold standard exists with which to compare the findings (Grills-Taquechel and Ollendick 2008). For issues related to the concept of validity, see Note 2 at the end of this chapter.

Key Points

- Issues related to engaging and treatment alliance are emphasized and centrality is given to the exploration of the presenting problem.
- There are questions and ways of questioning that foster the interviewing process, There are others that do not.
- Developmental sensitivity facilitates the technical aspects of the interview along the life arc from infancy to young adulthood.

Notes

1. *Unstructured interviews* give full discretion to the interviewer as to what, when, and how to ask questions, and how to record them. *Semistructured interviews* also allow leeway to the interviewer regarding the order in which questions are asked. The emphasis is on obtaining consistent and reliable information. Extensive training is required to ensure that clinical discretion is used judiciously. *Highly structured interviews* are more restrictive in the amount of freedom allotted to the interviewer, and all responses need to be recorded in a prespecified format. Clinical judgments are reduced, and no extensive training is required for their administration. Structured interviews are commonly administered by laypersons. The rigidity of these interviews renders them impersonal because the format hinders the creation of rapport. These protocols also interfere with reliability and validity by not giving the interviewee an opportunity to report all difficulties or to explore them in depth (Grills-Taquechel and Ollendick 2008). Examples of highly structured interviews include the Diagnostic Interview for Children and Adolescents (DICA) and the Diagnostic Interview Schedule for Children (DISC-IV). Examples of semistructured interviews include the Schedule for Affective Disorders and Schizophrenia for School-Aged Children (K-SADS), the Child Assessment Schedule (CAS), and the Interview Schedule for Children (ISC; Costello 1996, pp. 460–463). The Anxiety Disorders Interview Schedule for DSM-IV: Child and Parent Versions (ADIS-IV-CP) have been used frequently in youth anxiety disorders research. It covers all the anxiety disorders included in DSM-IV (American Psychiatric Association 1994), as well as most of the prevalent disorders of childhood (Grills-Taquechel and Ollendick 2008, p. 465). Comprehensive diagnostic instruments vary in the degree of training required to administer them and in their degree of reliability, sensitivity, and specificity for certain diagnoses. In clinical practice, the distinction between structured and unstructured interviews is blurred. For example, relatively inexperienced clinicians have administered semistructured instruments "in a highly structured fashion, with little variation from the suggested wording...and experienced clinicians have varied the wording of highly structured interviews without apparently changing the performance of the interview" (Costello 1996, p. 463). Lay examiners have also been able to make judgments about answers that rival the judgments made by clinicians (Costello 1996). The K-SADS-P IV, -E, and -PL are the most comprehensive in diagnostic categories when compared with the ADIS-IV-CP, DISC-IV, and DICA. The ranking from the most to the least comprehensive is K-SADS-P IV, -E, and -PL, DISC-IV, DICA, ADIS-IV (Grills-Taquechel and Ollendick 2008, p. 467). On the overall importance and

relevance of structured interviews, Angold (1994) commented, "Though structured interview techniques have many advantages, they will aid the clinical processes only when used skillfully and sensitively" (p. 54). Fisher, Chin, and Vidair (2015, pp. 419–435) review a variety of batteries and interview protocols, including specific measures for a number of diagnoses, and broad-based schedules aiming to determine psychopathology in many behavioral and emotional fields. The authors discuss indications and recommend particular protocols for certain conditions depending on age range.

2. A number of difficulties linger around the validity and reliability of diagnostic interviews: 1) One of the most consistent difficulties involves the use of parent-child diagnostic interviews, because the findings are commonly discordant. In general, symptoms and diagnostic agreements within and across multiple informants are usually poor. 2) The sequence of disorder presentation in the interviews affects the informants' reports. 3) The emotional state of the informants affects the quality of the responses. 4) The degree of structure affects validity and reliability. 5) The child's cognitive capacities affect validity and reliability. Some experts propose that children should be at least age 10 years to respond to highly structured instruments such as the Diagnostic Interview Schedule for Children—Revised (DISC-R). 6) Motives can affect responses. Individuals may deliberately overreport or underreport to get access to services, or children may suppress or deny problems. 7) The validity and reliability vary depending on the nature of the disorder or disorders that are being investigated. 8) Parental psychopathology may affect the nature of the reporting (Grills-Taquechel and Ollendick 2008).

Validity refers to how well a test measures what it is supposed to measure. *Content validity* refers to the degree to which questions (e.g., in an interview) explore all aspects of the domain under study (e.g., a specific disorder). *Criterion-related validity* relates to the degree to which a measure predicts an outcome on another measure such as adjustment; it is considered *concurrent* when the measures are obtained at the same time and *predictive* when one measure is obtained prior to the other. *Construct validity* measures how effectively the information obtained from the interview agrees with the theoretical construct being investigated (*convergent validity*). *Divergent validity* relates to nonsignificant associations with measures determined to measure theoretically diverse constructs (Grills-Taquechel and Ollendick 2008).

CHAPTER 3

Special Interviewing Techniques

This chapter addresses situations or circumstances during the psychiatric evaluation that require specific handling. A variety of diagnostic approaches can be used to circumstances in which standard protocols are ineffective and special knowledge and skills are required. Effective use of a variety of nonstandard diagnostic techniques expands the diagnostic and engagement "toolbox." When standard techniques fail to achieve the goals of obtaining useful clinical data and secure an engagement, the examiner needs to try alternative means to reach these goals. In this chapter we present techniques that may be used when common approaches are unfruitful.

Gathering Collateral Information

Examiners always gather collateral information from a child's significant others: parents, siblings, grandparents or other relatives. There are times when the examiner seeks information about a child from teachers, school counselors, and other school liaison personnel; probation officers or judicial representatives; and consultant physicians, therapists, alcohol/drug counselors, and the like. A child's friends are worth considering as sources when the presenting problem relates to suicide, homicide, or terroristic activities. Friends often know far more about what the child under examination is thinking or contemplating than anybody else.

Limit Setting During the Psychiatric Examination

Novice examiners have significant difficulty maintaining a safe and unencumbered diagnostic environment. Impulsive children frequently violate space or personal boundaries, and children may become destructive or aggressive during the diagnostic examination, posing a risk to the safety of the diagnostic process. In these circumstances, the examiner needs to convey unambiguously that these behaviors must stop.

The examiner needs to convey that he or she is in charge of the psychiatric examination process at all times. Inexperienced examiners fear that setting limits during the diagnostic interview will make the child less cooperative or that setting limits will decrease the chances for building a diagnostic and therapeutic alliance; this is a groundless concern. Rather than decreasing trust in the examiner, appropriate and opportune limit setting gives patients a sense of security. Children and adolescents with impulse-control difficulties hope to find someone who will help them to have a secure hold off themselves.

Appropriate structuring and timely limit setting are fundamental requirements in any diagnostic interview. Failure to assert limits and to delineate boundaries poses risks for the patient and the examiner and may imperil the entire diagnostic enterprise. The therapeutic alliance may be jeopardized if the patient perceives the examiner as not capable of establishing or maintaining a sense of safety during the examination. The following case example illustrates inadequate management of risk and boundary problems during a diagnostic interview:

Case Example 1

During the live patient interview portion of a mock oral board examination, a first-year fellow in child and adolescent psychiatry encountered a 13-year-old Caucasian female who displayed marked hyperactivity, impulsivity, and immaturity from the beginning of the interview. The adolescent started off by making fun of the fellow's name. She also began to smile inappropriately, fidgeted a great deal, and stared at one of the ceiling corners. The fellow kept busy writing down the child's answers to his questions missing important nonverbal behaviors.

The child kept squirming and tilting her chair backward. At one point, she got up, picked up a long stick that was leaning against the wall in a corner of the room, and began to swing it from side to side. The stick made contact progressively with a piece of furniture, the child's chin, and the fellow's boots, legs, and knees. Finally, the child pointed the stick at the fellow's tie, directly at his neck, in a teasing, provocative, and dangerous manner. In a bland and unconvincing fashion, the fellow said to the child that what she was doing was dangerous; however, he hesitated in asking her to put down the stick.

In the preceding case example, the hazardous development was predictable once this impulsive child picked up the stick. An experienced clinician would have anticipated the child's impulsivity, immaturity and escalating and inappropriate social behaviors and her potential for aggressive behaviors. The most appropriate and timely intervention would have been to ask the child to put down the stick as soon as she picked it up from the corner.

Many examiners have had experience with children who bring to the interview knives, lighters, and other potentially dangerous items. In one way or another, these children make the examiners aware of the presence of these items. These children sometimes display and use these weapons in a clearly provocative and dangerous manner. The examiner must indicate in an unambiguous and convincing voice and demeanor that the threatening and dangerous behavior needs to end at once. If necessary the examiner needs to call extra help to ensure the safety of the patient, the interviewer, and the diagnostic environment. (Issues regarding limit setting in a preschooler are discussed in the next section.)

Physical Holding During the Diagnostic Assessment

The examiner needs to hone in on different areas of family and parental functioning as well as different developmental acquisitions when assessing a preschool child. The examiner will attempt to determine the quality of the child's attachment to the parental figure and at the same time ascertain the degree of parental figure's emotional investment in the child. Does the examiner see evidence of the child's exploratory behavior in an unfamiliar environment? Does the child show evidence of separation anxiety? Does the child show behavior organization (see Chapter 8, "Documenting the Examination,")? Does the examiner observe the parent demonstrating a positive regard toward the child? Is the parent attuned to the child's biological, emotional and security needs? Does the parent attend to the child's safety and to his or her impulsivity? Does the parent display a capacity for sensitive and effective limit setting? Does the parent allow the child to do whatever he or she wants? Does the parental support the child's efforts at self-soothing, behavioral organization, or self-regulation?

Issues with continuity of upbringing need to be explored. "Have you taken care of your child all the time?" "Who else has been involved in the rearing of your child?" "Have you ever been separated from your child?" What were the circumstances?" "Who took care of the child while you were away?" "Has the child ever been placed outside of the family?" The examiner needs to inquire if Child Protective Services (CPS) has ever been involved with the family.

If so, what was the reason? Here is an example of an evaluation of and intervention for a 4-year-old boy.

Case Example 2

Rudd, a 4-year-old Caucasian male, was brought to the consulting psychiatrist for severe hyperactivity and impulsivity, low frustration tolerance, and aggressive outbursts. When he became angry, he threw things, such as toys, and overturned chairs and so forth. He had a history of significant developmental speech defects but was not receiving speech therapy at the time of the evaluation. Rudd would not listen to his mother and frequently became aggressive toward her and his 7-year-old sister. He did not seem to respond to time-outs, either. Rudd had no prior psychiatric treatments but had a history of developmental delays and a history of asthma and of a right polycystic kidney.

The biological mother was a 25-year-old, single parent who had four children from four different fathers. Her first child had died at 3 months, and the third child had been given away for adoption at birth. Mother was totally on her own: she had no extended family support (she received no support whatsoever from her own mother) and had no friends; she was not receiving child support payments, but her two children were receiving SSI [Supplemental Security Income]. Rudd's biological father was not involved in his life.

When the examiner came to the waiting area, Rudd was throwing a tantrum; mother was asking him to get up but he did not obey and persisted in his outburst. I asked mother to proceed with me to the office [*first intervention*]. When he saw that mother had gone beyond the reception door, he readily got up and joined mom and his older sister. In the office, Rudd began to fuss, and since he had no expressive functional speech, he started demanding by nonverbal means that he wanted this or that. Rudd did not show behavioral organization and lacked capacities for self-soothing and self-regulation; cognitive deficits were also likely. Rudd wanted to imitate or to do anything his sister did. For example, if his sister began to draw, he also asked for a sheet of paper and a pencil. Rudd did not utter any understandable verbalizations during the evaluation. A number of times Rudd got into what his sister was doing, and when his sister appropriately asserted herself, he started to whine; when his sister did not give in, Rudd's frustration escalated and he began to hit his sister, threw things, and started a tantrum. Commonly, mother would observe her children's misbehavior but she did not do anything about it. When mother acted, her interventions were weak and unconvincing. Her voice was soft and did not carry any sense of authority. Mother's demeanor did not carry instrumental aggression or parental effectiveness. The examiner called mother's attention to the fact that Rudd was bothering his sister. Mother told the examiner that telling Rudd to stop misbehaving did not work. Mother told Rudd in a very bland and ambiguous manner to stop bothering his sister and even told daughter to give in to Rudd's demands.

Because Rudd did not get what he wanted, first, he hit his sister and then he picked up a metallic toy car and threw it at his mother. Mother did not respond to this incident either. When he attempted to throw a number of books that lay on the examiner's round table, the examiner picked Rudd firmly up in his arms, lifted him over the table, and set him down in a corner near the door [*second intervention*]. The examiner asked mother not to make any eye contact with him [*third intervention*]. Rudd fussed and whined for about 3 minutes and then quieted down. Mother was amazed that Rudd had calmed down. The examiner explained to mother that she needed to convey conviction and authority every time she told him to stop. Once the child was calm, the examiner suggested to mother to make contact with the child and even to provide some comforting body contact [*fourth intervention*]. The child remained in good self-control for the rest of the evaluation. At the end of the interview, when the family was departing, Rudd came to the examiner and embraced him [*fifth intervention*]![1]

Confrontation as an Engagement Technique

Confrontation is not the technical approach that first comes to mind during a discussion of engagement. Using confrontation as an engagement technique appears to be either counter-intuitive or at best paradoxical. However, when sensitively used, confrontation is a very good and appropriate engaging technique.

Case Example 3

Casper, a 16½-year-old Caucasian male, was referred for an emergency psychiatric evaluation after he placed his head in a train track when he saw the train coming. He pulled himself back from the tracks shortly before the train passed, feeling a sense of shock that he had gone that far. Casper had also tried to hang himself some days prior to the rail track incident. During the initial assessment, the examiner learned that Casper had been feeling depressed for more than 3 years and had received no psychiatric treatment. Casper did endorse feeling anxious and preferred to be by himself. He reported that he had problems getting up in the mornings and that he also had difficulties concentrating; the latter difficulties went back to grammar school years. Casper said that it was hard for him to be around other people and that it was even harder to initiate conversations.

Regarding emotional issues, Casper stated that life was pointless, that life was a bother, that he did not see any point in going on, and that things had a predictable path: "You have to get up every morning, go to school…" He was not doing well at school and had heard from teachers that there was no chance he could go to college to become a psychologist (his professional ambition) with the grades he was making. Casper was a junior in high school and, previously, had participated in the Gifted and Talented program till the 9th grade; this was the time when he started feeling depressed and anxious and when his grades began to drop. Casper disclosed to the examiner that he had been feeling hopeless for a long time and that he had stopped caring. There was no history of physical, emotional, or sexual abuse, no history of alcohol/drug abuse, and no difficulties with the law. Casper was very defen-

---

[1]See Chapter 4, "Family Assessment," for further comments on this case.

sive during the initial interview, conducted in a hospital setting. He definitely looked depressed and displayed a very constricted affect.

During the second diagnostic interview, he said that there was no reason for him to be in the hospital and that his problems were not as serious as those of other children in the acute care unit; he stated that he wanted to go home. The examiner told him that in his many years of practice, he had never heard of an adolescent attempting to kill himself by putting his head on the train tracks! When Casper stated that he was not thinking about that anymore, the examiner reminded him that he had tried to hang himself some days before. Casper remained silent for a short while but then told the examiner that when he was brought to the hospital, he had been expecting to be seen by a therapist and had not thought of being put in the hospital.

On an early Monday morning, after his emergency admission on Sunday, the day before, Casper had already called his mother to complain about the facility and had demanded that his mother take him out. The examiner realized that significant separation anxiety was activating the patient's anxieties about being away from home. When the patient told the examiner that he was going to ask his mother to come to pick him up from the hospital, the examiner told Casper that he would not be released. He was also told that even though he had stopped caring for himself, the examiner still cared about him and that the examiner had professional responsibilities regarding Casper's care and his safety.

When the examiner asked Casper to tell him his three wishes, he rejected the request; he said he never wished for anything. The examiner pressed on this issue, Casper said he wished he could wish for everything he wanted. The examiner rejected that wish and told him that he expected him to continue in the task of creating three wishes. Casper then said that his first wish was to go home. The examiner prompted him, "And the second?" He answered, "To finish high school." The examiner was pleased with his second wish. The examiner prompted him again, "And the third? He said, "To go to college." The examiner was also supportive of his third wish. After hearing this, the examiner told Casper, "If I were you, I would have the following wishes: the first, I wish I would feel better about myself; my second wish would be to feel confident around people, and my third one would be to not feel depressed and anxious to the point that I want to kill myself." The examiner asked Casper, "What do you think of my wishes? He hesitatingly conveyed to the examiner in a nonverbal manner that he liked them.

The examiner confronted the child's suicidal behavior denials and his sense of hopelessness. The examiner used the three wishes technique to confront his hopelessness and to engage him; he also supported the child's adaptive and motivating wishes. Furthermore, the examiner used the three wishes to open areas of exploration that the patient had been reluctant to discuss.

The following day, Casper was a bit more open with the examiner; when the examiner asked him what he had been thinking, he said that he had been thinking about the examiner's wishes from the previous day; Casper told the examiner that he was going to work on trying to feel better about himself, and he apologized for having given the examiner such a hard time the day before.

It is clear that in spite of the therapist's firm and confronting stance toward Casper's dramatic suicidal behavior, hopelessness, and massive denials, the therapeutic alliance was maintained.

The confrontations were successful in breaking some of "the ice" and the denials and in prompting Casper to be more reflective and less defensive. Chapter 15 ("Diagnostic Obstacles [Resistances]") has many vignettes that illustrate the use of confrontation to overcome resistances during the evaluation process.

The Good and the Bad

If a sensitive confrontation does not break down defensiveness and denials, the authors recommend the following intervention: the examiner asks the patient to list what is good about the behavior in question (e.g., suicidal behavior, self-abusive behavior, anorexic/bulimic behavior, aggressive behavior). The examiner assists the child in seeking reasons why he or she would want to perpetuate this behavior. If the issues at hand were persistent suicidal behavior, for instance, the examiner will encourage the child to find reasons to continue acting self-destructively. Common reasons that are proposed are: "This is my body and I can do with my body whatever I want," "It makes me feel better," "I feel relieved; I get rid of my problems," "I feel I have control over myself," "I stop feeling depressed," "I get rid of my anger without hurting anyone," "I will make my family or my girl friend suffer," and so forth. The examiner strives to be exhaustive in this subject: "Are there any other reasons for you to hurt or kill yourself?" There may be some factors that have been missed and are worth noting.

After this, the examiner asks the patient to list all that is bad about killing himself or herself (or the like), and strives again to be exhaustive in discussing the bad things that could happen as a result of the patient taking his or her own life, or the consequences of the patient's persistence in his or her maladaptive behaviors. Thus the discussion could address how the parents and sibling will suffer as a result of his death, how he or she will not be able to reach his goals in life, how people will be shocked and in disbelief upon learning of the patient's actions, how he or she will be missed by friends and relatives, and how people will keep wondering what happened. What will people think of his actions? Pertinent issues to ponder may be brought into the discussion: impact on a romantic or broken relationship, feelings about after life or God, and so forth. Equally, the examiner will attempt to be exhaustive in this area. The contrasting of the ambivalent feelings about a particular behavior may open avenues to dissociative feelings or memories that may set the child's mind into alternative behavior and different ways of feeling and being.

Interviewing in Displacement

When interviewing preschoolers and early latency-age children, the examiner frequently encounters difficulties in exploring issues directly. When the examiner senses that the child is too self-conscious or too guarded, he or she may interview the child in displacement by addressing a fantasy character's issues rather than the patient's issues. The following case illustrates this point.

Case Example 4

Roland, a 9-year-old Caucasian male born with paralysis of the left side, was evaluated for aggressive behavior at home and at school. He initially refused to answer any questions regarding why he had been brought for a psychiatric examination. Roland's residual neurological sequelae were obvious: besides the paralysis, he displayed conjugated gazing to the left and nystagmus with rapid eye movements to the right. His voice was infantile and had an immature and unmelodious quality.

Roland was disgruntled and unhappy, and during the individual assessment he asked for his mother. The examiner empathized with Roland's distress over being away from his mother. Because Roland refused to indicate why his mother had brought him for the evaluation, and having announced that he wanted to talk about dinosaurs, the examiner went along with that idea.

Roland started by saying, "The baby dinosaur is angry." The examiner replied, "The baby dinosaur is angry at his mother." Roland agreed and continued, "The baby dinosaur is really mad and felt like hitting people." The examiner responded, "If the baby dinosaur loses control and hits people, he is going to get in trouble." The examiner added, "The baby dinosaur is angry, in part, because he is not with his mother," and she asked, "Are there other reasons why the baby dinosaur is so angry? While this interaction continued, Roland kept attempting to stretch the fingers of his paralyzed left hand with his right hand. Roland was angry as he attempted to move his limp hand. The examiner said, "It seemed that the baby dinosaur is angry at his mother because he has problems with his left arm and left leg." Roland responded, "I'm very angry at my mother." The child then began to bite himself, saying "It's better to bite myself than to bite my mother."

The examiner addressed issues of Roland's defective self-concept and his feeling of rejection; he also suggested that Roland blamed his mother for the problems he had with his left side. Roland acknowledged that he had problems controlling his anger and that this was one of the reasons that he had been brought for the psychiatric examination.

In the preceding case example, the child was resistant to discussing the nature of his problems. Once the examiner followed the child's lead and approached his emotional problems in an indirect manner, using the mechanism of displacement, the examiner was able to move into a direct exploration of the patient's painful subjective difficulties. In the next case example, the child was very uncommunicative and resistant at first but became more open after the displacement mechanisms were respected and utilized.

Case Example 5

Saul, a 7-year-old African American male, had been referred for a psychiatric evaluation because of aggressive and unruly behaviors. There was also a question regarding the presence of psychotic behaviors because he displayed a series of atypical behaviors at home and at school. He lived with his mother; a sister, who was a couple of years his senior; and his maternal grandmother. Saul had threatened to kill his sister, mother, and grandmother with a knife. Saul's parents had been divorced for over a year, and his father had broken off all contact with the children. Saul and his sister missed their father a lot and were very angry that their father did not seem to care about them anymore.

Saul reported seeing his grandfather, who had died 18 months earlier. Also, the family had overheard Saul talking to himself (as though he were talking to other people) when he was alone. Apparently he believed that people talked about him and that God was telling him to be good.

During the psychiatric examination, Saul was very unhappy. He appeared downcast and was overtly angry and defiant. He displayed poor eye contact and was uncooperative with the examiner. When the examiner asked him questions, he refused to answer them. He demonstrated unhappiness after each question, no matter how empathic the examiner tried to be. For instance, the examiner commented on how sad it must be for Saul that his father didn't show any interest in calling him. Instead of being more forthcoming with his communications, Saul became more defensive and less verbal.

Saul brought to the second diagnostic interview his school project on caterpillars. He began to talk about his project. The examiner picked up Saul's lead and followed the content and process of his narrative. Saul continued discussing his project and demonstrated an interest in the caterpillar's life. The examiner asked Saul what the caterpillar's family life was like. Saul explained that the caterpillar lived with his mother and sister alone. The examiner asked what happened to the caterpillar's father. Saul became sad and said that the father had gone away and had not come back. The examiner commented that the caterpillar must be very sad because it could not see its father anymore. Saul began to cry. At this point, the examiner said, "It is very hard for you not to see your father. You miss him a lot and you are very angry that you can't see him." This interpretation brought the child's concerns from the displacement to the reality of his life.

In these and similar cases, the examiner's comments and interpretations through displacement build a bridge to the child's emotional difficulties in real life and to the feelings the child has in diverse areas of his life. Issues that the child has refused to acknowledge directly are accepted via the comments and interpretations made through displacement. Interviewing through displacement is developmentally appropriate for preadolescents because this mechanism is prevalent among children in this age group.

Use of Role Reversal During a Child or Adolescent Interview

Role reversal, by which the therapist becomes the person with problems, is a useful diagnostic technique. First, the technique externalizes or displaces the child's problems onto the examiner. Second, the technique counterbalances the child's sense of helplessness and makes him or her an expert. Third, the technique explores the patient's capacity for empathy and his or her problem-solving skills, among others. The following case example illustrates the effectiveness of reversing roles with the patient.

Case Example 6

Damian, a 16-year-old African American male, was brought by his mother for a psychiatric evaluation because she felt she could no longer control him and was concerned that he was getting into progressive trouble. Damian's parents had divorced 6 years earlier. The father kept custody of Damian and his younger brother after the divorce, but the children regularly spent summers with their mother. Both parents had remarried.

Damian's father had sent him to live with his mother 4 months earlier. Damian had very serious difficulties with his father, including physical fights on four occasions. The father had called the police and placed both children in shelter homes for a couple of weeks. Damian also had difficulties at school: he was found with illegal substances on school grounds and was on probation. The father was so angry and frustrated with Damian that he did not want anything to do with him.

Since being with his mother, Damian had displayed problems at home and at school. He flunked the previous school year because of poor attendance and had been truant from school on a regular basis. At home he was unruly, defiant, and confrontational, and he sought isolation. Damian left home without permission whenever he felt like doing so. He frequently sneaked out at night and had stayed out all night a number of times. His mother had found spray cans in his room and suspected that he was using other drugs. Damian adamantly denied that he was abusing illegal substances. He had obtained a very well-paid summer job, but he was fired for unexplained absences.

The mental status examination revealed a very defensive and uncooperative adolescent who looked older than his stated age. He remained distant and uninvolved for most of the examination. He said at the outset, "I am not crazy. I am not hearing voices or seeing things." He added, "I don't need any help. I want to go home." He also said, "I want to go to Arizona," where his father lived. When the examiner asked Damian how he had felt when his father sent him to live with his mother, he became tearful. He said he had been surprised, adding, "I couldn't believe it." Damian mentioned several times that he missed his friends and indicated how unhappy he was living with his mother. The examiner asked Damian about his parents' divorce. He responded, "My life has been wrecked ever since the divorce." He felt that he could be mean to his parents because of the pain and misery they had put him through. Damian became even more tearful as he talked about how his parents' divorce had affected him.

When the examiner began to talk about options to handle Damian's problems, Damian became defensive again and asserted that he had no problems and that he wanted to go home. Because he did not seem amenable to any recommendations, the examiner opted to ask Damian for help. The examiner asked Damian to switch chairs with the examiner. After the chairs were exchanged, the examiner said to Damian, "Now you are the doctor. What would you do to help a child who is getting in trouble all the time? How would you help a youngster who cannot get along with either parent and flunked the previous year? How can you help a child who doesn't like school?" Damian became reflective and then suggested that the child has to learn to get along with his mother, has to stay at home, has to ask permission to leave, and so on.

Although Damian had been negative about receiving any psychiatric services, he now agreed to come back for an extended evaluation.

Psychiatrist's Role Enactment During the Psychiatric Examination

Equally helpful is role enactment, in which the examiner impersonates an important person in the child's life, as illustrated in the following vignette.

Case Example 7

Richie, a 15-year-old Caucasian male, had undergone a heart transplant 1 year prior to the psychiatric evaluation. Richie got into a conflict with his mother because he broke a house rule, a curfew, and was given consequences; to retaliate he told mother that he was going to stop the anti-rejecting medications; actually he had stopped his medications all together for a number of days before. He persisted in this medication refusal no matter how much his mother and his immediate and extended family begged and pleaded with him to start his medications again. When the transplant team heard of this development, they initiated a referral for a prompt psychiatric evaluation. Surgeons and transplant team physicians made it very clear to the evaluating psychiatrist that if Richie did not start taking the anti-rejecting medications right away he was going to die. Since the patient's life on the line, he was hospitalized.

The psychiatrist attempted to understand the patient's aggressive and self-destructive behaviors without success; it appeared that any attempt to bring up the issue of the medications intake gave Richie a renewed stimulus to persist in his refusal. The psychiatrist opted for exploring who persons in Richie's life he did care about, and asked him, who was the most important person in your life? Without hesitation Richie responded, "My youngest brother!" The psychiatrist took advantage of that disclosure and pulled a chair in front of Richie and told him that the psychiatrist was going to play the role of his youngest brother. The psychiatrist sat close and in front of Richie and in a pleading tone asked Richie, "Brother, why do you want to kill yourself?" Richie's response was dramatic. He was perplexed and bewildered. He said he was going to start taking his medications. He went to the nurse to request his medications, took them, and continued taking them during the few days he remained in the hospital.

The point in this example is that the psychiatrist, respecting the patient's autonomy, and without using patronizing or power manipulations, was able to find a way to influence the patient to revert his lethal refusal course. The psychiatrist was able to find a meaningful point of leverage to influence the patient's refusal by mobilizing an area of emotional investment that had a significant impact or connection with the symptom.

That the younger brother was extremely meaningful to Richie was indicated by the fact this sibling was present in his immediate awareness but had been dissociated from his self-destructive ideation; a positive connecting bond was reestablished when the brother was represented to Richie's awareness, thus breaking down the dissociation. The technique reactivated a supportive bonding (a positive introject) that had been dissociated or split off from Richie's awareness. To a certain extent, the technique produced a narcissistic repair.

Double Chair Technique

The double chair technique is used to externalize and confront the patient's presenting problems, to assess the patient's internal conflict, and to determine the degree of ambivalence the patient has about his or her symptoms. In the example below, psychodramatic techniques are used to explore nonverbalized feelings between the patient and his parents.

Case Example 8

Chen, a 17-year-old mixed-race Korean American male, was evaluated for suicidal ideation with a plan to shoot himself or to run his car against a wall. He had a long history of depression and had been thinking about suicide for over a year. His academic performance had deteriorated, and he had become progressively irritable, aggressive, and destructive; he had lost over 40 lbs. during the previous 6 months. He was also unable to sleep or to stay asleep. When Chen was asked what sort of thing he worried about, he said that he worried about his parents' health: his father had gotten a liver transplant, and he did not know how many more years his father had to live, and his mother had a bad case of rheumatoid arthritis.

The examiner started the examination with Chen by himself. The parents were in their way to the examiner's office. The examiner was in an advanced stage of the individual interview with Chen when his parents arrived. When the parents joined the examiner and their child, the examiner addressed father by saying: "I heard that you had a liver transplant." He said he had non-alcohol cirrhosis of the liver and that he was also diabetic. Father, a 53-year-old Caucasian ex-military, said that the liver was doing fine; he had received the liver about 18 months before the evaluation and that he felt very well. The examiner addressed the Korean native mother by saying that he had heard she had a bad case of arthritis. Mother, who had limited English skills, was aided by her husband a great deal both in understanding what was being communicated and in expressing herself. She spoke in broken English, saying that she had a problem with her joints and that she also had significant pain.

The examiner placed a chair in front of Chen and asked father to sit there. Then, he asked Chen to tell father how worried he was about his health. Chen did so. Father said that he was feeling OK and that the transplant was doing well. Father told his son not to worry. After this, the examiner asked mother to switch chairs with father and told Chen to tell mother how worried he was about her health. Chen did so. When mom was struggling to articulate in English how she was doing, the examiner overheard Chen talking in a low voice in what appeared to the examiner to be an Asian language. The examiner wondered if Chen was speaking Korean; Chen assented but clarified that he was not fluent in it. Knowing that Chen could understand mother, he told mother to speak to his son in Korean. She did so. While mother was speaking in her native tongue, Chen demonstrated a great deal of deference and respectful listening. Father and Chen stated that mother asked Chen not to worry.

Father was asked to switch chairs again and to tell Chen what things he worried about in regard to his son. Father became emotional and told Chen that he worried about his depression, his poor performance at school, and his progressive anger. Mother was asked to go back to the chair and to address her worries. She stated that she expected him to grow to be a strong man to marry and to have a family. Since the parents had not addressed the suicidal behavior, the examiner put the father back on the chair and asked him to tell Chen how he would feel if Chen were to kill himself. The father was overcome by emotion and asked to have the tissue box that was nearby the examiner. He said that if Chen were to kill himself, life would cease having any meaning for him and that there would be no incentive for him to keep living. Then, the examiner asked mother to take the chair. At this point, Chen objected and said he did not want his mother to be subjected to more pain. Father told Chen to let her speak, and after she sat down, the examiner encouraged her to speak in Korean. Apparently the mother said that if Chen were to kill himself, she would feel death inside and that she would go through a great deal of pain. She also hinted that she might kill herself. She was visibly moved and tearful. After this, the examiner asked Chen to respond to the parents' worries. He appreciated his parents' love and concerns and felt sorry that he was causing them pain. When the examiner wondered why he wanted to kill himself, he stated that he wanted to kill himself "because I feel that nothing I do is right and that everything I try turns out to be wrong." Father became supportive, telling Chen "that everybody makes mistakes and that we need to learn to overcome obstacles and to learn from our mistakes." The examiner told the parents that it was possible that Chen had stopped sharing his worries with them because of their serious health issues. Father understood and agreed with that proposition and passed it on to mother.

Following that, the examiner asked Chen put his chair close to his parents. He chose to put his chair in between his parents, and immediately mother and son embraced for a long time, displaying affection and mutual concern. After this emotional reunion, the examiner left.

This technique was successful because it reopened the channels of communications between parents and the adolescent. The child was able to voice his worries, and the parents were able to express theirs. The examiner broke the silence regarding Chen's suicidal behavior and allowed mother to air her feelings in her own language [a culturally sensitive intervention]; she was able to voice her anxieties and worries about her son. The technique succeeded in airing the child and the parents' mutual concerns and ended in a positive empathic and emotional "family reunion."

In the following family session (3 days later), when the father was asked what was his view of the previous session, he said that it had been very helpful, that it put the family back together, and that there was a better understanding about what the family members were going through. The examiner picked up on mother's difficulties in expressing herself and in her probable sense of isolation and loneliness. As it turned out, she did not have any friends and had limited contacts with the local Korean community. In this session the examiner explored the family's anxieties about Chen leaving home and going to college. Father stated that he had been telling his wife, "You are holding on to Chen too tightly and that it is time for her to let go." The session further explored what parents needed to do for Chen not to worry about them, and the things Chen needed to do to avoid parents worrying about him.

Case Example 9

Natalie, a blond, blue-eyed 16½-year-old Mexican American female, was brought for a psychiatric evaluation for persistent suicidal behavior, self-abusive behavior, and mood instability. Natalie had no prior psychiatric history and had been in CPS custody for 7 years; she was removed from her mother's custody after it was found that her mother's husband, the child's stepfather, had raped Natalie. She had a history of promiscuity since age 12, including 6 months of prostitution, and an extensive history of polysubstance abuse, including cocaine, speed (her favorite drug), crack, acid, meth, and others. She had refused to attend school and was academically behind 3 years. Natalie had been arrested a couple of times for drug possession and shoplifting.

Natalie was an attractive Anglo-looking adolescent who displayed conspicuous inappropriate smiling. She stated that she smiled even when cutting and hurting herself; she pretended she was happy all the time. In spite of this affective display she declared that she was suicidal and that she was determined to kill herself. She said that life was pointless and that she would kill herself any time and any way she could. She smiled when she said that. Natalie revealed that she had flashbacks about the rape and that she thought about the rape on a daily basis; she also had recurrent dreams about the rape. She had strong homicidal ideation toward the stepfather. The examiner told Natalie that her surname did not match her Caucasian features; to this Natalie replied that her mother was an American blond.

When the examiner asked details about the rape, Natalie became silent; she said she could not say. The examiner wondered how many times it had happened, and Natalie revealed that the stepfather had raped her from ages 5 to 10. The examiner wondered where her mother had been during all these years; she said, "She was working." The examiner attempted to extract more information about the rape or about her mother response's to the rape, but both attempts were met with defensiveness and silence.

The examiner attempted to explore how mother responded to the raping; Natalie said that both mother and maternal grandmother told her that she was lying. She added she did not want to talk about it. When the examiner asked Natalie who the most important person in her life was, she said, "My younger sister." The examiner proceeded, "And after your sister?" Natalie responded, "My brother." Examiner asked once more, "After your brother?" "My mom," she said.

Since Natalie was very ambivalent about her mother and the way she had responded to the disclosure of the ongoing rape, the examiner used the double chair technique. The examiner placed "mother" in the empty chair and told Natalie to tell mother that her stepfather had raped her for many years. When Natalie took her mother's place and attempted to articulate her mother's words, with hesitation she said, "I don't believe you." Natalie got upset. She was asked to go back to her chair and to talk back to her mother. Natalie became downcast and struggled to proceed, but said she couldn't do it. She was given emotional support and was told, "It must have been very hard for you to hear that neither your mom nor your grandma believed you." Natalie was visibly sad and upset; she became silent.

Since Natalie had felt unsupported by her own mother, Natalie was given support regarding the abandonment, neglect, and rejection she experienced from her real mom. Natalie was prompt to excuse and to forgive her mother and was eagerly expecting to become 18 to have the freedom to reunite with her. Natalie had unrealistic and idealized views of how thing were going to be like when she had the chance to be with her mother again. Those unrealistic fantasies were challenged systematically.

Nonverbal Techniques When Interviewing Children and Adolescents

The child must be encouraged to express problems in his or her own words—to verbalize psychological, family, and social problems in her own personal way. According to Warren et al. (1996), "Understanding the child's experience is important for a comprehensive diagnosis and for designing treatment programs" (p. 1331).

As an alternative to verbal exploration, the examiner occasionally needs to use nonverbal techniques to access the child's psychological world. The value of nonverbal diagnostic techniques varies in relation to the effectiveness of each technique in drawing out relevant information from the child's internal world. Nonverbal techniques may enhance trust and communication between the child and the examiner. The specific techniques used depend on the interviewer's style and the child's developmental level. For example, some interviewers prefer diagnostic activities in the microsphere (the circumscribed therapeutic playing space of the office), whereas others prefer the larger field of the macrosphere (including space outside the office, e.g., in the playground). Some examiners select artistic media, whereas others prefer sports-oriented activities. The best choice seems to be one that best stimulates the child's skills or talents, that is most appealing to the child, that is closest to the child's favorite activities, or that is most appropriate to the child's developmental state. A developmental fit will be the most motivating to the child.

Nonverbal techniques are productive when 1) new material is revealed, 2) the nonverbal productions complement prior verbalizations, or 3) the nonverbal productions add depth or new dimensions to the evaluation. Nonverbal techniques are particularly helpful when the child's capacity to speak is markedly inhibited (e.g., in elective mutism) or when the child is very anxious or very resistant to disclosing private feelings or a secret such as abuse; in these circumstances pressing for verbal communication may be counterproductive.

Although verbal engagement is the most desirable technique, nonverbal engagement becomes a stepping-stone in the process of building trust to develop a diagnostic and therapeutic alliance. The following case example illustrates this point.

Case Example 10

Pedro, a 5-year-old Hispanic male, was referred for a psychiatric evaluation for aggressive behavior. He was also unruly and oppositional. He had been in the care of his maternal grandmother since he was 2 years old. Pedro's mother was conspicuously neglectful and abusive; she would leave her children unattended for prolonged periods of time. Pedro's grandmother and other relatives would find the children unkempt, soiled, and malnourished on a regular basis. A number of times, his grandmother picked up the children from the streets, where Pedro's mother had left them.

The examiner learned that during the first 2 years of Pedro's life, he had endured frequent maltreatment and neglect. A 7-year-old sister had decided not to stay with the mother any longer because "I got tired of acting like a mom." The mother frequently put her daughter in charge of her two younger siblings. The grandmother was the legal custodian of the two older children and had cared for the two younger ones. Although tired and emotionally exhausted, she could not bear the thought of leaving the younger ones in the care of Pedro's mother.

Pedro was small for his age. He looked a bit scraggly and was very inhibited and submissive. During the individual interview, he was completely silent and remained distant, apprehensive, and reserved. Because he did not respond to simple questions such as "What is your name?" and "How old are you?" the examiner made an effort to engage him in play. Pedro was offered a set of animals, a group of dinosaurs, and a number of dolls. He did not show any interest in the toys. In an attempt to engage Pedro, the examiner began to place the animals in a circle, hoping Pedro would join him in the play; that did not happen. After a while, the examiner left the animals alone and began to play with the dolls; Pedro did not join in this play either. The examiner then attempted to engage Pedro in the squiggle technique: he picked up a sheet of paper; put a pencil on the table, closer to Pedro; and invited Pedro to draw something with him; Pedro refused. After Pedro refused a number of invitations to engage in an interactive nonverbal communication, the examiner collected all the items from the table.

The examiner had a tennis ball on top of the desk. He picked it up and rolled it to Pedro. Pedro picked up the ball and rolled it back to the examiner. The examiner rolled the ball again, and Pedro rolled it back in return. The ball was rolled back and forth many times. At one point, the distant, unanimated child began to smile. Shortly thereafter, he began to throw the ball progressively more forcefully and somewhat aggressively: on two occasions he hit the examiner in the chest and began to get more emotionally involved, if not excited, in the rolling and catching the ball game. After throwing the ball back and forth a number of times, the interview was concluded. Pedro was told, "Next time we will play some more."

This engagement attempt lasted for about 45 minutes; at no point during the interview did Pedro utter a word. Significant anxiety, language disorders, and cognitive limitations may have contributed to the child's elective mutism.

The preceding case example illustrates nonverbal engagement after unsuccessful attempts to involve the child in verbal interactions. Recognizing the child's mistrust, the examiner made plans to take the child to the courtyard for the next diagnostic appointment to play in the playground, and told so to Pedro. The novelty and intimacy of the office and the private nature of the examination (i.e., having to stay alone with the examiner behind closed doors) may have been too threatening for the child. A history of anxiety disorders, abuse, developmental language disorders, or cognitive limitations is common in children like Pedro and may contribute to difficulty responding verbally during an interview.

Drawing Techniques

If verbalization is gold, drawings are silver. Drawings, complemented with a sensitive exploration of their content, can illuminate the child's major issues or concerns. Drawings also give a good indication of the child's level of intelligence and creative and artistic talents and may indicate whether neuropsychological deficits are present. In addition, drawings aid in identifying body image difficulties and a variety of psychological conflicts or psychosocial stressors.

An added advantage of drawings is that they may serve as visible and concrete evidence that may be presented to parents who do not want to believe that anything is wrong with their child. A drawing may be used as a springboard for a discussion about sexual abuse or violence within the family when the drawing clearly represents or suggests these themes. When the examiner analyzes drawings, he or she needs to keep in mind that "drawings by young children are representations and not reproductions, that they express an inner and not a visual realism. The drawings make a statement about the child himself and less about the object drawn. The image is imbued with affective as well as cognitive elements" (Di Leo 1973, p. 9). Table 3–1 lists the types of drawings used in a diagnostic interview, in the order in which they are solicited.

Male children regularly draw male figures when they are asked to draw a person; if a boy draws a female figure, sexual identity conflicts should be explored. This is not the case for girls. The family drawing, called the *kinetic family drawing*, offers the examiner insight into family dynamics and particularly into the child's perceived role within the family. Whereas the person drawings may indicate the child's cognitive development, the family drawing elicits "mobilization of feelings that, while rendering the family drawing less valuable as an indicator of intelligence, confers upon it significance as an expression of the child's emotional life. The family drawing, then, can be viewed as an unstructured projective technique that may reveal the child's feelings in relation to those whom he regards as most important and whose formative influence is most powerful" (Di Leo 1973, p. 100).

In the following case example, the use of drawing was instrumental in breaking through a mother's denial about her child's problems.

Case Example 11

Tom, a 9-year-old African American male, was referred for evaluation because he was becoming progressively aggressive at school, both with teachers and with peers. Tom had been suspended many times because of this behavior and was frequently sent home, creating significant disruption for his mother, who was on active duty with the military. Tom's mother could not understand the school's concerns; she declared categorically that her son did not have any problems at home. Tom had been given the diagnosis of attention-deficit/hyperactivity disorder before and had taken medication for a short time without any benefit.

Tom's parents had divorced a year before the evaluation, and Tom missed his father a great deal. Tom's mother described the child's father as very dependent and unreliable.

During the family interview, many aspects of the child's overall functioning were explored systematically. When asked how Tom was doing at home, his mother responded in a protective and defensive manner. To his mother's surprise, Tom reported, without prompting, that on one occasion he had pulled a knife on his brother when the latter found him attempting to harm himself with the knife. Tom added that he had thought about killing himself many times. He then revealed that he frequently abused himself by punching himself in the face or by throwing himself to the ground. This information alarmed his mother. Throughout this portion of the assessment, Tom remained

Table 3–1.   Sequence of requested diagnostic drawings

1. Free drawing

2. Draw a person

3. Draw a person from the opposite sex from the previous one

4. Draw the family doing something together (kinetic family drawing)

5. Draw a tree

6. Optional drawing: draw a house, a car, the last dream you had

Source.   Modified from Cepeda 2010, p. 81.

very quiet and calm. He looked affectively frozen, if not emotionally blunted. Tom did not show any evidence of hyperactivity nor of overt distractibility during the examination.

When the examiner asked Tom about the things that he enjoyed doing, he said that he liked drawing a lot. The examiner pursued this interest by giving Tom some white paper and pencils and asking him first to draw whatever he wanted. He was then prompted for additional drawings.

Tom's first drawing was of a big, female figure with an open mouth and pointed teeth; this figure was holding a child's head in her right hand. The female figure had beheaded the child, whose head was dripping blood. One of the child's eyes had popped out, and the female figure was eating the other eye. Tom narrated all of this without emotion.

Tom's second drawing, in response to the examiner's request that he draws a person, was of a male person in profile who was using a machine gun to shoot at a smaller figure. The smaller figure appeared to be scared. The examiner asked Tom, "Why is that big guy shooting the smaller one?" Tom replied, "The small one 'crossed' the other guy."

Tom's third drawing, in response to the examiner's request that he draw a female or a girl, was, again, of a big, female figure, this time strangling a child. The female figure was smiling, and the child was faceless.

Tom's fourth drawing, a family kinetic drawing, showed Tom's five family members, all holding weapons in both hands. Each family member had a different pair of weapons: knives, axes, pitchforks, small saws, and big saws. The family had killed someone, whose body lay in front of the group, and was posing in front of an automatic camera that was set to take a picture of the whole scene.

Tom displayed no emotion as he explained his drawings. The morbid content and preoccupation with violence reflected in Tom's drawings were alarming. After Tom's mother saw her son's drawings, it was not difficult to persuade her that Tom was a very disturbed child. She was shocked after seeing the drawings and hearing Tom's descriptions of them. Tom's drawings broke through his mother's denial, and she became receptive to therapeutic recommendations.

The following case example demonstrates the effectiveness of using drawings to evaluate an electively mute preadolescent girl.

Case Example 12

Tina, an 8-year-old Caucasian female, had been referred by a counselor from the nearby mental health mental center because of concerns about her regressive behavior. The counselor noted that Tina rarely, if ever, spoke. Three months before the evaluation, it was brought to Tina's mother's attention that Tina's 12-year-old sister had been sexually molested by the mother's fiancé. After this disclosure, the mother broke off her engagement. Tina's mother also learned that her former boyfriend had fondled Tina. At the time of the evaluation, charges had been filed against the former fiancé in connection with the sexual abuse he perpetrated against Tina's sister.

Since the time of the disclosure, Tina had exhibited significant regressive behavior: she had become very clingy, shadowed her mother everywhere, and refused to sleep in her own bed. There was no evidence of other regressive behavior such as enuresis or encopresis. At school, Tina was known as a quiet child who seldom spoke, which had been a concern to her teachers. Tina was a very good student and had kept up her grades, even during the time of the observed regressive behaviors.

Tina's father had been physically abusive toward her mother in front of the children; he also had problems with alcohol. Although contact between Tina and her father was irregular, she seemed to enjoy his sporadic visits.

Tina was a very pretty girl with freckles and big inquisitive eyes. Her eye contact was intermittent. She clung to her mother, clutching her mother's hands throughout the interview. The examiner attempted to engage Tina in a verbal exchange, but whenever she was addressed, she would signal her mother to answer for her. She never spoke spontaneously. Although Tina didn't respond verbally, she gestured to the examiner when she was asked a number of questions during the mental status examination. She denied that she had ever thought of suicide or that she ever had any hallucinatory experiences.

Tina's mother reported that Tina also had problems talking to her counselor. When her mother said that Tina spent a great deal of time drawing, the examiner asked Tina if she would like to draw. She showed interest immediately. Tina's drawings helped the examiner to understand the reasons for her regressive behaviors and the effect of the recent fondling.

For the first drawing, Tina was asked to draw whatever she wanted. She drew a big house with two curtained windows (Figure 3–1). Tina drew a girl at the right side of the house, holding a flower in one hand and a lollipop in the other. The girl in the drawing seemed to be smiling. The sky was sunny (actually, the sun was smiling), three birds were flying around, and there were a few clouds. At the other side of the house was a tree with fruit on it, and hanging from the tree was a bird feeder with three birds feeding. This was an altogether happy and positive drawing.

For the second drawing, Tina was asked to draw a person. She drew a good-sized girl who was smiling. On the girl's abdomen she drew a large black dot that she identified as the girl's bellybutton (Figure 3–2).

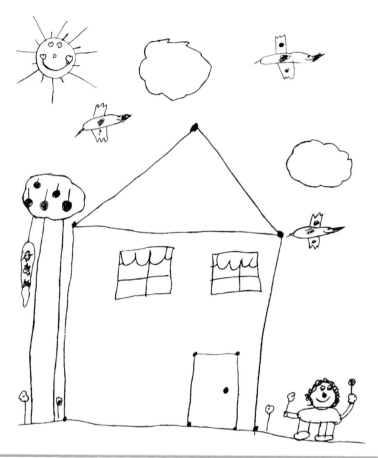

Figure 3–1. Tina's first drawing; she was asked to draw whatever she wanted.

Source. Reprinted from Cepeda C: "Nonverbal Techniques for Interviewing Children and Adolescents," in *Concise Guide to the Psychiatric Interview of Children and Adolescents.* Washington, DC, American Psychiatric Press, 2000, p. 75. Copyright 2000, American Psychiatric Press. Used with permission.

For the third drawing, Tina was asked to draw a boy. She had problems drawing the figure; she erased the head a couple of times. The boy was clearly smaller than the girl in the previous drawing. She didn't draw a bellybutton on the boy, and he had a rather pleasant smile (Figure 3–3).

For the fourth drawing, Tina was asked to draw her family doing something together. The examiner also asked the mother to draw, in parallel, the same drawing. Tina's drawing was full of movement: the family members were holding hands while watching TV (Figure 3–4). In an interesting parallel, the mother drew herself and her children watching a movie at the theater (drawing not shown here).

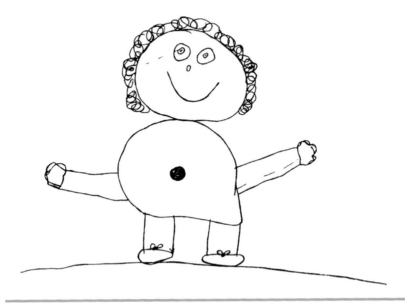

Figure 3-2.   Tina's second drawing; she was asked to draw a person.

Source.   Reprinted from Cepeda C: "Nonverbal Techniques for Interviewing Children and Adolescents," in *Concise Guide to the Psychiatric Interview of Children and Adolescents.* Washington, DC, American Psychiatric Press, 2000, p. 76. Copyright 2000, American Psychiatric Press. Used with permission.

The examiner went back to the second drawing and asked Tina why the bellybutton was visible. Because Tina remained mute, the examiner ventured to say that the little girl felt pretty bad about what had happened to her when her mother's boyfriend touched her on her private parts and that she feared that everybody knew or was going to know about it. The mother answered for Tina, saying that her daughter had told her how ashamed she felt about what happened. Because Tina didn't verbalize how she felt about the abusive incident, the examiner asked her to draw the way she was feeling about what had happened. Tina's mother was asked again to draw in parallel to Tina. Tina drew a girl crying, tears running down both of the girl's cheeks (Figure 3–5). The mother again drew a picture similar to Tina's: a woman crying and looking quite sad (Figure 3–6).

The drawings were useful in getting information about Tina's sense of herself and in exploring the feelings she could not put into words. The drawings also showed that the girl was intelligent and creative. The first drawing demonstrated a positive self-image and the fourth demonstrated a good family relationship. The examiner felt that the regression was limited and that with ongoing counseling and maternal support, the impact of the fondling could be minimized. The examiner took into account that the elective mutism had preceded the abuse. Furthermore, Tina was demonstrating good evidence of resilience: she liked school and was doing well in her classes. Fea-

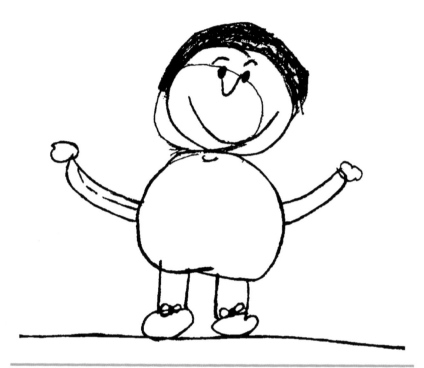

Figure 3–3. Tina's third drawing; she was asked to draw a boy.

Source.   Reprinted from Cepeda C: "Nonverbal Techniques for Interviewing Children and Adolescents," in *Concise Guide to the Psychiatric Interview of Children and Adolescents.* Washington, DC, American Psychiatric Press, 2000, p. 76. Copyright 2000, American Psychiatric Press. Used with permission.

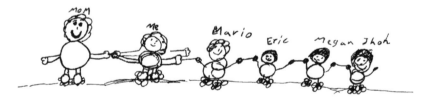

Figure 3–4. Tina's fourth drawing; she was asked to draw her family doing something together.

Source.   Reprinted from Cepeda C: "Nonverbal Techniques for Interviewing Children and Adolescents," in *Concise Guide to the Psychiatric Interview of Children and Adolescents.* Washington, DC, American Psychiatric Press, 2000, p. 77. Copyright 2000, American Psychiatric Press. Used with permission.

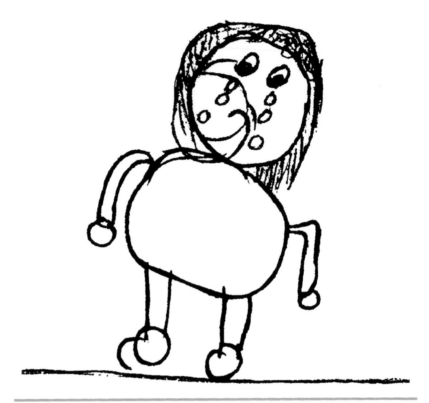

Figure 3–5. Tina's fifth drawing; she was asked to draw the way she was feeling about the abusive incident.

Source. Reprinted from Cepeda C: "Nonverbal Techniques for Interviewing Children and Adolescents," in *Concise Guide to the Psychiatric Interview of Children and Adolescents.* Washington, DC, American Psychiatric Press, 2000, p. 79. Copyright 2000, American Psychiatric Press. Used with permission.

tures of separation anxiety disorder were present, but features of a mood disorder were not. Tina was mandated back to her individual counselor, who was told that Tina could be reevaluated if her regressive behaviors worsened or if other signs of emotional or behavioral deterioration appeared.

In the preceding case example, the parallel content of the mother's and daughter's drawings was remarkable. It was also interesting that the examiner involved the mother and the daughter in the process of drawing; the convergence of themes and feelings helped the examiner determine that the child was receiving good maternal care and that the mother was attuned to the child's needs.

In the following case example, drawing helps the examiner to discriminate diagnostic issues in a late adolescent girl with complex symptomatology.

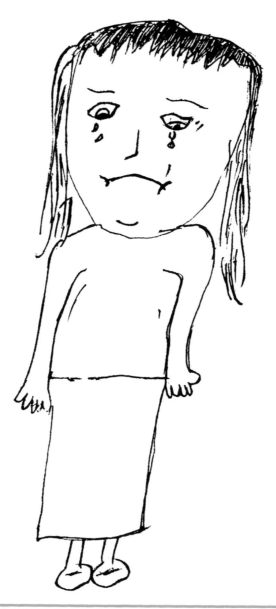

Figure 3–6. **Tina's mother's drawing in response to being asked to draw in parallel to Tina's fifth drawing.**

Source. Reprinted from Cepeda C: "Nonverbal Techniques for Interviewing Children and Adolescents," in *Concise Guide to the Psychiatric Interview of Children and Adolescents.* Washington, DC, American Psychiatric Press, 2000, p. 79. Copyright 2000, American Psychiatric Press. Used with permission.

Case Example 13

Serena, a 17-year-old Caucasian female, was evaluated because she was, in her parents' view, "a very picky eater" and they were concerned about the long-term repercussions of her eating habits. Mother stated that Serena had a very long history of being a picky eater since she was started on solids. Mother stated that her concerns were increasing because she would be graduating from high school in a year, and the family was wondering if she would be able to adapt to the larger world. Serena had a long history of nail biting, twirling her hair and massaging herself when she felt stressed. She used to even chew her toenails, and when she was tried in summer camps she cried every night. At the time of the psychiatric interview, she was not dating and had never been sexually active. Although, she was a social butterfly in middle school, she had become progressively more reserved; however, Serena said she had a number of good friends.

Mother reported that Serena was a full-term baby and that the pregnancy and delivery had been uneventful. There was no history of developmental delays. She had always been a very good student and was planning on going into genetics and psychology. Mother stated she had a good marriage. Serena's mother came from a physician's family; mother came across as a strong parent who had very high expectations for her daughter. Serena had a 15-year-old brother who was in 10th grade and doing well. Serena's father was in an import business and had an autoimmune disease. No history of mood or anxiety disorders on either side of the family was reported. Nor was there a history of mental illness in either side of the family.

During the interview, this petite and attractive adolescent kept on biting her nails and displayed multiple anxious features. Serena informed the examiner that she frequently felt sad and down whenever she felt she was not angry. She stated she felt irritable and angry most of the time and that this had been going on for a very long time. "I get easily pissed off." Serena disclosed that she had been cutting herself for the last year. She added that she procrastinated a lot and that she had a low energy level. She stated that she was unable to feel pleasure and that she felt very lonely. Furthermore, she had a poor image of herself: she thought that people thought that she was worthless and felt that nobody liked her. She thought that she was fat and had issues with her stomach, thighs, hips, and her sides. She also thought that people thought that she was a "bitch," that she "had no heart, and that she was ugly." She also felt watched and was afraid of what was under her bed. When the examiner told Serena that it seemed that her mother put more pressure on her than her father, she said, "That's the understatement of the day!" She affirmed that there was nothing wrong with her eating habits. When the examiner asked Serena what was her attitude toward sex, she responded with vehemence, "I would not dare to show my ugly body to a man. No! No!"

The examiner asked Serena to draw some pictures (Figures 3–7, 3–8, and 3–9), corresponding to a person, a boy, and a tree, respectively.

The drawings show major problems with self-esteem and a deep sense of shame, hesitation, and self-doubt. The examiner concluded that mood and anxiety/panic issues of her case were more destabilizing for her than the concerns about the picking of her food. The drawing spoke louder than her words about her major issues with self-esteem and self-concept and self-

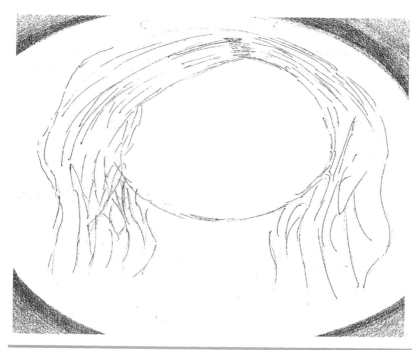

Figure 3–7.   Serena's first drawing: a person.

doubt. Serena's presentation fulfilled criteria for a mood disorder, a number of anxiety disorders, and of an eating disorder, unspecified.

The following illustration has forensic implications.

Case Example 14

Lucero, a 7-year-old Hispanic female, was evaluated 2 months after she made an outcry to her therapist that her father had sexually abused her; the child had been with biological father for the last 3 years. Parents had had joint custody until 2012, when Lucero's oldest sisters, 18 and 16 years old, got upset with their mother and went to live with her father, the alleged abuser. Father became the sole custodian of Lucero then. CPS gave mother a temporary custody over Lucero, since the outcry, till the agency completed the investigation. Mother informed the examiner that at the time of the forensic evaluation of the alleged sexual abuse Lucero recanted.

Mother said that since Lucero had come back home, she had been aggressive toward her brother and to other students at school, and that she had been disrespectful toward her mom and grandparents. She also displayed oppositional and defiant behaviors. Furthermore, Lucero had told another student that she was going to stab other students and had also stated the she wanted to kill her brother. Lucero had problems with anger control, and when she got upset, she threw things around, slammed the doors, and banged the table. Mother stated that her daughter did not seem to show remorse after her aggressive and inappropriate behaviors.

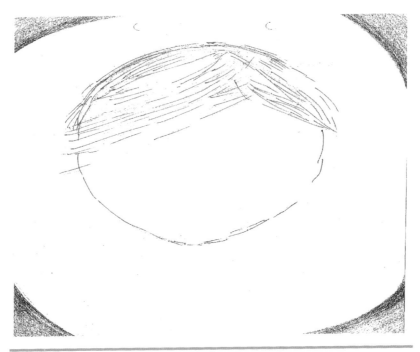

Figure 3-8.   Serena's second drawing: a boy.

Mother confided that, every night, Lucero would ask mother to put A&D ointment on her vaginal area, something mother used to do when Lucero complained of a "vaginal" rash when she was far younger. Mother had found that behavior "odd" and had given the ointment to Lucero for her to apply it herself. Mother was also concerned that Lucero would always kiss her on the lips and that she was preoccupied/infatuated with breasts to the point that she would put paper towel under her shirt to pretend she had breasts.

Parents had broken up their relationship some years before; mother claims father had been physically abusive to her son before they separated. Father had been reported to CPS for paddling his son so hard he left bruises on him. Mom also reported that during the time that mother and father were together, father used to degrade her in front of the children. Mother asserted that father had problems with anger control and that he believed he was always right; she said that father was very controlling. Mother believed that father had alienated her daughters from her.

Mother asserted that after Lucero made her outcry, she asked her second youngest daughter if she was aware of any inappropriate behavior between her father and Lucero; she answered that she had not seen anything but she revealed that father had had a sexual relationship with her for about 5 years.

As the mother was revealing the most recent events and the investigation of sexual abuse by CPS, the examiner asked Lucero what father did to her. Since she hesitated the examiner asked Lucero to draw what happened.

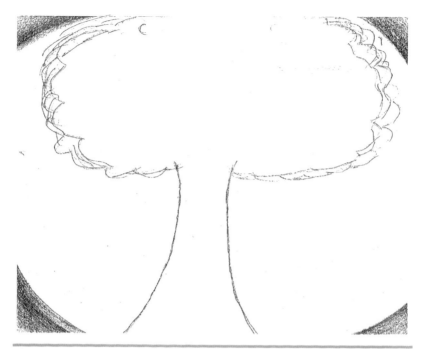

Figure 3–9. Serena's third drawing: a tree.

Lucero said that father had done things with her two times. On the top of her first drawing (Figure 3–10) she wrote: "When I got to the Hous he told me to tack my clos off But then in 2 days it Stop the and…,"with the writing continuing on the top of the second page (Figure 3–11), "He tole me to get in the Bed with Hm…He tole Me to tust Hes Penis."

On the next drawing (Figure 3–12), at the very top of the page, there is a series of numbers that seem to correspond to a local phone number. Underneath and on the left side of the page, she drew a home and wrote "2 tam" [second time], and in the upper right side of the page she wrote, "Becaze tath is How you tuch hes Hes Penis Do we they and tayts it," with the wording continuing on the next page (Figure 3–13): "Wey she ast me to tack my pans off so she kan like My Butt."

Inside of the house she drew a very crowded picture of her father and her. Since, it was difficult to make sense of the drawing, the examiner asked Lucero if she knew what a magnifier was, and she said she knew. The examiner then, traced a rectangle over the part of the drawing that needed clarity (as seen in Figure 3–12) and asked Lucero to draw that part of the drawing, keeping the magnifier in mind. She then made another drawing (Figure 3–14), with explicit sexual content.

The mother was stunned by seeing the drawings with explicit content and what Lucero had written. It's hard to accuse the examiner of leading the witness. The evidence thus gathered could bear scrutiny in court and could stand counter-examination.

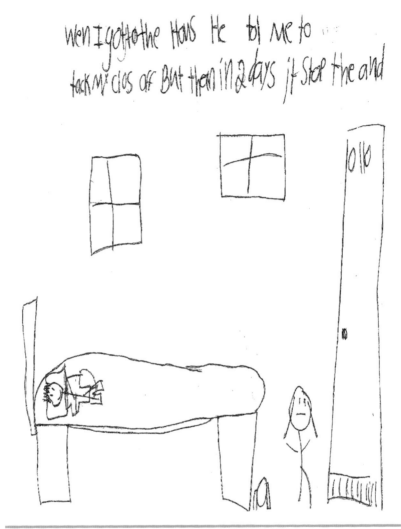

wen I got to the Haus He tol me to ...
tack mi clos off But then in 2 days it stop the and

Figure 3–10. Lucero's first drawing: first page.

He tole me to get in the Bed with
Hm He tole MC to tust hes penis.

Figure 3–11. Lucero's first drawing: second page.

Rectangle inreD
dove by examiner
Lucero was asked
To magnify area within.

2 10 4356269

Becaze ta th is How you thch Hes
Hes Penis Do we they and tay ts it

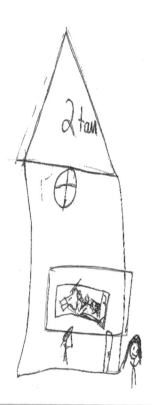

2 tan

Figure 3-12. Lucero's second drawing: first page.

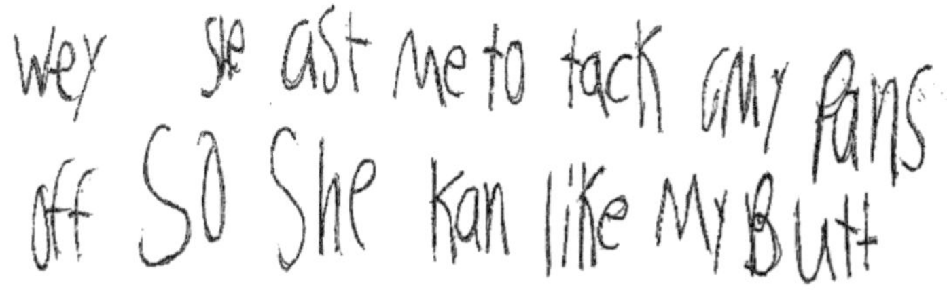

Wey she ast me to tack any Pans
off so she kan like My Butt

Figure 3-13. Lucero's second drawing: second page.

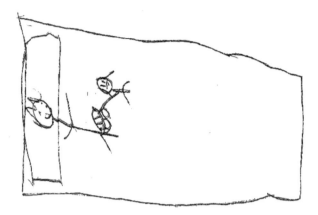

Figure 3–14. Lucero's drawing of a portion of her second drawing (when asked by the examiner to "magnify" the content in the portion of the drawing that the examiner enclosed in a rectangle).

Play Techniques

Play offers the examiner a unique insight into the psychological conflicts experienced by preschoolers and young preadolescents. Although a diagnosis can be derived by interviewing the child, the data obtained lack information regarding the ongoing psychological conflicts that contribute to the child's overall destabilization. Why is play a window to the child's subjective world? Table 3–2 summarizes aspects of the child's internal world that can be inferred during diagnostic play.

Russ (2008, pp. 179–180) describes four broad functions of play: a) play is a natural form of expression in children, "the language of play"; b) children use language to play, to communicate with the therapist; c) play is a vehicle for working through and insight; and d) play helps to regulate emotions. In addition, play gives the child multiple opportunities to practice a variety of ideas, feelings, behaviors, interpersonal behaviors, and verbal expressions.

Children enact their underlying anxieties and ongoing conflicts in play. Conflicts could be secondary to developmental delays, internalized conflicts, or difficulties with the child-rearing environment. Frequently it is easier for the child to express, through the medium of play, psychological difficulties he or she is unable to communicate otherwise. Often the difficulty is not a matter of revealing something that the child knows; children may be totally unaware or unconscious of the factors influencing their psychological and behavioral problems.

Table 3–2.   Elements of the child's subjective world

Conflicts, problems, and fears

Wishes and fantasies

Prior life experiences

Traumatic experiences

Ongoing experiences

    a. Home

    b. School

    c. Friends

    d. Boyfriends/girlfriends

    e. Looks, health and other body concerns

Problem-solving strategies

Creativity

Verbal capacity

Level of intelligence

Capacity for engagement and object relations

Concerns about the future

Source.   Modified from Cepeda 2010, p. 100.

According to Ablon (1996), "Play in itself allows the child to bring forward and explore feelings that are most troublesome and important" (p. 545). He also emphasizes the importance and salience of play in children's lives: "Play is a vehicle for symbolism and metaphor which the mind in turn utilizes to provide scaffolding for structuralization, integration, and organization of affectively charged experience" (p. 545). Summarizing the overall functional importance of play, Ablon notes, "The innate capacity of play for organization, synthesis, and promoting self-regulatory process provides a powerful therapeutic element" (p. 546). In the next three case examples, play sheds light on the child's underlying problems:

Case Example 15

Joel, a 5-year-old Caucasian male, was reassessed after he was released from an inpatient acute psychiatric preadolescent program. He had been admitted to the program after he became unmanageable at the day care center and at home. At the day care center he was hyperactive and impulsive and frequently was aggressive and abusive to his peers. At home he was restless and defiant, talked back to mother, and displayed ongoing jealousy and aggressive behavior toward his 8-month-old sister. Joel's mother also reported that her son often displayed unusual behaviors such as precocious sexual behavior and strange verbalizations, including statements that there was a bad Joel inside of him. At times Joel appeared to be self-absorbed; at other times he seemed to be in a frenzy and unable to sleep. His mother reported that Joel experienced fluctuating moods; at times he looked miserable, cried easily, and said that he was a bad child.

These problems had been reactivated by the time the reassessment was conducted. When Joel's mother was asked about a possible history of physical or sexual abuse, she became indignant. What was striking to the examiner was the emotional distance between the child and the mother. She was eager to attribute the child's dysfunction to a biological problem and proposed that the child probably had a chemical imbalance; she disregarded other possibilities. The examiner's efforts to gather information about the child-rearing environment were met with noncontributory, vague, and evasive responses.

Joel's mother had recently separated from the child's father. She gave no importance to this event, even after reporting that Joel and his father seemed to have a good time together. She reported that when Joel spent time with his father, he did not seem to display any of the troublesome behaviors she complained about. She had begun dating a man whom she believed was getting along well with Joel, and she hoped Joel would look up to him as a father, stating explicitly, "I wish Joel would forget about his real dad."

During the family interview, Joel made no contact with his mother. He displayed familiarity with the examiner, and at times he sought affection from him. When Joel's mother talked about Joel, she displayed no concern or sense of empathy for what he might be experiencing.

When Joel was evaluated alone, he asked to play with toys. He was offered a set of small animals, including a polar bear and a panda bear. Joel picked the polar bear and assigned the panda bear to the examiner; the polar bear was the mother, and the panda was the child. Joel told the examiner to make the panda bear call for its mommy. The examiner said, "Mommy! Mommy!" repeatedly, but the polar bear appeared to be completely indifferent to the panda's distress. When the examiner, in the role of the panda bear child, asked Joel, as the polar bear mother, why the mother didn't come to see him, Joel shouted, "Shut up," and added, "The mother is dead." He ordered the panda bear to continue crying and calling for its mommy.

This was a puzzling enactment (see Chapter 2, "General Principles of Interviewing," for more on the interpretation of enactments). When the examiner met again with the mother, he asked her to help him understand Joel's enactment. When she was told the content of the child's play, she confessed with great hesitation that she had been separated from Joel from the time he was 4 months old until he was 13 months old. She had been in prison for drug-related problems, and her mother had taken care of Joel. When she returned, Joel didn't recognize her, so she had attempted to gain the child's love, but for a long time she had felt that Joel didn't love her.

In the preceding case study, the revelation resulting from the child's play helped to explain the child's distance, the mother's emotional blandness, and the mother's parental inconsistency. The child's bonding with his mother was called into question. This developmental disturbance needed is much attention as the other disorders with which the child had been diagnosed (i.e., attention-deficit/hyperactivity disorder, oppositional defiant disorder, and probable bipolar disorder).

In the next case study, the child represents in play his concerns about body function and conflicts about elimination besides obvious problems with anger.

Case Example 16

Chad, a 5-year-old Caucasian male, was brought by his mother for evaluation. They had been staying at a shelter for battered women, where his mother had sought refuge with her two children from her husband's abusive treatment. Chad had attracted the attention of the shelter's administrators because of his hyperactive, disruptive, and aggressive behaviors toward his brother and even toward his mother. When it became clear that Chad was unresponsive to limits and discipline, his mother was advised to seek psychiatric consultation.

Chad's mother reported that his mood was very changeable. He had threatened to kill her, had voiced a desire to die, and had also made veiled statements that he would kill himself. Chad had become progressively withdrawn, had lost weight, and repeatedly expressed wishes to see his father. Chad seemed to be preoccupied with defecation. His mother had overheard him singing gleefully, using words such as "ca-ca" and "butt hole." Chad had problems sleeping and at times appeared sad and withdrawn; at other times he seemed happy and hyperactive. His mother denied that Chad had been physically or sexually abused; however, Chad had witnessed his father abusing his mother many times.

During the session with the mother, Chad showed a significant degree of behavioral organization (see Chapter 9, "Evaluation of Internalizing Symptoms"). He asked permission to use a number of toys and explored playing materials appropriately. Chad's mother was amazed to see him behaving so adaptively. She was equally amazed that after Chad finished playing, he picked up the toys and put them back where he had found them. At some point during the interview, Chad began to sing, using words such as "ca-ca," "butt," and "butt hole," as his mother had disclosed earlier. He seemed to be singing those words with a sense of joy.

Chad was a handsome boy. His speech was fairly well articulated; however, on occasion he exhibited speech difficulties. Although he appeared euthymic, he displayed some constriction in the affective sphere. Except when he was singing the scatological words, his affect was mostly appropriate. At times, the examiner sensed that Chad exhibited short-lived clang associations.[2] No psychotic symptoms were demonstrated, and no further evidence of thought disorder was observed. Chad moved around the office with a sense of famil-

---

[2]*Clang associations* refer to the expression of words that rhyme (e.g., dog, fog, log). It is usually a serious symptom of thought disorder.

iarity and explored many toy boxes and other items without any hesitation. Mother attempted to guide and control him by telling him to ask permission before touching things. She was far more anxious than Chad was. Although Chad made contact with many play objects, he didn't concentrate on any item or use the toys to enact any elaborated themes.

During the individual assessment, Chad first played with animal toys. Sometimes his playing behavior was calm and sometimes it was playfully aggressive. He often paired off the toys for play. When he turned to the dinosaurs, he picked up the Tyrannosaurus rex first. This dinosaur attacked the other dinosaurs. From time to time, Chad would find delight in sticking another dinosaur's tail or one of its limbs into the T. rex's mouth. After he enacted some aggressive scenes, Chad (still holding the T. rex) turned to the examiner and asked, "Where does the food the dinosaur eats go?" He asked if it went to the legs or to the bones. He seemed puzzled and intrigued. He repeated these questions a number of times, each time making direct eye contact with the examiner.

During the interpretive phase of the interview, Chad's mother added information of particular interest. She revealed that Chad had a history of chronic constipation. He would "hold on," not moving his bowels for long periods of time. He would indicate a need to defecate by holding his legs together tightly and showing facial discomfort, but even then he would not go to the toilet. Finally, when Chad did go, his mother would help him in the act of releasing the hardened feces. She would hold and separate his legs (while he was sitting on the toilet) until he would painfully relieve himself. Chad had been encopretic from time to time.

In the preceding case example, the short play session shed light on the child's struggles in understanding the transformation of food, his corresponding difficulties with elimination, and his preoccupation with body functioning. What was the importance of this symptom in the overall psychopathologic picture? What was the connection between the constipation, encopresis, and the other symptoms? The potty-training battle and other conflicts over control still seemed very active. How were the diagnoses of oppositional defiant disorder, attention-deficit/hyperactivity disorder, and a probable affective disorder related to Chad's encopretic behavior? Certainly the forceful child-mother transactions at the toilet and the child's own preoccupations with food intake and elimination provided a good starting point in understanding the strong power struggle between the child and his mother.

The next case example shows how descriptive psychiatric observations, regular exploratory questions, and psychodynamic inferences from play observations are accomplished concomitantly and complementarily.

Case Example 17

Suzy, an adopted 8-year-old Hispanic female, was referred for psychiatric evaluation for severe aggressive behavior. She had bitten a teacher's breast and had scratched some of her peers' faces to the point of bleeding. She had also been very obstinate and disruptive in the classroom.

Her adoptive parents were divorced. Suzy lived with her adoptive mother and other foster children (Suzy's mother had served as a foster mother to many children). Suzy was reported to be hyperactive, impulsive, and defiant. She had been adopted at age 5 years by the family that had cared for her since early infancy. She had not been expected to live because of severe respiratory difficulties shortly after birth. Her adoptive parents had been described as very inconsistent in limit setting and discipline. Suzy had been given a number of psychotropic medications, including stimulants, but none of them effectively controlled her behavior.

During the play session, Suzy selected a playhouse, a number of small dolls (a mother, a father, a son, and a daughter), and miniature furniture. As she opened the house and began to explore its contents, she would start to say something but never finish. This happened several times. When the examiner asked Suzy about this behavior, she appeared preoccupied, as if she were experiencing internal perceptions. Suzy did not respond to the examiner's comments. The examiner said, "I wonder if you are hearing something." When Suzy continued to be unresponsive, the examiner said, "It seems that you are hearing voices. Can you tell me what the voices are telling you?" She acknowledged that she was hearing voices but did not reveal anything about their content. Suzy also became distracted several times by noises that were coming from outside the office. She would ask the examiner where each noise came from and what was happening outside the office. Suzy asked if her mother was coming.

After Suzy explored some other elements of the playhouse (she particularly enjoyed turning on and off the working house light), she began to play with the dolls. She picked up the daughter doll and said it was her. She gave the father doll to the examiner and the mother doll to the female resident who was observing.

Suzy brought her doll to the examiner's father doll and made her doll "kiss" the father doll and whisper something in its ear. The examiner asked Suzy what her doll was saying to the father doll, but she refused to tell. Suzy then took her doll to the mother doll, which the resident had placed on the house patio, and made her doll "kiss" the mother doll. Suzy's doll whispered something in the mother doll's ear and again refused to tell the examiner what the whispering was about. Suzy used her voice in an endearing manner and showed significant excitement during these dramatizations.

Suzy's doll then wanted to get into the pool on the patio, but she said the water was too cold. She stated a number of times that she wanted to get into the pool and each time she would touch the water and say that it was cold. Suzy took the father doll from the examiner and put it in a reclining chair on the patio. She sat the mother in another chair. Suzy then placed her doll upstairs in the playhouse and turned the light off, saying that it was night. She said, "It was scary," more than once, but she would not tell the examiner what was scary in that room. She put her doll into bed and soon after brought the son doll (representing her brother) to sleep in the same bed. The examiner commented on the boy and the girl sleeping in the same bed, but Suzy did not respond.

Suzy then said it was morning time and she brought her doll back downstairs, where she began playing with the mother doll. Suzy had the mother doll ask the daughter doll to go upstairs to fix the bedroom because she had "made a mess." The daughter doll refused to go, and with a commanding voice, Suzy made the mother doll go upstairs and fix the mess herself. The examiner asked Suzy what was going on. Suzy made the daughter doll begin to whine and fret and laid the doll down on the floor. The examiner asked Suzy if the daughter doll was having a temper tantrum, and she agreed readily. The doll continued to lie on the floor, fussing and whining. The examiner restated that the doll was having a temper tantrum, and again Suzy agreed. After this, Suzy made the daughter doll go to the mother doll and kiss her. The daughter doll said she wanted to go to McDonald's. She displayed another temper tantrum when the mother doll said no. At this point, the examiner noticed a number of scabs and scars on Suzy's arms and asked her what had happened. She said that she had scratched herself. The examiner said, "It seems that you scratch yourself when you have temper tantrums." She agreed.

Suzy's next play scenario related to going to school. Her doll exited the house by the front door, was picked up by the school bus, and then came back home. Her doll kissed the mother and father dolls again. After 30 minutes of playing, the examiner said, "We are going to stop playing." Suzy continued to play as though the examiner hadn't said a word. The examiner said, "We have to stop. We need to pick up now." Again, Suzy didn't seem to listen. In a firmer manner, the examiner said, "We are not playing anymore. We need to pick up." Suzy protested and asked, "Why?" The examiner began to help her to put away the house and other toys. Only then did she acknowledge that the playing was over.

In the preceding case example, the enactment of this child's strong oppositional traits was apparent throughout the session. In particular, observations during this session hinted to the presence of psychotic features. The child's play also hinted at the child's fears (e.g., possible sexual abuse), her affectionate manipulations, and her difficulties with mood dysregulation and anger dyscontrol.

Prospective Interviewing

Patients sometimes refuse to talk about the past. Children who have been heavily traumatized are very apprehensive about, if not resistant to, "opening up old wounds." In these situations, the examiner may attempt to carry out a prospective interview, in which the questions are addressed towards the patient's future. Even though the patient refuses to reveal anything about the past, as the patient begins to talk about the future, he or she will provide informative clues about his or her problems and personality organization. Consider the following case example.

Case Example 18

Harold, an African American male, was 2 months shy of 18 years of age at the time of the psychiatric evaluation. He had a horrible childhood history, including gross neglect and frequent physical abuse by his alcoholic and drug-abusing mother. His father had been in and out of jail for theft and other crimes. Harold had received serious and extensive burns on one occasion when his mother threw scalding water on him because he wet his bed. Harold had moved frequently between his mother's house and his maternal grandmother's house. He yearned for his mother's love and couldn't understand why she didn't show any affection for him. His poverty and problems with enuresis led to frequent teasing by his peers; the enuresis also led to frequent whippings by his mother.

From a very young age, Harold felt different, "sort of unique," among his peers. Peers remarked that he didn't "speak like blacks." He remembered feeling depressed all his life. He was 14 years old when he started thinking about suicide. He had a number of psychiatric hospitalizations after suicidal attempts. His middle adolescence had been quite stormy: he had frequently been depressed and suicidal and had begun drinking, taking drugs, and stealing. He continued to crave for his mother's love.

At the time of the evaluation, Harold was living with a maternal aunt but still hoped to live with his mother. He described himself as a deep thinker and was actively involved with music, writing, and poetry. He had begun to understand that the lack of his mother's responsiveness probably was not his fault.

Harold was able to develop rapport with the examiner and was able to display some degree of relatedness during the interview. His eye contact was intermittent, but he didn't use body language when he spoke. Harold had a British-like accent that was somewhat unusual given his background. His mood was euthymic (Harold was taking venlafaxine and had a very positive response to the medication). His affect was markedly constricted in both range and intensity. He was not suicidal and did not exhibit signs of psychosis. He was articulate and seemed thoughtful in his responses. Sensorium was intact, and intelligence was judged as average if not better.

Although Harold would talk about any topic proposed for discussion, the examiner felt that a prospective interview would provide significant information about his ego strengths, resilience, and ideals. The examiner asked Harold to discuss his future plans. He said that he wanted to finish regular high school instead of opting for a GED. He wondered if he could become a social worker or a counselor to help other kids. He also discussed his interests in music and in writing. He didn't have any close friends but had begun to appreciate that different people have different things to offer. Efforts to gain his mother's love were still a high priority, even though he realized that his mother was a very troubled person and that he was not the reason why his mother had failed to love him. When asked to express his feeling about having a family, Harold said he would like to have a family of his own. Then, he became more thoughtful and added that he worried about having a son because he didn't know what kind of father he would be. He said he was scared of becoming angry and losing control. In the past, when he felt very angry, he had felt like killing someone.

Harold verbalized his inner preoccupations in a matter-of-fact way, exhibiting prominent isolation of affect and a lack of affective modulation in his speech. He credited the antidepressant for improving his mood. The adaptive pragmatics of communication (he had to learn to appear normal, although deep inside, he was depressed) at the beginning of the interview began to fade, and as the interview proceeded he became progressively apathetic and downcast. Harold appeared to be making good strides; however, he was at high risk for psychiatric relapse and future maladaptation. He required close psychiatric follow-up.

It is impossible to talk about the future without disclosing problems in the present and difficulties from the past. With the prospective interview strategy, the patient's defensiveness or resistance may be bypassed (see Chapter 10, "Evaluation of Externalizing Symptoms").

Key Points

- The examiner needs to have in the diagnostic "tool box" a number of strategies or logistic plans to meet the needs of children of different developmental levels, with a variety of clinical presentations.
- The different techniques described in this chapter represent different modalities of diagnostic engagement.
- Alternative diagnostic approaches are necessary when standard diagnostic approaches are unsuccessful.
- Interviewing in displacement, playing, and nonverbal techniques are more suitable with preschoolers or early-latency children.

CHAPTER 4

Family Assessment

A guiding principle for family assessment is that behavior problems by a child or young adult can never be understood devoid of their relational context of the family. From a systems point of view, any family member's problems are best understood as manifestations of dysfunctions within the broader family unit (McHale and Sullivan 2008).

The following are essential family system tenets (McHale and Sullivan 2008):

1. Systems are organized wholes, and their constituting elements or subsystems are interdependent.
2. Interconnected subsystems have their own integrity, are organized hierarchically, and are separated by boundaries.
3. Patterns in a system are circular, not linear.
4. Stable patterns are maintained over time through homeostatic processes.
5. Open systems do adapt, change, reorganize, and develop.

Most schools of family therapy agree that families function best when they are cohesive—that is, when they freely, openly, and directly exchange information and attend to the members' developmental needs at changing points of the life cycle. In addition, most school therapy perspectives view families as adaptive when they show flexibility, adapt to shifting circumstances, solve problems effectively, maintain a hierarchical structure, and support individual autonomy and growth of all members (McHale and Sullivan 2008). However, given the vast array of different family approaches and the different emphases represented by the different schools of thought, no standard or universally agreed on set of assessment practices or techniques for evaluating families has been developed (McHale and Sullivan 2008).

What has been said regarding the assessment of the child is equally applicable to the assessment of the family—that is, the examination of the family begins at the examiner's first contact with the family. The examiner may first connect with family members via the telephone, correspondence, e-mail, or some other way. Through these preliminary contacts, the examiner makes incipient hypotheses regarding the matter of concern, the degree of the family understanding of the presenting problem, and the degree of the family commitment to deal with it.

Parents' reports typically play a critical role in the diagnostic process, because the symptoms of a child's disorder wax and wane, preventing the clinician from directly observing the child displaying the cardinal signs of the disorder, and because many children, especially younger children, may lack the insight or cognitive skills to report symptoms (Vitiello 2008). In addition to emphasizing the explicit seeking of information and clarity about certain critical life events, such as domestic violence, sexual abuse, extramarital affairs, and drug and alcohol abuse, most family systems approaches give special credence to the behavioral sequences and interactions that are revealed during early contacts with the family (McHale and Sullivan 2008).

Presenting Problem

The examiner seeks to understand how family members view the identified problem(s), what causes they attribute to the problems, what measures or interventions have been attempted, or what they plan to do about the problematic issues. The examiner notices how rigidly the family conceptualizes the problem or how open their system is to alternative explanations. Of equal importance is determining the degree of scapegoating or the flexibility to consider that other family members may be playing a role in the ongoing family functioning (dysfunction), or that other members might be in as much need of help as the identified member.

The examiner should approach the theory of illness from all the family members. The examiner gives each family member an opportunity to express his or her view regarding the nature of the problem and its possible causes. The examiner notices any convergences or differences of views in the explanations of the nature of the presenting problem and its presumed origins. The examiner also notes if various family members identify different members as being in need of psychiatric help and attempts to understand the reasons they feel this way. Along the way, the examiner observes the presence or absence of parental alliance, as well as the presence of coalitions that undermine the parental alliance. The examiner attempts to determine where the family is in the family life cycle and how the family copes with transitions in the life cycle and with current life tasks or demands.

In certain cultural milieus, families might seek traditional religious assistance (e.g., from a rabbi, priest, pastor) or nontraditional indigenous practices (e.g., voodoo, *barrida*, or other forms of supernatural influence). The examiner will strive to understand the system of beliefs underlying these practices.

Marital Subsystem

The examiner determines the strength of the marriage and the degree of family cohesiveness. Basically, the examiner observes for evidence of love and respect, understanding and caring, compassion, and empathy between the parents. The examiner attends to their marital and parental roles, as well as their sharing of efforts in caring for the children and maintaining the home environment. In the same vein, the examiner notes how the family resources are used and how equitable decision making is.

When exploring a presenting problem, an examiner often detects parental tension, lack of parental agreement regarding the nature or severity of the problem, or disagreement about the need for psychiatric help. The examiner strives to elucidate the source of the disagreements and, when necessary, to refocus the parents' digression about their own problems back to the child's present concerns.

Intergenerational Boundaries

Establishing the degree of harmony or conflict between the parents' generation and the previous and future one(s) is clinically important. The examiner observes or makes inferences about how each parent relates to his or her own parents and in-laws. The examiner must be attentive to trans-generational boundary transgressions. Prior generations (i.e., a child's grandparents) may have a great deal to say about the kind of life their children have or the manner in which the parents should raise the new generation, among other things. Some grandparents make misalliances with the grandchildren and undermine parental discipline and home rules, either overtly (by openly criticizing parents) or covertly (by condoning the violation of rules). A number of grandparents are averse to psychiatric interventions or the use of psychotropic medications. The examiner needs to identify these covert barriers and attempt to understand and overcome them. The examiner also needs to note how much the parents depend on grandparents for emotional or financial support and determine whether the parents have ever been able to achieve independent functioning on their own.

When the family is estranged or cut off from a previous generation, the examiner can help by exploring the source for such alienation and will attempt to build bridges or to repair broken relationships. The same is applicable to other important relationships in the past.

Family Organigram

The *family organigram* is a visual diagram that shows the members of the nuclear family and their extended families; the organigram displays the lineage of the family and marks or highlights the members affected by psychiatric illnesses (see Note 1 at the end of this chapter).

The time spent in the creation of a family organigram will pay a variety of clinical dividends. The visual scheme of the family is a resource the clinician goes back to when there are events within the nuclear or extended family or when there are conflicts either within the nuclear family or between and/or among other generations. The examiner needs to start the exploration within the nuclear family and will ask directly each parent if they have history of emotional or psychiatric illnesses. For instance, the examiner may ask the mother, "Have you ever had issues with anxiety? depression? psychosis?" "Is there any history of suicide in the family?" "Have you ever had psychiatric treatment? What kind?" The examiner may probe deeper depending on the responses to the preliminary inquiry. After this, the examiner addresses similar questions to the other spouse or significant other. Then, the examiner asks history of psychiatric illnesses in the siblings of each parent followed by an inquiry into the parents' background in both sides of the couple; frequently, the exploration goes as far as probing into the great-grandparents of the identified child or adolescent, again, in both sides of the spouses' families. If the parents do not have knowledge of their parents' background, this becomes a task that each parent needs to complete before the next diagnostic appointment.

Completing the organigram provides the examiner with important information regarding family connections and family cut-offs. In the latter case, the examiner will attempt to ascertain the cause of the family's cut-off. Besides mood, anxiety, and psychotic disorders, it is important to extend the inquiry into areas of alcohol, drug abuse, suicides, and incarcerations.

Organigrams for two identified patients and their families are shown below. In the first (Figure 4–1), the identified patient, Al, was 15 years old when he was evaluated for depression and suicidal thinking. Al's father, Bob, had a history of depression. Bob's mother had history of depression. A maternal grandmother's sister had suffered from depression and had a nephew with history of depression.

In the second organigram (Figure 4–2), the identified patient, Tim, was 15 years old when he was evaluated for depression, suicidal ideation, and ex-

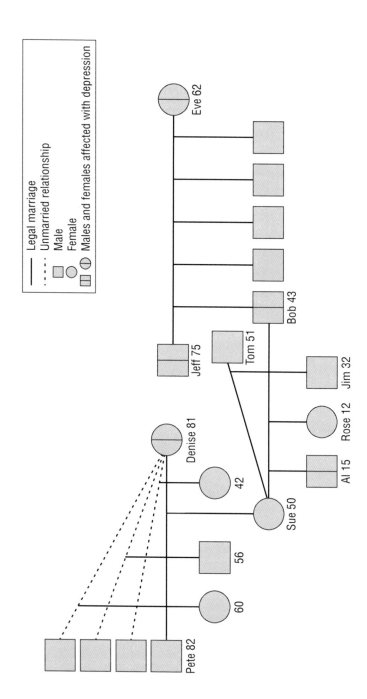

Figure 4-1. Family organigram/genogram for identified patient Al.

treme anxiety. Tim's mother had two children with Gus in and out of wedlock relationship: Tess (18 years old) and Tim. Gus had problems with drugs and alcohol. Ron was Tim's stepfather. Eighteen months prior to the evaluation, Ron, a 37-year-old impaired veteran, shot his wife Liz in the face and then turned the gun on himself and killed himself. Liz survived and was left with no disfigurement or physical incapacities. Ron suffered from PTSD and problems with alcohol and drugs, and had a violent temper, prior to his suicide. He had been physically abusive to Tim and had been very abusive to his wife, Liz. Ron Sr., Ron's father, had overdosed with heroin.

Deaths in the Family

History of deaths in the immediate family is common in psychiatric patients. Death destabilizes the family hierarchy and support systems. If the lost one is a parent, the psychosocial impact is more direct and detrimental. The child experiences an immediate loss of care, nurturance, and support, and if the dead parent is the main breadwinner, the survivors may experience devastating financial and social status consequences.

Serious psychological sequelae endure when the death is not the result of natural causes but rather the consequence, for instance, of a car accident that occurred while the parent was under the influence of alcohol or drugs, or worse, if the death is caused by suicide. Depression, persistent anger, guilt, and blame are common complications for children following parental suicide. Children feel responsible for the parent's suicide or may feel they are to blame for the parent's demise. Suicide of a sibling is equally devastating. Experiences with suicide have negative and long-lasting consequences.

Deaths of a significant family friend may have as great an impact as a death within one's own family. The suicide of a child's friend has a major negative impact on the child's psychological life. Guilt and self-blame are pervasive responses. When a child's friend has died by suicide, the examiner needs to explore the possibility of a suicide pact or of the presence of suicidal intentions based on the need to atone for the perceived blame (see the section "Evaluation of Suicidal Behaviors" in Chapter 9, "Evaluation of Internalizing Symptoms.")

The loss of a friend could be more destabilizing for an adolescent than the death of a family member. Research indicates that "losing a close friend and having family with a drug or alcohol problem were the only specific proximal risks significantly associated with adolescents' current total difficulties. Adolescents who reported that someone in their families had died in the past month appeared to score lower on the total difficulties than those without this experience, which appears counterintuitive" (Flouri and Kallis 2007, pp. 1651–1659).

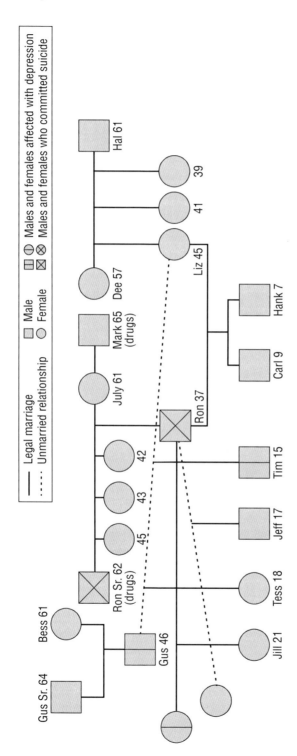

Ron and Ron Sr. both killed themselves. Ron Sr. overdosed on heroin. Ron shot Liz in the face, before turning the gun on himself. Liz survived. Ron was a Vietnam veteran who suffered from PTSD and alcoholism. Tess was 16 and Tim was 13 when Ron shot Liz and killed himself. Gus, Tess and Tim's father, was a drug abuser. Tim was the identified patient. He had a major depressive disorder and a very severe social anxiety disorder.

Figure 4–2. Family organigram/genogram for identified patient Tim.

Maternal Depression

For new mothers and for mothers who become pregnant again, maternal screening for psychiatric illnesses is now recommended. Detrimental effects of psychiatric illness, and of depression in particular, are becoming a major focus in infant and in child psychiatry, and in public health in general. The U.S. Preventive Services Task Force issued the recommendation to institute, at the beginning of 2016, screening mothers for mental illnesses, during pregnancy and after childbirth. The task force recognized that depressed pregnant women take poor prenatal care of themselves and that depression causes ill effects in infants and children. This recommendation was extended to 1 year after delivery. This screening is covered under the Affordable Care Act. Depression, anxiety, obsessive-compulsive disorder (OCD), and psychosis are disorders that need to be identified. The group recommended the Edinburgh Postnatal Depression Scale for screening purposes. This scale has 10 questions (Belluck 2016, p. A1, 13) (see Note 2 at the end of this chapter). Most women do not harm their babies, but mothers' level of stress can undermine their ability to care and can affect children' emotional well-being, social behavior, and cognitive skills. In as many as half of postpartum cases, depression starts during pregnancy and symptoms may start any time within a year after the baby is born. Some women experience depression after their first child, some with subsequent births, and some with every pregnancy. Studies suggest that 1 in 12 women, and as many as 1 in 5 women, develop depression, anxiety, bipolar disorder, OCD, or a combination, during pregnancy or after childbirth (Belluck 2016, A13).

Illnesses in the Family

Chronic parental illness results in serious developmental disturbances in the offspring. Chronic parental illnesses (medical or psychiatric) impact the organization and support system within the family. In the case of parental illness, a reversal of roles may occur: the child becomes parental and attends to the parent's needs instead of his or her own. In these circumstances, the child experiences neglect and emotional deprivation.

A negative impact also results when the family has to contend with a child's chronic medical or psychiatric illness. The other children in the family may resent the attention the ill child receives. A variety of negative impacts on the family and on the other siblings are common consequences.

Similar negative consequences occur when a parent or parents are deemed incompetent to take care of the offspring because of neglect or poor parental supervision, or when children are placed in the care of the extended family (grandparents or other relatives) or outside of the family. Children cannot understand the rationale of a social agency's decisions; commonly, children ally with the parental figures against the external agents (e.g., Child Protective Services, judiciary, school) that threaten the family integrity.

When failures occur in the executive system of the family—that is, when the parental figures are incapable of providing care, safety, and supervision for their children—the sibling subsystem develops compensatory organizations; in general, the oldest child takes a parental role. The elevation of the oldest child to a parental role is resented by the younger siblings and becomes a source of power conflict between the impaired parent and the parental child. Commonly, a child stuck in a parental role abrogates to herself or himself the right to set her or his own rules and to challenge or disregard the parental ones.

The following case is an example of a child's problems resulting from severe illness in a parent.

Case Example 1

Shon, a 12-year-old Asian American male, was evaluated for disruptive behavior at school and aggressive behavior at home. He had not had previous psychiatric treatment. Shon had been aggressive toward his sisters and also had been destructive at home. He had become increasingly rebellious, and his father complained that Shon took things from his sisters and from him. Some minor shoplifting had been reported, and he had a history of ongoing enuresis and episodic encopresis. The school had not complained of aggressive behavior.

Shon's father was Asian American and his mother was of Portuguese descent. As the mother entered the room, the psychiatrist noticed her wide base and labored walking. The examiner asked her what was the matter. She started by saying that she was recovering from a very serious ankle fracture in her right leg 2 years before; as she continued, she mentioned that she had a bad case of diabetes and advanced retinal disease, and a history of a right-side stroke 5 years before. She suffered from left-side hemiparesis and had a residual aphasia. She was disabled because of her multiple medical conditions.

The father reported that Shon talked back to his mother and that he had been progressively verbally abusive to her. The father was fearful that Shon might become physically aggressive with his mother. Shon's problems had become progressively worse over the previous 2 years, a period of time that coincided with his mother's surgery. The child acknowledged being sad for the previous 5 years.

The mental status examination of Shon revealed an overweight male child who appeared his chronological age. He was shy and nonspontaneous and talked with a low tone of voice; some degree of "baby talking" was discerned. Shon had difficulties warming up to the interviewer. He denied suicidal or homicidal ideation. He endorsed hearing voices telling him to do bad things. Shon frequently would ask his mother whether she heard what he did. He would also tell his mother that somebody was trying to get into the home and felt that people said bad things about him. He endorsed a history of self-abusive behavior in the past: he had scratched himself two times before.

The family was unaware of the impact that the mother's extended illness had had on Shon's emotional life. His mother recollected that when she was in the hospital, Shon was 7 years old; then, he pleaded insistently for her to return home, saying, "Mom I need you." When the examiner explored the impact of the mother's illness in the family, Shon began to cry.

The family had not been able to appreciate that Shon's deteriorating academic and behavioral course ran a parallel course to his mother's deteriorating medical condition. Shon's behavioral adaptation suffered markedly after his mother had a stroke 5 years before. His mother's illnesses were a severe threat to Shon's strong dependency needs. Shon felt helpless without his mother around. Furthermore, his mother's medical condition had changed the dynamics between her and the child in such a way that she needed care and was incapacitated to provide the nurturing for which Shon was so hungry.

Financial Stressors

Financial stressors can affect families in a variety of ways. Some parents attempt to work longer hours or obtain multiple jobs to produce additional income, especially when the provision of basic necessities is at stake. Additional work means more parental time away from the family, with a negative impact on the family's emotional atmosphere. Often, consistency of enforcement of family rules suffers. When both parents work, children may be left unsupervised for hours and experience more keenly parental deprivation. Financial stressors create tensions between parents and cause the children to have a sense of material and emotional deprivation, particularly if parents cannot meet the children's basic needs

Family Conflicts With Other Systems

As an open system, the family is always transacting with other systems: schools, health organizations, religious groups, social agencies, and others. The transactions of the family with other systems evolve from the natural or intrinsic relationship of the family with those systems. The family is embedded in and regulated by large social systems; that is, the family is influenced by other systems at all times. The family is expected to transact with other social agencies along the evolution of the family life cycle.

A functional family system carries out the basic responsibilities of caring for, protecting, and supervising the offspring successfully while transacting with other systems. A family system gains autonomy from the influence of other systems on the basis of its success in fulfilling these basic tasks. Simply, a functioning family unit transacts with other systems without undue conflict and is open to the positive influences of the larger systems. On the other hand, a dysfunctional family is pressed by other systems to do a better job in fulfilling the basic family tasks. The more the family deviates from the expectations and influences of the larger systems, the greater the resulting conflict will be between the family and the parallel or superordinate systems.

Ultimately, adolescent outcome appears to depend on the contextual cumulative risk rather than on specific risks, and the relationship between proximal contextual adversity and psychopathology is monotonic (Flouri and Kallis 2007). An alternative or complementary explanation derives from the concept of *allostatic load* (see Chapter 14, "Symptom Formation and Comorbidity" for details). As Flouri and Kallis (2007) note, "This suggests that increments in the number of proximal adverse life events experienced increase psychopathology scores, which highlights the importance of protecting those at risk from further risk exposure. Finally…reasoning ability moderates the association of proximal cumulative adversity and psychopathology" (p. 1657).

Observations of Family Behavior During the Family Interview

The examination of the family begins when the examiner meets the family in the waiting room, or even before if there had been any communications between the examiner and any members of the family. The examiner should invite into the office any family members who have come to the appointment and extend an invitation to any significant others the family has brought along; the family has the choice to select who attends the meeting. Once in the office and after the family members and significant others have been accommodated, the examiner introduces himself to every member of the family.

The examiner will pay notice to who is the family's spokesperson and what are the family's hierarchical rules of power and control. In general, the family spokesperson is the gatekeeper of the family—that is, the person with power and through whom all major family decisions are made. This is the member the examiner needs to "win over" for diagnostic and therapeutic success. The examiner needs to be sensitive to family cultural issues in family social deportment. For example, in dealing with Latino and Asian families, addressing the father first and then the mother is the accepted practice. In Latino families, fathers and husbands "are supposed to be in charge," and unlike in most European and African American families, sleeping with and hand feeding of children well through the preschool years are normative behaviors in many Asian families (McHale and Sullivan 2008).

The examiner pays attention to the seating arrangements and to the verbal and nonverbal communication of the family members. The examiner should pay special attention to nonverbal behavior, including nonverbal communication and body contact between and among the members. Frequently, what the parents are expressing in words is contradicted by their nonverbal behavior. For instance, a parent may express disgust with a child's behavior, but at the same time the same parent or the other parental figure makes affectionate contact with the child, thus cancelling the verbal disapproval. Also, a common observation is that when a parent asserts himself or herself in enforcing a rule or establishing a new rule, the child may attempt to make body contact with that parent to weaken the parent's resolve or to convey to the parent, "You do not really mean to do what you're saying, do you?"

The examiner observes the affection and respect among the family members and notes if a child respects parental authority. Of equal importance is observing the level of hostility among the members (e.g., between the parents, between the parents and children, among the children). From the very beginning of the interview, the examiner can observe evidence of separation anxiety in a child (e.g., close proximity to a parent, lack of spontaneity, frozen expression, timidity, anxious pragmatics of communication), open defiance and rebelliousness against parental authority, or other intergenerational conflicts. In the same vein, the examiner may observe evidence of depression, mania, developmental abnormalities, or oddities or unusual behaviors in the identified child or any other member of the family. An alert examiner attends to clues of alcohol or substance abuse in the parents or other family members.

Family assessments differ depending on the child's developmental stage, as demonstrated in the following two subsections.

Observations of the Family When the Identified Member Is an Adolescent

During adolescence, psychiatric problems are complicated by conflicting family and adolescent issues related to autonomy and control. The adolescent's unfolding needs for individuation and for exercising autonomy and developing a supportive nexus outside of the nuclear family (including romantic attachments and sexual exploration) collide with the family's need to exercise protection, vigilance, and supervision of the child.

In addition to the parents' concern regarding the presenting psychiatric problem(s), the psychiatrist needs to observe the parents' empathy for the child's developmental needs. Are the parents' rules too restrictive? Are the rules too liberal and inconsistent? Is discipline disproportionate, even abusive? Are parents attentive to the child's growing sexuality? Are they negligent about this developmental imperative or, on the contrary, too preoccupied with this issue? How sound is the parents' supervision over the child's social life? Are they vigilant about the child's sexual or substance abuse behaviors? The examiner needs to explore the family's attitudes toward sex, birth control, use of alcohol and mind-altering substances, and so on. The examiner needs to understand the family's rules regarding curfews, dating, driving, and other issues. The examiner should ask questions such as the following: "Has there been any violence in your home?" "Have the police ever come to your home?" "Has the family had any legal issues?" "Do any family members have alcohol or substance abuse problems?" "Has a Child Protective Services agency been involved?"

At all times, the examiner needs to be respectful of the families' religious leanings and philosophy of life. For certain religious groups, mores of contemporary American life, particularly regarding adolescents' privileges, are considered totally unacceptable. The following is an example of observations of a family with a suicidal adolescent.

Case Example 2

Mark, a Caucasian male a few months short of his 18th birthday, was evaluated for planning to kill himself. He had made a suicide pact with his girlfriend, had gotten hold of a couple of his father's handguns, and had driven toward a coastal city 200 miles from his hometown, with the clear intent of killing himself. Fortunately, he had difficulties finding ammunition and loading the guns.

Mark had a long history of depression and had been entertaining thoughts of killing himself for over 2 years. He felt estranged from his family and felt totally alienated from society as a whole. He felt that he did not fit anywhere and felt utterly hopeless about his family and his future.

At the time of this crisis, Mark's girlfriend had gone through a parallel emotional and existential crisis: she had recently attempted suicide and had been in an acute psychiatric program. The girlfriend had also been estranged from her family for a long time.

According to Mark's parents, Mark had been a very bright student and was multitalented; however, his academic interest had faltered, and Mark was struggling to finish high school in a magnet school. In the past, he had excelled in athletics and had been in the gifted and talented program. At the time of this evaluation, he had no career plans and going to college was the farthest thing from his mind.

Mark's family reported no prior psychiatric treatment. However, the family had previously participated in family therapy for a few months, and that experience, in the parents' view, had "left Mark with a negative perception of psychiatrists and therapists."

Mark was a white-haired adolescent with a rather quiet demeanor. He was articulate and used words with precision but sparingly. He was ostensibly depressed and somewhat downcast and kept limited eye contact. He endorsed the already described plan to commit suicide and acknowledged the plot to shoot himself. Mark admitted that he had ingested mushrooms prior to activating the suicide pact. He had also abused marijuana in the past. The rest of the mental status examination was irrelevant to the present discussion.

Issues with hopelessness were explored. He verbalized a sense of futility about life and about going to school in particular. He felt that it made no sense for him to go through life's daily requirements and to settle into a professional career. He wanted to travel, to see the world, and to meet new people.

Obviously, he wanted to move from under his parents' control and to make his own life.

The mother's side of the family had a three-generation history of mood disorders. Mark's mother had a history of chronic depression and was taking duloxetine at the time of the evaluation. His mother was keenly sensitive to the presence of a mood disorder in her son. After graduating from college, she had opted for a position as a flight attendant with one of the major airlines, and she was very happy with her job. Mark's father was a musician and made his living from an assortment of manual jobs. His father was inclined to attribute his son's recent crisis to the mushroom abuse and minimized the role of depression in his son's ongoing difficulties. The couple disagreed about their son's need for psychiatric treatment or psychotropic medication.

Mark's mother was mildly depressed but easily engaged; she kept a very active role during the diagnostic interview and became the spokesperson for the family. The father was warm but not very talkative; he listened attentively to the ongoing discourse and became verbally engaged at appropriate times.

In a conjoint meeting with Mark and his parents, held the same day as the initial evaluation, Mark expressed that he felt his parents had lots of expectations for him and specific plans for his future. He felt very constrained. Mark felt his parents wanted him to go into some professional career, but he emphasized that what he really wanted to do was to travel. His parents were prompt to respond to the represented expectations. His mother said that she did not have any specific plans for him. She was concerned that Mark was depressed and wanted him to be happy. His father asserted that what he wanted for his son was for him to be able to use his talents and potentials and for him to give himself options for his future. He particularly wanted him to be happy.

Mark was surprised by his parents' views and felt moved by his parents' concerns regarding the ongoing crisis and his apparent lack of motivation. Mark acknowledged that he had created some grief for his parents and felt bad that he had not given enough recognition to their concerns and efforts. Mark was visibly moved by his parents' affectionate expressions, voicing that he had felt distant and unable to communicate with them for a long time, in part because he believed they had a pre-established plan for him. As he articulated these thoughts, his demeanor softened, his affect expanded, and he became tearful, expressing the wish to have a closer relationship with both parents. The whole family was emotionally touched. This was an "emotional reunion" for Mark and his parents.

During the family meeting, Mark and his parents became emotionally engaged (reengaged), given the perception that some ice had been melted and that some walls had come down. In fact, when Mark was interviewed at the following session, he said that he was feeling better—that he was feeling more connected to his family—and he no longer saw the future to be as threatening or bleak as he used to. He also felt that his self-esteem had improved. When reflecting about his girlfriend, Mark stated that he did not know what was going to happen with that relationship. Mark did not know whether his girlfriend was interested in feeling better or was still considering suicide. He recognized that he had been dealing with his girlfriend's depression and suicidality for a long time and that this had been emotionally draining for him. He stated, "I am not going to allow her to pull me down."

Through the diagnostic interview, the examiner helped the identified and alienated family member to feel supported and understood and to reconnect with his family. By clarifying the adolescent's misperception and facilitating the family engagement (reengagement), the diagnostic interview helped to tear down Mark's emotional distancing from his parents and rekindle a caring and loving relationship between him and his parents. Mark's reengagement with his parents during the family meeting became a breakthrough, a turning point in his pervasive sense of hopelessness, alienation, and interpersonal isolation.

The following is another example of observations of a family during the interview involving an adolescent threatening suicide.

Case Example 3

Wanda, a 17-year-old Caucasian female, was evaluated after she barricaded herself in the bathroom following an altercation with her mother. Wanda's sister, 3 years her junior, broke down the door and found Wanda with a loaded gun aimed at her temple. Wanda was admitted to an acute inpatient adolescent program.

Wanda was concerned that she was pregnant and had taken some money from her mother's purse to buy a pregnancy kit. Her mother was upset when she found that Wanda had taken money from her. This initiated the argument that preceded the suicide attempt. Wanda had a problematic history of chronic depression and mood instability and had tried to kill herself a number of times before. She stated that she felt unattractive and ugly. She also had used drugs, and her academic performance had deteriorated. Because of Wanda's acting out and her persistent unruly behaviors, she had been placed in a residential treatment program for close to a year and had returned from that program about 6 weeks prior to the present crisis. Apparently, Wanda had confided to her younger sister that she was sexually active but swore to her mother that she was not, even though Wanda's boyfriend confessed to the contrary. The mother had an anxious relationship with Wanda; she felt that her daughter could not do anything without her help and that Wanda was markedly impulsive and unstable. Mother and daughter engaged in frequent power struggles, and according to the mother, Wanda wanted to get her way all the time and badgered her mother to no end in her effort to make her mother change her mind.

Wanda stated that she felt like killing herself when her mother discovered that Wanda had taken money (less than $20) from her purse. She felt that her mother was going to send her away to another treatment facility, because "that is the way of fixing problems with me, to send me away." Wanda represented her mother as controlling and uncompromising.

Thirty-six hours after the hospital admission, staff members were informed that the mother was coming to discharge the patient. Apparently, her mother was upset that Wanda had been allowed to call home without her consent and that Wanda had been allowed to leave the unit to go to the cafeteria without notifying her. Wanda did not feel ready to leave the hospital yet. Her mother was so upset at the hospital that she refused to consider talking to the psychiatrist. Once in the hospital, however, the mother agreed to talk to the attending psychiatrist. She stated that the psychiatrist had not seen her daughter; actually, the psychiatrist had already had two extensive interviews and a third short one with Wanda. The mother demanded discharge, basing her decision on the advice of the child's previous therapist and the staff of the previous residential treatment program. The psychiatrist was unsatisfied with the mother's safety plan and with the lack of qualified mental health providers following Wanda's discharge. The mother became upset with the psychiatrist and complained about the examiner's tone of voice. The examiner explained that the hospital needed to organize a solid outpatient team of mental health providers before Wanda could be discharged. The mother was asked to come the following day and to bring her husband and younger daughter. Before the mother left, she recognized some of her misunderstanding and felt comfortable about leaving her daughter in the hospital for another day. When the psychiatrist shook the mother's hand, she shook the examiner's hand with both hands and demonstrated a positive rapport.

The next day, Wanda's parents and younger sister came to the hospital. The whole family was present. The sisters sat close together, and the younger sister held Wanda's hand. The examiner, desiring a change in the sitting arrangement, asked Wanda's sister to move to the right side of the father; the mother then took the place previously occupied by the sister.

When the examiner asked Wanda's sister how she had felt when she found her older sister with a gun to her head, she became so emotional and moved that she could not talk; she gestured that she was unable to talk about the scene, while at the same time she displayed a spring of emotion and a stream of tears. Wanda was unmoved.

Following the silence related to the sister's emoting, Wanda's father said that Wanda had certainly crossed the line. He discussed with a well of emotion that "all my blood went to my legs" when he received the call from his wife. He could barely stand up and walk. Wanda's father said that he sped home, almost getting hit by an 18 wheeler, and kept wondering along the way what he was going to find as he entered his home: Was he going to find his wife shot? Was his younger daughter dead? Did Wanda commit suicide? He asserted that these moments were the worst of his life. Wanda did not show any emotional response to her father's revelation.

The mother, who could barely hide her resentment, said that from now on things were going to change. Wanda would be in total lockdown after discharge and would not be allowed to talk to her boyfriend. Wanda's persistent concern was for the family not to send her to another placement center, and she attempted to negotiate the lockdown and restrictions from her boyfriend in exchange for not being sent away. The father did not make any deals. Both parents were surprised at how soon the recent crisis occurred after the extended residential treatment placement, and reiterated how little Wanda could be trusted.

Throughout the session, Wanda showed no change of affect and expressed no apologies or regrets. She deflected any invitation to respond to her sister's reactions, to her father's revelations, or to her mother's visible disappointment in her. Wanda displayed a bland demeanor and was unable to empathize with the family's grief and resentment.

She only voiced that although the lockdown was going to be hard, she felt she was going to make a big effort to make it through. Once the aftercare plan was discussed and the parents were satisfied with the aftercare contingencies, Wanda was discharged.

In this vignette, Wanda dissociated the emotional impact of a dramatic suicide attempt. Wanda was unable to recognize the emotional impact that her actions had on her family. She was very narcissistic and manipulative and had no regard for the impact of her behavior on her family. Even though she had claimed that her younger sister was the most important person in her life, she was incapable of expressing any regret or sympathy for her.

Observations of the Family When the Identified Child Is a Preschooler

When assessing a preschool child, the examiner needs to focus on different areas of family and parental functioning and different developmental acquisitions than when assessing an adolescent. The examiner attempts to determine the quality of the child's attachment to the parental figure and to ascertain the degree of the parental figure's emotional investment in the child. Does the examiner see evidence of the child's exploratory behavior in an unfamiliar environment? Does the child show evidence of separation anxiety? Does the child show behavioral organization? Does the examiner observe the parent demonstrating a positive regard toward the child? Is the parent attuned to the child's biological, emotional, and security needs? Does the parent attend to the child's safety and impulsivity? Does the parent display a capacity for sensitive and effective limit setting? Does the parent allow the child to do whatever he or she wants? Does the parent support the child's efforts at self-soothing, behavioral organization, or self-regulation?

Issues regarding the continuity of the child's upbringing need to be explored. The examiner should ask questions such as "Have you taken care of your child all the time?" "Who else has been involved in the rearing of your child?" "Have you ever been separated from your child?" "What were the circumstances?" "Who took care of the child while you were away?" "Has the child ever been placed outside of the family?" The examiner needs to inquire about whether Child Protective Services has ever been involved in the family and, if so, for what reason.

The case of Rudd was discussed in Chapter 3, "Special Interviewing Techniques" (Case Example 2), as an example of physical holding and limit setting during the diagnostic assessment of a preschooler. The following is another example of a preschooler evaluation.

Case Example 4

Daphne, a 3-year-old girl, was referred by a local military hospital after an extensive comprehensive pediatric evaluation—involving developmental pediatricians, a pediatric neurologist, and consultant child psychiatrists—determined that no objective reason accounted for her perplexing symptoms. A week before, the girl had been taken to the emergency room in an intense and protracted tantrum; she had screamed for hours without stopping, had refused to eat or talk, and would not open her fists. At the military hospital, Daphne displayed persistent mutism and would not release the clenching of both hands. She also displayed a number of regressive behaviors. To the hospital observers, the mother was very anxious and unduly solicitous of the child's attention.

Daphne had a history of a willful temperament and threw tantrums when she did not get her way. She had a previous history of hunger strikes and had once gone a whole week accepting only fluids.

Daphne reportedly got along well with other children and was able to play pretend games, but she needed assistance with dressing and bathing. She also wanted to be fed. Daphne had been sleeping a lot throughout the day and night and had become very clingy. She had always been a difficult child and reportedly had difficulties with transitions. Her regressive behavior had begun shortly after Daphne and her mother had returned from visiting the child's biological father in another state; the child had not known her father before. Apparently, the child idealized her father and carried her father's picture everywhere. She had been toilet trained, but after a visitation with her father, she had some accidents. Because of Daphne's dramatic change in behavior, some clinicians wondered if the child had been abused during the visit with her biological father and contacted Child Protective Services.

Daphne had been breastfed until age 2½. Her mother slept with Daphne, rationalizing that a stranger could break into the house at night. Also, when the mother showered, she would take the child into the bathroom. The child had difficulties separating from her mother.

During the time Daphne was in the pediatric hospital, she made repeated references to not letting the germs in and had focused on hand washing for the previous 3 months. During the hospital stay, she would not go to the bathroom by herself; her mother had to take her, sit her at the toilet, and wipe her. During her multiple screaming episodes, Daphne would yell that she wanted her mommy, and when her mother attempted to comfort her, Daphne would scream to her, "Go away!" She was uncooperative and combative with the hospital staff.

During the psychiatric assessment, Daphne's mother excused herself to go to the bathroom, but she did not go without taking her child. The examiner learned that the mother had severe anxiety, some phobias, and paranoia and that her side of the family had a history of depression, anxiety, and bipolar disorder. The mother reported that she had always been anxious and that she would vomit when especially anxious. She disclosed that her anxiety got so severe that she was unable to calm herself. The mother was afraid to drive and wondered if the child had inherited her anxiety. When the mother was a child, she had witnessed violence between her parents. Daphne's mother reported that she and her child were very close. The mother had not received any psychiatric treatment.

In this clinical case, the examiner determined that developmental interferences had promoted and maintained the child's regressive behaviors. The mother obviously had a severe anxiety disorder that needed identification and treatment. At the time the child was discharged from the diagnostic psychiatric hospital, the child's regressive episode had resolved. The Child Protective Services agency was informed of the findings and discharge planning. The agency was to monitor parental behavior and assist the mother in procuring treatment for her own anxiety disorders. The mother was referred for a psychiatric evaluation and received treatment with fluoxetine. A follow-up of the child indicated that the elective mutism and regressive behaviors had resolved and that the hand movements had normalized.

Sometimes during a psychiatric assessment, the examiner needs to intervene to ensure the safety of the child, the examiner, or the persons attending the evaluation, or to preserve the integrity of the evaluation environment. In Rudd's case (described in Chapter 3, "Special Interviewing Techniques" [Case Example 2]), the examiner gave hints to ("coached") an insecure and ineffectual mother about how to stop reinforcing a tantrum (by asking her to leave the situation and proceed to the office), modeled effective parental behaviors by putting the child under control, suggested affectionate support once the child regained self-control, and accepted reparation (affectionate contact) at the time of departure. Thus, the examiner challenged the mother's beliefs that limit setting did not work.

Areas of Family Assessment That Need Specific Inquiry

Almost any topic can be explored within a family meeting, but some issues should be approached more privately. At all times, the examiner should respect the parental choice regarding what issues need to be addressed, who may be privy to such discussion, or what will be the most appropriate therapeutic venue for such exploration. At all times, the examiner will attempt to understand the parental decision-making process. In principle, marital issues should not be discussed in front of the children or in front of prior-generation members.

In general, when a major psychiatric disorder is identified in a child, the family undergoes a great deal of soul and generational searching for the origins of the disorder. Frequently, families become revealing and share family secrets or information about the family they have not previously discussed with others, or they begin to question older relatives about histories of relatives who may have had related psychiatric issues.

The examiner should begin the inquiry by asking each parent specifically about his or her history of mood or anxiety disorders, alcohol or substance abuse, relevant legal history, or any condition related to the presenting problem. If the responses are positive, the examiner further explores response to treatment, complications, relapses, and so forth (see section "Family Organigram" earlier in this chapter).

Key Points

- The family is the essential system for optimal upbringing.
- The examiner needs to engage all the family participants and win over the support of the "gatekeeper."
- The examiner needs to assess how the family provides love, care, support, and discipline. This is the preeminent function of the family.

Notes

1. The authors understand that the electronic medical record makes it difficult to construct a family diagram. In many cases; a narrative description is the second best substitute. In cases in which the family is "loaded" with psychopathology—that is, when there are many members afflicted—a manual diagram will be the most helpful alternative.

2. The Edinburgh Postnatal Depression Scale (Cox et al. 1987) has 10 questions that explore happiness, capacity for humor, capacity for enjoyment, guilt, anxiety, inability to cope, difficulty sleeping related to unhappiness, feelings of sadness, crying, and suicidal ideation; items are rated from 0 to 3. The cut-off score ranges from 9 to 13. A score of 13 or more is considered to be an indicator of serious depression. Women with scores of 9 or above should be referred for further assessment and treatment if the score on suicidal ideation is 1 or more (Belluck 2016, A13).

CHAPTER 5

Providing Post-evaluation Feedback to Families

A Word of Caution

Providing post-evaluation feedback is a critical part of the psychiatric interview. A number of principles guide the examiner's professional deportment during this important phase of the interviewing process. The examiner needs to demonstrate expertise, empathy, and sensitivity and to show his or her educational abilities and skills. The examiner needs to keep an open and exploratory mind, even at this late phase of the interview, and be sensitive to the nature of the feedback, to anticipate the parents' or the child's reactions to it, and be prepared to deal with its repercussions.

A good way to start the post-evaluation phase of the interview is for the evaluator to ask the child and family if they have any topics that have not been discussed that would be helpful for understanding the presenting problem. Someone may bring up a new issue about the child or the family; this may shed additional light on the presenting problem.

Legal/Custody Concerns

If the parents are divorced, the physician needs to clarify who is the custodian and who has the medical decision rights over the child. In the case of divorced or separated parents, the psychiatrist must make efforts to involve the non-custodial parent. If the custodial parent has reasons to believe that the noncustodial parent would refuse consent to non-urgent psychiatric treatment, providing treatment over that parent's objections is legally questionable and clinically unwise. Both parents' input is valuable for a variety of reasons: involving both parents 1) provides greater opportunity for more information concerning behaviors in a variety of contexts and perspectives; 2) helps ensure that less bias and less one-sided information will be presented; 3) increases the chances for treatment planning and implementation; and 4) likely results in better medication management and more effective therapy (Mossman and Weston 2008, pp. 64, 66). Briefly, listening to both parents' sides increases the likelihood of compliance with the treatment plan.

Confidentiality

The psychiatrist needs to clarify the nature of confidentiality and inform the child and family about which communications are bound by confidentiality rules and which ones are not. The family needs to know that the examiner is not bound to confidentiality rules when circumstances of neglect, physical abuse, or sexual abuse are evident, or when the patient is at imminent risk of harming someone.

Opportunities to Educate the Patient and Family

During the post-evaluation feedback phase, the psychiatrist educates the family about the current standards of care for a particular disorder. What Vitiello (2008) wrote about bipolar disorder is equally applicable to the diagnosis and treatment of most child and adolescent psychiatric disorders:

> Parents should be informed of the current state-of-the-science of [diagnosis and] treatment for bipolar disorder [or the disorder in question] and made aware that, though there is expert consensus that children with bipolar disorder [or other psychiatric disorders] should receive pharmacological treatment [or other interventions] to stabilize mood, the effectiveness of treatment in preventing recurrences and improving ultimate prognosis remains to be documented [demonstrated]. Because response to treatment is highly variable across individuals, finding an effective treatment regimen for a patient is still very much a process of trial and error. It is important for patients and parents to be aware of these limitations. (p. 393)

Consideration Regarding Health Resources/ Finances and Other Family Issues

In making therapeutic recommendations, the psychiatrist needs to be cognizant of the family's mental health and financial resources, as well as the local mental health resources, so he or she can present options that are affordable and available to the family. Also, good therapeutic recommendations take into account the religious, cultural, and other ecological aspects of the family. No recommendations are likely to be implemented by a family if they contravene the family's religious or cultural norms. In a similar manner, the therapeutic recommendations are more likely to be implemented if they agree with the family's theory of illness.

In determining a diagnosis and establishing a therapeutic plan, the psychiatrist should strive to involve the child in the process, especially if the subject is an adolescent. At the same time, the psychiatrist should make an effort to promote an understanding of the child's pathology.

Avoiding Premature Diagnostic Closures

The examiner should avoid making premature closures and should be tentative when presenting professional diagnostic opinions. As Nurcombe (2008a) noted, "Given the fuzzy nature of clinical data, medical decisions have to be probabilistic" (p. 2). (For Nurcombe's strategies of diagnostic reasoning, see Note 1 at the end of this chapter.) Before giving a serious diagnosis, such as a severe psychotic disorder, the examiner may suggest to the family that the preliminary impressions indicate the possibility of a serious diagnosis but that a number of steps are needed before committing to a definitive diagnosis: 1) conducting further diagnostic interviewing; 2) completing a number of diagnostic procedures and consultations to further elucidate the case (lab studies, drug abuse testing, psychological testing, speech and language assessment, neurological and other medical consultations); 3) observing the response to sensible treatment trials targeting major psychopathological dimensions; and 4) giving opportunity for a period of longitudinal observation. The examiner needs to avoid making either overoptimistic pronouncements or negative and pessimistic prognostications.

Except when a patient demonstrates clear manifestations of an indisputable psychiatric syndrome and a categorical diagnosis is imperative, the examiner may consider prioritizing the most salient psychopathological dimensions of behavior that are currently interfering with successful adaptation. A categorical diagnosis tends to remove the parents from the circular causality of the psychopathology and from other issues that need to be considered in the understanding of precipitating or maintaining factors.

A Balanced Stand Regarding Nature and Nurture

Despite the growing consensus that a number of psychiatric disorders have clear biological underpinnings, the importance of family stability and a warm parental ambiance cannot be overemphasized. For instance, Tillman and Geller (2008) reported that the likelihood of relapse in children diagnosed with bipolar disorder depends on maternal warmth; those children whose mothers were warm had less incidence of relapse than the ones whose mothers were not.

Parents often project onto the other spouse responsibility for whatever is wrong with the child, particularly when the psychiatric condition is severe. The psychiatrist needs to be attentive to the emergence of such conflict and attempt to help the parents understand the irrationality of their projected blame and guilt. The psychiatrist needs to educate the patient and family about the nature of the disorder(s) in question.

During post-evaluation feedback, the examiner should monitor any reaction of the child and family indicating ambivalence and covert or overt disagreements with the treatment recommendations. The examiner should attempt to deal with the reservations or ambivalence over the diagnosis or treatment plan.

Safety Issues

When issues regarding safety are apparent, these concerns need to take priority over everything else. The examiner needs to convey to the family that any indication or hint of suicide needs to be taken seriously. If suicide is considered a risk, the examiner needs to implement a safety plan with the family. Depending on the immediacy of the risk, the plan may include the consideration of an acute hospitalization. Basically, hospitalization is indicated when the patient expresses in words or behavior that he or she is determined, if not driven, to end his or her life. If the examiner believes that the child's life is at stake, it is imperative that he or she make every possible effort to persuade the family to seek hospitalization for the child. If the family is not supportive of this therapeutic recommendation, the psychiatrist should take steps to ensure that the child is taken to a nearby psychiatric unit by facilitating an order of protected custody or by issuing a medical certificate for involuntary commitment. Furthermore, if the psychiatrist feels that the child is in serious danger of hurting himself or herself, and the family opposes the psychiatrist's safety plan, the psychiatrist needs to contact Child Protective Services (CPS) to report the family for medical neglect.

The physician needs to be clear and convincing regarding the nonavailability of arms (knives and particularly guns) around the house. About half of the total number of suicides in the United States—21,000 in 2014 for example—were caused by fire arms. According to Ash (2008), only a quarter of families follow the recommendation that guns be removed from the home. That being the case, the psychiatrists need to monitor this risk is paramount.

Similar considerations apply when the child poses a risk to others. Homicidal behavior requires emergency psychiatry intervention. Nowadays, because schools' zero tolerance for violence, schools demand a psychiatric evaluation every time a student makes overt or veiled threats to hurt somebody or to carry out a terroristic threat. The psychiatrist needs to assert the implementation of a safety plan and take steps similar to those discussed above regarding suicidal crises. The psychiatrist must also remember the obligation to warn potential victims, as established by the 1976 *Tarasoff vs. Regents of the University of California* precedent. Too many school tragedies have occurred in which students and teachers have lost their lives at the hands of mentally ill students. Many of these tragedies resulted from multi-systemic failures of the duty to protect; the mental health system and psychiatrists, schools, peers, parents, and others failed to take assertive steps to deal with the psychopathology that was detected or suspected. In the case of suicide, the non-availability of arms should be made a serious goal. The patient's access to potentially suicidal weapons needs to be monitored on an ongoing basis.

Dealing With Abuse Issues

One of the most difficult issues for the psychiatrist to handle during the feedback phase concerns physical or sexual abuse. The psychiatrist needs to be straightforward and determined when addressing issues of potential physical and sexual abuse. The examiner is obligated to report to CPS any circumstance of suspected abuse in any form. When the family takes responsibility for a child's claims of physical abuse, the psychiatrist may guide the family to call CPS to open a case, with the goal of ensuring the safety of the child (or other children) and of establishing a therapeutic program for effective discipline without the use of abusive punishment. That initial call to CPS can be made at the physician or mental health professional office.

Families are less open to accepting responsibility for claims of sexual abuse (see Note 2 at the end of this chapter). Mothers often disregard or disbelieve their children's claims, in part because such an acceptance would mean the end of the marriage or a relationship; the mothers may be financially dependent on the perpetrators and cannot risk breaking off the dependent relationship. For some mothers, the awareness that they failed in protecting and caring for their children is very painful and unacceptable. The psychiatrist needs to anticipate the complications surrounding the disclosure and assist the child and whatever is left of the family in dealing with the complex consequences of sexual abuse.

Because the disclosure of sexual abuse has multiple implications and legal ramifications, the psychiatrist must contact CPS. This governmental agency is in charge of implementing a safety plan to spare the child from further traumatization and to protect the child from retaliation for the disclosure of abuse.

If the psychiatrist makes an assessment requested by a third party, he or she needs to make it clear to the parents that feedback or information will be shared with the interested parties (CPS, judicial system, noncustodial parent, and maybe others). The examiner should similarly handle the detection of parental neglect or related circumstances that imperil children's physical and mental well-being.

Psychiatrist Interface With School and Other Systems

Regarding issues related to special education and other ancillary services, including psychological testing, speech therapy, occupational therapy, and so on, the psychiatrist should advise the family to pursue a deliberate advocacy. Increased roadblocks have been placed to children with special education needs. At times, not even expert assessment and recommendations have any sway (see Cepeda 2007). Frankly stated, schools neglect the timely identification of speech and learning disorders and delay implementation of necessary services. Parents unhappily learn that the decisions and recommendations of the ARD (admission, review, and dismissal) committees are hollow promises.

Issues With Alcohol and Illegal Drugs

Most families are very concerned when they learn that their children are involved with drugs or alcohol. Parents might want to know details about their child's abuse or addiction, but if the child does not want to share this information with parents, the psychiatrist has to oblige. The psychiatrist should inform the family that federal law (Confidentiality of Alcohol and Drug Abuse Patient Records 2005) stipulates that issues related to substance abuse are confidential, regardless of the child's age (see Note 3 at the end of this chapter). The examiner might explain the situation as follows: "One important recommendation I have for your daughter is that she attend a chemical dependency program; unfortunately, your daughter has not authorized me to share the nature or extent of her problem with you. You may find this strange and inadmissible, but the law prevents me from discussing a child's alcohol or drug abuse with parents. I advise you to talk with your daughter about these issues."

Families' Reaction to Diagnostic Feedback

Families are often ready to seek affirmation for an affective disorder, such as bipolar disorder, which is frequently discussed in the media. On the other hand, families are typically apprehensive about certain psychiatric diagnoses, including psychotic disorders. Many families have difficulty believing that children could experience hallucinations or harbor paranoid thinking. The examiner can take several actions to decrease the family's reservations about some of these disorders: the examiner can carry out the child's mental status examination in the parents' presence or, as suggested in Chapter 2, "General Principles of Interviewing," the examiner may allow the parents to take an active role in the exploration of these controversial symptoms.

The Option of Doing Nothing

In discussing therapeutic recommendations, the psychiatrist needs to present the option and consequences of doing nothing. If the parents choose this alternative, the psychiatrist, always respectful of the parents' choice, should request that the family notify him if the child's symptoms change. The psychiatrist should emphasize that he or she would like to know if the child gets better or worse. If the child's symptoms worsen, the psychiatrist needs to reconceptualize the case and to consider therapeutic options anew.

The Need for Combination of Treatments

The psychiatrist should stress the importance of combined treatments. Accumulated expertise indicates that combined treatments have a larger therapeutic impact than isolated treatments. Even though the effect size for a number of psychiatric disorders in children and adolescents favors psychotropic medications, the importance of psychosocial interventions for those disorders should not be underestimated. For a number of psychiatric disorders, such as posttraumatic stress disorder, anxiety disorders, and mood disorders, psychosocial interventions are fundamental.

Some parents are apprehensive about psychopharmacological recommendations. They are wary of potential side effects, including a medication's impact on level of alertness, cognitive dulling, drug dependency, impact on growth (see Note 4 at the end of this chapter), puberty and reproductive life, and so forth. These parents prefer to defer psychotropic intervention and advocate for psychosocial interventions first. After educating the parents about the benefits and risks of an intended medication and presenting the benefit/risk ratio of the recommended medications, the psychiatrist needs to respect the parents' decisions on this matter. The psychiatrist also can consider recommending that the family seek a second opinion to buttress his or her case on the importance of interventions about which the family is apprehensive.

When discussing psychotropic medications, the psychiatrist needs to clearly state the target symptoms and the medication's side effects, present the benefit/risk ratio, and give the parents and child ample opportunity to ask questions and clarify issues. Asking the parents to repeat what they heard gives the psychiatrist the opportunity to correct misunderstandings and to stress issues that seem ambiguous.

The psychiatrist must stress the need for parents to monitor medication compliance and attend to potential side effects, emphasizing the possibility of serious untoward side effects for each particular medication. The psychiatrist is obligated to discuss, for example, the increased risk of suicidal ideation with antidepressant medications, antiepileptic medications, atomoxetine, and many others; cardiological side effects with stimulants and ziprasidone; serious dermatological reactions with carbamazepine and lamotrigine; and severe metabolic side effects with atypical antipsychotics. For patients with a history of substance abuse, the parents need to be extra cautious about storing and administering medications (particularly, painkillers like opiates and the like) and be vigilant about strict compliance.

When recommending psychotropic medications to adolescent females, the psychiatrist must make the patient and family aware of hormonal risks (menstrual irregularities), polycystic ovarian disease, and teratogenic risks. In the same vein, the psychiatrist needs to alert the patient that some psychotropic medications, such as carbamazepine, may interfere with the effectiveness of oral birth control, increasing the risk of unwanted pregnancies. It is desirable that all sexually active adolescents receive birth control protection.

Basic Care Issues

The psychiatrist needs to take the opportunity to advocate for recommended health care (regular pediatric and odontological care), dietary changes, and gynecological consultations and to promote necessary levels of exercise and hygienic sleep, as well as cultural and spiritual activities. These basic aspects of health promotion should be a common generic recommendation for every child and family. The same is true regarding an open discussion of sexual behavior and contraception, as well the parental need to monitor alcohol and drug abuse.

Last but not least, the examiner needs to advise the family that having a child with behavioral or emotional problems is a source of stress for the marriage. Although the child's emotional needs must take a higher priority, improving and nurturing the marriage need to be considered important priorities for optimal family functioning.

Key Points

• The examiner needs to take multiple factors into account when giving feedback about the diagnostic assessment.
• The examiner needs to be tactful, sensitive, deliberate, and forthright when giving feedback to the child and family.
• The examiner needs to anticipate complications during the feedback phase and should be prepared to deal with them.
• Safety of the child and family is a paramount concern when providing feedback.

Notes

1. Nurcombe (2008a, p. 6) recommended the following strategies of diagnostic reasoning:

   • Tolerate uncertainty; avoid premature closures and consider alternatives.
   • Separate cues from inferences. Refer inferences to salient cues.
   • Be aware of personal reactions to the patient (countertransference).
   • Be alert to fresh evidence that may demand a revision or deletion of a hypothesis or diagnosis.
   • *Value negative evidence above positive evidence.*
   • Be prepared to commit to a diagnosis when enough evidence has been gathered.

2. Generally, a disclosure of sexual abuse within the family has devastating consequences for the family and the parental relationship. If a parent is involved, the parents' relationship is unlikely to survive the consequences of such a transgression. Furthermore, the consequences of the disclosure add further trauma for the abused child: the family is fragmented and a family rift may occur, and depending on the mother's response, the child could lose both parents and the family as a whole when the child is separated from his or her siblings and home; unfortunately, this may occur at a time when the child needs the most support. In addition, some family members may become accusatory toward the child; under these conditions of immense pressure, the child may begin to think that the disclosure was wrong and that he or she is being punished for a wrong deed. Under these circumstances it is not surprising that many children recant.

A mother's response may be strongly emotional when the disclosure is new. We have witnessed serious and dramatic reactions when mothers first learn about the abuse by their husbands. Mothers have exhibited a variety of reactions, including acute psychosomatic responses (e.g., sudden and intense vomiting), panic attacks, sudden depressive reactions, and intense rage accompanied by homicidal urges toward the spouse.

3. If a minor is acting alone, only he or she can provide written authorization to disclose medical records, including disclosure to the parents. Individual states have their own laws concerning minors seeking treatment. The Texas Commission on Alcohol and Drug Abuse Web site compares the Health Insurance Portability and Accountability Act of 1996 (HIPAA), 42 CFR 2.14 (Confidentiality of Alcohol and Drug Abuse Patient Records 2005), and state regulations. Texas state law does not require parental consent for drug abuse treatment, and written authorization is required for disclosure of confidential information to parents. Under the same provisions, if a minor signs himself or herself into treatment, he or she may consent to examination and treatment for chemical dependency or any condition associated with chemical use.

4. Intake of conventional stimulants (methylphenidate or dextroamphetamine derivatives) is associated with a small but statistically significant reduction of height and weight gain rates in children over many years. The magnitude of the impact is dose related, and height and weight rates increase when the stimulants are discontinued. Studies show that after 2–3.5 years of stimulant intake by children, they have a decrement in height of 1–2.5 cm and a decrement in weight of 0–5 kg (0–10 lb) compared with prestimulant treatment predictions (Towbin 2008, p. 977). The Pediatric Advisory Committee recommends strong warnings regarding the use of stimulant medications in patients with underlying structural cardiovascular defects or cardiomyopathies (Towbin 2008). The guidelines are not clear regarding whether an electrocardiogram baseline should be requested prior to initiation of stimulants. A small subgroup of children with cardiac disorders carry an elevated risk for pediatric sudden cardiac death, regardless of whether they receive stimulants or not. The American Heart Association notes that most cardiovascular disorders or congenital heart diseases are not absolute contraindications to stimulant use (Towbin 2008, p. 979).

CHAPTER 6

Evaluation of Special Populations

In this chapter, we discuss some brief general principles about evaluating children who have certain medical conditions or who live in specific socio-economic circumstances. In general, children who grow up in adverse circumstances or endure traumatic incidents (e.g., natural catastrophes, burns) experience clear developmental interferences (see Chapter 13, "Comprehensive Psychiatric Formulation"). The psychiatrist needs to recognize the nature of the developmental interferences and attempt to correct or ameliorate the developmental environment.

Children With Serious Acute or Chronic Medical Illness

A chronic medical illness constitutes a true developmental interference. Children with severe acute medical illnesses may not understand the seriousness of their predicament. They might feel sick and be aware that something is wrong, but they rarely consider the possibility of death or the implication of the disease as the parents do. Parents of children who face a sudden or fulminating illness go through an acute stress reaction, if not a state of shock, and may have to contend with the possibility of the child's death. This experience is very traumatic. Parents need a great deal of emotional support and ongoing sensitive feedback about how the medical condition is unfolding:

"Parents should receive a full explanation of the cause, nature, treatment, and prognosis of the disease. They may have a false, unhelpful sense of responsibility for the illness, particularly if they are carriers of what proves to be a genetic disease" (Nurcombe 2008b, p. 677).

In cases of a child's impending death, parents need assistance with the forthcoming loss and guidance as to how to communicate with the child. As Nurcombe (2008b) notes, "Regression is a normal reaction to acute physical illness. Physically ill children become more dependent, clinging, and demanding. Younger children may revert to bedwetting and immature speech. Preschool children may interpret the illness as a punishment for something they have done" (p. 675). Parents with a prior psychiatric history are particularly vulnerable to responding to the child's health crisis by reverting to previous psychopathological conditions (e.g., depression, anxiety) or by relapsing into alcohol or drug abuse. "Some parents react initially with denial. Others react by becoming overprotective, by having unrealistic expectations for improvement, by withdrawing, or by rejecting or abandoning the child. Latent tensions between parents can be aggravated and, at times, separation or divorce [is] precipitated" (Nurcombe 2008b, p. 677). The psychiatrist should be attentive to these parental reactions and attempt to deal with them in a timely and pertinent manner.

Children With Burn Trauma

Of all people who experience burns in the United States, 34% are children (Stoddard et al. 2006). Fire-related injuries are the third leading cause of unintentional injury. Posttraumatic stress disorder (PTSD) is a frequent result of burn injuries in children. Burns are also associated with a number of other psychiatric conditions, including overanxious disorder, phobias, and enuresis (Saxe et al. 2005). Saxe et al. (2005) found two pathways to PTSD following burns: from acute separation anxiety and from dissociation. The magnitude of the trauma, or the size of the burn, was not related to PTSD directly but exerted influence through both pathways. The pathway mediated by separation anxiety was influenced by the acute pain response and the burn size and was inversely related to the child's age. The pathway of dissociation was influenced only by the size of the burn. The independence of the anxiety and dissociation pathways suggests that different biobehavioral systems contribute to PTSD (Saxe et al. 2005). Two biological theories explain children's response to trauma: the fight or flight response (a response involving the sympathetic nervous system and the hypothalamic-pituitary-adrenal axis) and the freeze/immobilization response (controlled by the parasympathetic system) (Saxe et al. 2005).

The nature of the burn and the prolonged recovery process impose stressful separations between the child and the parents when the child has a great need for help and comfort. Children who experience the greatest anxiety on separations are the most likely to develop PTSD. The implication is that burn trauma, like all trauma, has a very important interpersonal component (Saxe et al. 2005). The degree of dissociation shortly after the burn is a predictor of PTSD (see Note 1 at the end of this chapter). The implications of the cited study are that in the treatment of burn children, the parents should be encouraged to be around their children for comfort and reassurance, and optimal treatment of pain with opiates could forestall the development of PTSD (Saxe et al. 2005).

In a study of 52 children younger than 48 months, Stoddard et al. (2006) found that the rate of acute stress disorder was 29%: 80% of the children had symptoms that met the criteria for re-experiencing, 62% had symptoms that met the criteria for avoidance, and 39% had symptoms that met the criteria for arousal. The authors found two direct pathways to acute stress symptoms: from pulse rate ($\beta = 0.43$) and from parents' symptoms ($\beta = 0.47$). Pulse rate was a mediator between total burn surface area and acute stress symptoms, and parents' symptoms were a mediator between pain and acute stress disorder. Pulse rate, which increased as a result of a hyperadrenergic state at the time of trauma, has been shown to be predictive of PTSD. The hyperadrenergic state may be involved in the consolidation of traumatic memory manifested in memory intrusion and reexperiencing. Recall leads to a re-release of catecholamines and stress hormones, resulting in an enhancement of the traumatic memory (Stoddard et al. 2006). Level of pain has repeatedly been associated with PTSD in children with burns and nonburn injuries. Pain seems to exert its influence via the parents' acute stress symptoms. If the caregivers become symptomatic themselves and are less able to provide soothing and reassurance because they are overwhelmed, or if the parents use avoidance or other mechanisms, they may have a deleterious influence on the child (Stoddard et al. 2006).

The child psychiatrist needs to assess how the child and parents are dealing with the burn injury and how they are participating in and coping with medical care. The psychiatrist needs to be sensitive to the child's pain and separation anxieties, as well as other forms of distress, such as eating or sleeping problems and emotional withdrawal. Furthermore, the psychiatrist needs to be attentive to the parents' emotional state and to their availability to the child's needs of succor, comfort, and reassurance. Equally important for the child psychiatrist is his or her role as liaison with the burn treatment team to maximize optimal comprehensive healing so as to minimize physical and emotional scarring.

Children With Neurodevelopmental Disorders

Neurodevelopmental disorders, which are typically diagnosed during childhood, cause lifelong and characteristic impairment of socialization, communication, intellectual abilities, and behavior (Posey and McDougle 2008). Because optimal functionality is a desirable outcome, some comments about functional assessment are included; this assessment is necessary for a comprehensive rehabilitation program for children with neurodevelopmental disorders. Brief descriptions are provided of intellectual disability, cerebral palsy, and a number of neurogenetic disorders.

Categorization of developmental disabilities has been narrow and has left out significant dimensions of the persons with these conditions. These "classification procedures and standards fail to regard the whole person; they produce only a limited picture of the person and thus also fail to identify the ways in which the person can function and participate in various activities with and without reasonable accommodations or individual and appropriate services" (Turnbull et al. 2007, p. 24). Persons with disabilities have the right to empowerment and participatory decision making, service coordination and collaboration, liberty, protection from harm, autonomy, privacy and confidentiality, integration, productivity, contribution, family integrity and unity, family-centered services, culturally responsive services, accountability, personal, professional and system capacity development, and prevention (Turnbull et al. 2007). In assessing an individual with a neurodevelopmental disorder, the examiner has two equally important goals: 1) to identify the individual's deficits and limitations and 2) to determine his or her functional capacities.

In working with children with neurodevelopmental disorders, the child psychiatrist attempts to identify the nature and extent of the deficits and the psychological and compensatory reactions to them. The child psychiatrist attempts to elucidate how the child and family cope with the deficits and what evidence of resilience they demonstrate in dealing with the impacts of their limitations. The psychiatrist also monitors the child's and family's compliance with therapeutic and medical recommendations and identifies any barriers to compliance with the rehabilitation program.

Children With Intellectual Disability

Intellectual disability (intellectual developmental disorder) (ID/IDD) is classified in DSM-5 (American Psychiatric Association 2013) as a neurodevelopmental disorder that is characterized by deficits in intellectual and adaptive functioning in terms of conceptual, social, and practical domains originating in the developmental period (Munir 2016, p. 95).

Sundheim et al. (2006) warned about two frequent pitfalls in the diagnostic process of individuals with intellectual disability: 1) *diagnostic overshadowing*, which refers to using the diagnosis of ID/IDD as the explanation for whatever is wrong with the patient instead of using standardized diagnostic criteria, and 2) *diagnostic presumption*, which refers to the assumption of a psychiatric diagnosis based exclusively on the association with ID/IDD.

Psychiatric disorders are more easily diagnosed in patients with mild to moderate ID/IDD than in those with severe ID/IDD. In the group with co-occurrence of disorders there are more subjects with three or more disorders than one would expect if the disorders were independently distributed (Munir 2016, p. 96). Multiple disabilities and disorders are more common among children with severe ID/IDD (Munir 2016, p. 97). Early studies showed high comorbidity of ID/IDD with autism spectrum disorder, childhood psychosis, attention-deficit/hyperactivity disorder (ADHD), and stereotyped disorders among study participants with moderate ID/IDD with an IQ of 50 or lower; the rates more than double in persons with brain damage or epilepsy (Munir 2016). The prevalence of autism is 5%–10% in individuals with mild ID but 30% in those with moderate ID. The prevalence of ADHD in persons with ID is about 8.7%–16%, compared with 5% in the general population. The rates of major depressive disorder in ID subjects are 1.5- to 2-fold higher than in the general population, and it is estimated that the rates of bipolar disorder and schizophrenia are twice the rates in the general population (Aggarwal et al. 2013, p. 10). The diagnostic difficulties stem from the atypical presentations and assessment difficulties due to communication barriers and lack of diagnostic tools appropriate for this population. The accuracy of the diagnosis is affected by language skills and the severity of ID/IDD (Aggarwal et al. 2013, p. 11). Collateral information in the evaluation of individuals with ID/IDD is invaluable. It is important to screen for physical causes of anomalous behavior such as unrecognized pain (reflux, otitis, urinary tract infections, dental pain, fractures, constipation, and others), endocrine causes, seizures, and adverse reaction to medications (Aggarwal et al. 2013, p. 12).

According to Sundheim et al. (2006), patients with ID have trouble verbalizing their difficulties. They might express their reaction to some illnesses that cause pain with irritability, aggression, and self-abusive behaviors; these ailments demand timely identification and treatment. Sundheim et al. stressed that optimally, the neuropsychiatric assessment for persons with intellectual disability should be carried out in the context of a diagnostic team: pediatricians and other physician specialists, educators, and behavioral specialists. Although most people with developmental disabilities can communicate with words, when working with patients with ID, the examiner may need to modify the interview to work around the linguistic limitations. Nonverbal patients develop ways of expressing themselves, and the strategies they use may be troublesome enough to be the reason for the referral. Collateral information is necessary. However, systematic observation of the patient is fundamental for understanding the behaviors in question and for developing an effective communication and a correct diagnosis. This means that even for patients with communication difficulties, the mental status examination remains indispensable. In lieu of verbalization, the individual with ID may be able to use sign language, respond to yes-no questions, answer structured questions, or use a picture book or other media to facilitate the interview. Subjective experiences may be cautiously inferred from facial expressions and body language (Sundheim et al. 2006).

Children With Cerebral Palsy

Cerebral palsy is a permanent, nonprogressive disorder of movement and posture that is due to a neurological insult that occurs during fetal or infant development. Associated features include abnormal cognition and communication, epilepsy, and musculoskeletal problems. The causes of cerebral palsy include injury to the developing brain (stroke, hypoxia/ischemia, malformations, early traumatic brain injury), infection, and prematurity (Nickels 2015, p. 679). Cerebral palsy is characterized by changes in muscle tone (mostly spasticity or rigidity), muscle weakness, involuntary movements, ataxia, or a combination of these abnormalities.

Cerebral palsy is neither episodic nor progressive; the full extent of the motor disabilities is evident by age 3–4 years. Intellectual, sensory, and behavioral difficulties may accompany cerebral palsy but are not included in the diagnostic criteria. Of children with cerebral palsy, 52% have intellectual disability, 45% have epilepsy, 38% have speech and language disorder, 28% have ophthalmological defects, and 12% have hearing impairment. Preterm infants constitute 50%–60% of all infants with cerebral palsy (Swaiman and Wu 2006). Prevalence of psychiatric disorders in individuals with cerebral palsy is three to five times higher than in control subjects, but no one psychiatric disorder is typical (Nurcombe 2008b). Cerebral palsy needs to be differentiated from developmental delays and developmental plateau. If there is a clear failure to acquire a milestone even slowly, or if there is a loss of a previously acquired milestone, this is not cerebral palsy, a static encephalopathy; developmental plateau or regression is suggestive of progressive neurological disease due to metabolic, infectious, autoimmune, or genetic causes (Nickles 2015, p. 680).

The child psychiatrist is commonly involved in the evaluation and treatment of the emotional and behavioral problems of children with cerebral palsy. The psychiatrist plays a major role in the comprehensive assessment of the multiple deficits of these children and in the coordination of care, including physical therapy, occupational therapy, speech therapy, neurological follow-ups, specialized education, and pertinent diagnostic and psychiatric care (including individual and family psychotherapy and psychotropic medication monitoring).

Major issues for the child with cerebral palsy are problems with self-image and sense of competence, and issues and problems with socialization. The psychiatrist needs to explore broad issues of family functioning, paying special attention to how the family copes with the child's multiple needs and how the family complies with treatment plans and the implementation of multiple interventions. The psychiatrist also needs to monitor how the family handles the ambivalence of dealing with a child with special needs and multiple handicaps and how the family manages emotional and financial resources in dealing with the nonhandicapped children.

Children With Neurogenetic Disorders

Behavioral neurogeneticists look for etiologically defined and relatively homogeneous genetic syndromes, including fragile X syndrome, Prader-Willi syndrome, Turner syndrome, Williams syndrome, and Rett syndrome. The neural mechanisms underlying the maladaptive cognition, psychiatric symptoms, and abnormal behaviors of these syndromes can be systematically investigated (Gothelf 2007). The child psychiatrist assists in a prompt identification of these syndromes and in fostering a timely and coordinated treatment of the identified disorder.

A number of behavioral phenotypes have been identified as originating from specific gene deletions or mutation syndromes that result in genetic neurodevelopmental disorders. These disorders represent distinctive patterns of cognitive and behavioral features and congenital medical sequelae (Feinstein and Singh 2007). *Endophenotypes* refer to measurable traits associated with underlying susceptibility genes. The traits are associated with illness, are heritable, are state independent (i.e., they are present even when the illness is not active), and cosegregate within families of probands (Feinstein and Singh 2007).

Fragile X Syndrome

Fragile X mental retardation 1 gene (*FMR1*) mutations are associated with autism or autism spectrum disorders. The full mutation typically causes methylation of the promoter region of *FMR1*. The mutated gene causes transcription disruption, translation, and *FMR1* protein production (FMRP) impairment. It is the lack or deficiency of FMRP that leads to fragile X syndrome. The range of overall intellectual abilities is correlated with the levels of FMRP: individuals with a mild deficiency present with normal or borderline IQ, learning disabilities, social deficits, and anxiety; this group represents about 15% of males and 70% of females with fragile X syndrome. Individuals with very low levels or no production of FMRP experience moderate to severe intellectual disabilities, and autism at the lower IQ level. Approximately 30% of subjects with fragile X syndrome have autism and another 20%–30% have autism spectrum disorders. The remainder of fragile X syndrome subjects do not have presentations that fulfill criteria for autism spectrum disorder but exhibit autism-like features, including, hand flapping, hand biting, and poor eye contact (Hagerman et al. 2011, p. 801).

Fragile X syndrome is the most common inherited cause of ID and developmental delays. It is present in 1 in every 4,000 boys and 1 in every 6,000–8,000 girls and is caused by an expansion mutation of *FMR1* at the X chromosome. Symptoms are more severe in boys than in girls. The social phenotype in boys consists of social withdrawal, anxiety, high emotionality, poor eye contact, atypical speech, and theory of mind impairment. A substantial proportion of boys with fragile X syndrome (25%–47%) have a presentation that meets the criteria for autism (Feinstein and Singh 2007).

Down Syndrome

Down syndrome was first described by Jean-Etienne Esquirol in 1838, and promulgated by John Langdon Down in 1866 as a condition with a recognizable phenotype and limited intellectual endowment due to extra 21 chromosome material. The long arm of chromosome 21 contains more than 400 genes, and it is a subset of those genes that have been implicated in Down syndrome; this area has been designated as the "Down syndrome critical region" located at 21q22 to qter. Nondisjunction of chromosome 21 is responsible for the majority of Down syndrome cases (about 95% of trisomic Down syndrome with approximately 90% of maternal meiotic origin; this form is not inherited). In about 4%–5% of cases, the Down syndrome is caused by translocation, with attachment of the long arm of chromosome 21 to the long arm of chromosome 14, 21, or 22 being the most common translocations. The translocation may have a 10% chance of occurring again in a future pregnancy (Nehring 2010, p. 447).

Down syndrome is the most common chromosomal cause of ID and occurs in 1.3 in 1,000 live births. Approximately 4,000 children with Down syndrome are born every year (Nehring 2010). The incidence of Down syndrome increases with maternal age at the time of pregnancy. Risk for a woman in the twenties is about 1 in 1,667 births; by age 35, the risk is about 1 in 30 live births. Parental age increases the prevalence too (Nehring 2010, pp. 447–448). Down syndrome is associated with distinctive facial features, congenital heart disease, duodenal stenosis, congenital megacolon, tracheo-esophageal fistula, and ID. Children with Down syndrome tend to be affectionate and engaging. Adults with Down syndrome, compared with age- and IQ-matched adults with learning disabilities, have a lower prevalence of aggression, antisocial behaviors, property destruction, night disturbances, attention seeking, untruthfulness, hyperactivity, and excessive noise. Despite having language impairment, adults with Down syndrome have social communication and relationships that are comparable to those of adults with learning disabilities. Of children with Down syndrome, 7%–10% have symptoms that meet the criteria for autism (Feinstein and Singh 2007).

Prader-Willi Syndrome and Angelman Syndrome

Loss of function of maternal or paternal genes in the imprinted chromosomal region 15q11–q13 causes Prader Willi syndrome and Angelman syndrome. Prader Willi syndrome is a multigenic syndrome involving 10 imprinted genes. In Angelman syndrome, 70% of the patients carry a large maternal deletion of the 15q11–q13 region and display a severe phenotype; however, mutations of a single gene, *UBE3A*, are sufficient to cause major clinical manifestations of the syndrome. *UBE3A* encodes for E6-AP, an enzyme that has ubiquitin ligase and transcriptional coactivator activities (Hsiao et al. 2011, p. 944).

Prader-Willi syndrome is a genetic disorder that usually involves a deletion or uniparental disomy in chromosome 15. It has a prevalence of 1 in 10,000–15,000 births and is characterized by hyperphagia, hypotonia, hypogonadism, ID, short stature, small hands and feet, developmental delays, and distinct facial features. Behavioral traits described in Prader-Willi syndrome include stubbornness, tantrums, aggressive behaviors, disobedience, talkativeness, and antisociality. Compulsive behaviors not related to food have been identified, as have asociality, argumentativeness, and verbal and physical aggression (Feinstein and Singh 2007).

Children with Prader-Willi syndrome frequently display excessive daytime sleepiness, and sleep studies indicate a more than 50% incidence of obstructive sleep apnea. Individuals with Prader-Willi syndrome also display rapid-eye movement abnormalities (severely shortened rapid-eye movement latency). Prader-Willi syndrome has been associated with narcolepsy (Cvejic 2015, p. 822).

Persons with Angelman syndrome, otherwise known as the "happy puppet syndrome" (due to frequent paroxysms of unprovoked laughter), have problems with sleep maintenance and nocturnal seizures. Individuals with Angelman syndrome suffer from balance problems, wide-based gait, puppet-like movements, and a cheery disposition (Cvejic 2015, p. 822). Angelman syndrome has an incidence of less than 1 in 10,000. There is a disproportionate lack of speech that is not commensurable with the ID. Seizures are common (Menkes and Falk 2006, p. 241).

Smith-Magenis Syndrome

Smith-Magenis syndrome is a genetic disorder associated with a deletion of band 17p11.2 in the gene *RAI1*. The typical phenotype includes brachycephaly, midface hypoplasia, prognathism, hoarse voice, speech delay, psychomotor and growth retardation, and behavior problems. The syndrome is estimated to occur in 1 in 25,000 births. Maladaptive behaviors include emotional lability, argumentativeness, destructiveness, attention seeking, and physical aggression (Feinstein and Singh 2007).

Subjects with Smith-Magenis syndrome have a severe disrupted sleep-wake pattern caused by an inverted pattern of melatonin secretion. Facial features are distinctive, with multiple dysmorphisms such as brachycephaly, a flat midface, and a down-turned mouth. In early infancy, children may be very friendly and easygoing and often display excellent sleep. By the first or second year parents begin to complain of frequent awakenings and daytime naps indicating a short sleep cycle. By childhood, children start displaying temper tantrums that may progress to severe self-injurious behaviors (Cvejic 2015, pp. 821–822).

Turner Syndrome

Turner syndrome is a genetic disorder associated with partial or complete absence of one of the two X chromosomes in a phenotypic girl. The phenotype includes short stature, webbed neck, renal dysgenesis, and heart malformations. Females with Turner syndrome have difficulties in social maturity, social cognition, social relationships, and self-esteem (Feinstein and Singh 2007). Other physical characteristics include high arched palate, wide spaced nipples, hypertension, and kidney abnormalities. The Turner syndrome phenotype is variable and may be subtle in girls with mosaicism. Turner syndrome may be diagnosed in infant girls at birth: they are small and may exhibit lymphedema. Females with Turner syndrome have an increased risk of aortic coarctation (11%) and bicuspid aortic valve defects (16%). Emotional disorders are common. Affected women are prone to autoimmune disease. These women have hypogonadism: primary amenorrhea, in 80%, or early ovarian failure, in 20% (Fitzgerald 2015, p. 1178).

Williams Syndrome/Williams-Beuren Syndrome

Williams syndrome, also know as Williams-Beuren syndrome, is a rare genetic disorder caused by a microdeletion on chromosome 7q11.23. The incidence has been estimated to be as high as 1 in 7,500 or as low as 1 in 20,000 live births. Clinical features include atypical craniofacial morphology (pouting lips, wide mouth, spaced teeth, broad brow, full cheeks, short upturned nose, flat nasal bridge, full nasal tip), growth retardation, and cardiovascular abnormalities (supravalvular aortic stenosis and a narrowing of the aorta) (Santos and Meyer-Lindenberg 2011, p. 537). It is also characterized by hypercalcemia, hyperacusis, and abnormalities of muscle and kidneys, and, in addition, mild to moderate ID (Feinstein and Singh 2007). Hypersociability is a hallmark of the Williams syndrome social phenotype. Individuals with Williams syndrome are also socially anxious and by adult age have failed to develop and maintain friendships and suffer from unsatisfying peer relationships (Feinstein and Singh 2007).

Chromosome 22q11.2 Deletion Syndrome/ Velocardiofacial Syndrome

Chromosome 22q11.2 deletion syndrome is the most common microdeletion, affecting one in 2,000–4,000 live births, and involves a haploinsufficiency of about 50 genes causing a multisystem disorder. Individual with this deletion are at increased risk of developing several psychiatric disorders, such as anxiety disorders, ADHD, and autism (Swillen 2016, p. 313). Schizophrenia spectrum disorder is diagnosed in up to 25%–30% of adults with this deletion (Swillen 2016, p. 134). Most cases are de novo mutations. Symptoms include cleft palate, velopharyngeal insufficiency, cardiac defects, distinctive facial features, reduced intelligence, and a dramatic delay in early language development. Individuals with velocardiofacial syndrome have receptive and higher-order language deficits, as well as abstract reasoning and visual-spatial deficits. Younger children display mood lability, social withdrawal, awkwardness, shyness, ADHD, anxiety, and disinhibited behavior. Approximately 30% of individuals with velocardiofacial syndrome develop psychosis (schizophrenia, schizoaffective disorder) by adolescence or young adulthood, accounting for about 2% of the schizophrenia cases (Feinstein and Singh 2007).

Recent longitudinal studies on the cognitive development of children and adolescents with 22q11.2 deletion syndrome reveal substantial diversity in cognitive trajectories through childhood and adolescence: a relative stable IQ trajectory over time (trajectory of delay), a "growing into deficit" trajectory, and a trajectory of absolute decline in IQ (Verbal IQ in particular). The latter trajectory precedes psychosis (Swillen 2016, p. 136).

Rett Syndrome

First reported by Andreas Rett, an Australian pediatrician, in the 1960s, Rett syndrome has been shown to be caused by mutations in the gene encoding methyl-CpG-binding protein 2. Rett syndrome is a rare condition affecting 1.09 per 10,000 females by age 12 years. There has been an increased interest in this disorder because clinical features found in Rett syndrome are also seen in a number of other neurodevelopmental disorders as well as in adult neurological and psychiatric conditions, including autism, Angelman syndrome–like features, intellectual disabilities in boys with associated neuropsychiatric features, and neuropsychiatric features such as anxiety and depression in women (Neul 2011, p. 776).

Rett syndrome is a severe X-linked dominant neurodevelopmental disorder affecting postnatal brain growth. It is the second most common cause of genetic intellectual disability in girls and the first pervasive developmental disorder with a known genetic basis. Usually, mothers of girls with Rett syndrome have an uneventful pregnancy and delivery, and the daughters develop normally until about age 6 months. A deceleration of head growth from around age 4 months onward usually results in microcephaly. This period is followed by a developmental regression that includes social withdrawal, loss of purposeful hand usage coinciding with the appearance of stereotypic hand movements, and loss of acquired speech and language abilities. Gait apraxia and ataxia are common (Ben Zeev Ghidoni 2007). The main diagnostic criteria for Rett syndrome are as follows:

1. Partial or complete loss of acquired purposeful hand skills
2. Partial or complete loss of acquired spoken language
3. Gait abnormalities: impaired (dyspraxic) or absence of ability
4. Stereotyped hand movements such as hand wringing/squeezing, clapping/tapping, mouthing, washing/rubbing automatisms

Supportive criteria include the following:

1. Breathing disturbances when awake
2. Bruxism when awake
3. Impaired sleep pattern
4. Abnormal muscle tone
5. Peripheral vasomotor disturbances
6. Scoliosis/kyphosis
7. Growth retardation
8. Small cold hands and feet
9. Inappropriate laughing/screaming spells
10. Diminished response to pain
11. Intense eye communication–eye pointing

In spite of the identifiable genetics, the diagnosis is made on the basis of clinical findings (Neul 2011, p. 777). Acquired microcephaly is a preamble and should raise suspicion for the diagnosis. Epilepsy is reported in 90% of girls with Rett syndrome.

Linkage to the Xq28 region has been demonstrated, and *MECP2* has been identified as the gene responsible for Rett syndrome. Mutation of this gene has been observed in up to 95% of classical cases (Ben Zeev Ghidoni 2007).

Children Living in Poverty

Children who live in families at the poverty level experience a multiplicity of adversities that become major developmental interferences, such as inadequate nutrition, poor pediatric care, low-quality schooling, family stress, and abusive discipline. The core interference for children with poverty is deprivation in a variety of forms. Poverty is associated with atypical development of a number of brain areas (see Chapter 12, "Neuropsychiatric Interview and Examination").

For economically disadvantaged youths, the psychiatrist may become their primary physician. As a result, he or she needs to be attentive to these children's basic health needs and help their families navigate the complex health care system. Recognition of and assistance in overcoming barriers to access of care are essential in the implementation of an effective treatment plan for these children. Basic nutrition and hygienic habits should not be assumed. The psychiatrist cannot take for granted that these children receive basic pediatric or odontological care. The psychiatrist needs to make efforts to help these families procure such services. In the same light, the psychiatrist needs to know that poor families depend on public and arranged transportation services and often need to provide a flexible schedule of appointments to meet their needs.

Another hurdle that poor families must surmount involves special education services for their children. Educational systems often delay the provision of specialized services or deprive poor children of needed services they require. The psychiatrist must begin with a psychoeducational role regarding the options and rights to special education services and may need to take an active advocacy role to secure the special services that these children need.

Children From Minority Populations

A major developmental interference for children of minority populations is centered on overcoming scapegoatism and stereotyping. These children struggle against powerful social barriers and are under an ongoing need to prove themselves and to fight discrimination. Middle Eastern children have the added burden of being perceived as being associated with terrorism.

Minority status is often associated with socioeconomic disadvantages, such as poverty, mediocre schools, and lack of access to medical care. Therefore, the child psychiatrist needs to be attentive to this population's satisfaction of basic needs, such as food and shelter, medical care, and quality of education. The psychiatrist also needs to be diligent about detecting neglect or physical or sexual abuse while maintaining respect for the mores or culture of each particular family. The child and adolescent psychiatrist needs to be vigilant about cultural developmental practices that are not condoned or are even proscribed in the United States.

The minority child is frequently ostracized by peers and has particular difficulties in building friendship bridges with members of the dominating majority group. The psychiatrist needs to systematically explore with a child any issues of identity, problems with self-esteem, issues with self-doubt, and concerns with belonging and lovability.

Adaptation and acculturation to a new society can be especially complicated for families from non-Western cultures. The child psychiatrist needs to be sensitive to the process of acculturation and, in dealing with children and their families, must attempt to implement culturally sensitive interventions. Implementing specific culturally sensitive treatments is difficult in working with patients from different cultures. Some studies have found that tailoring interventions for specific populations can increase their effectiveness, but other studies have found that cultural adaptations of interventions dilute the effectiveness of the original treatments, even though retention is improved (Ngo et al. 2008). Important cultural issues that need to be integrated into any treatment include help-seeking preferences, expressions of distress, communication styles, migration experiences, family values, and sociopolitical history. These concepts are central to understanding the experience of specific populations (Ngo et al. 2008).

Children in Out-of-Home Placement

A fundamental need for every child is to grow in a family environment surrounded by loving parental figures. This is the sine qua non prerequisite of the indispensable process of attachment, without which working models of adaptive behavior are unlikely. In the soul of most children living away from home is the unending longing to return to the family of origin. This craving for the family is expressed in daydreaming, in fantasy life, and above all in the relationship with the parental substitutes. Many of these children develop tenacious attachments to the original parents, no matter how negative their life experiences were with them. Children with tenacious attachments to the original parents keep a strong loyalty to them and refuse emotional investments in parental substitutes.

The number of children living in foster care has declined substantially over the last decade, from 800,000 in 2005 to about 650,000 in 2014. This trend has been true across most racial and ethnic groups, but the rate has increased among mixed-race children (Scheid 2016, p. 16).

A distinction could be made between children living outside of their home environments temporarily and those permanently living away from the family of origin. For those living away from home for only a limited time, the separation from the family may cause only a temporary emotional pain (but may leave enduring negative consequences). These children hope and expect that they will return home. The situation is different for children separated from their families permanently—that is, those whose parents' rights have been terminated. Some of these children dream of turning age 18 to exercise the freedom to reunite with their progenitors. The examiner needs to keep the strength of this bond in mind. Only by understanding the nature of such an attachment can the examiner decipher the problem the child displays with substitute parents and living in alternative home environments. A related dynamic is commonly present in many failed late adoptions.

The factors that motivated the removal from the family of origin influence the children's psychological organization and rationalization of the events. Many children defend their parents' abusive or neglectful behaviors by minimizing or rationalizing the behaviors or by denying parental misconduct all together. Children removed for sexual abuse are left with a number of psychological scars: the guilt that they caused the family breakup, and the sense that they were violated and that their abuse is not aggrieved. The impact of the abuse is worse when girls disclose the abuse and their mothers do not support them or do not believe their claims (these events, unfortunately, are not uncommon). These children feel betrayed, violated, and utterly alone, firmly believing they cannot trust anybody. For these children, exploration of abusive issues is strongly opposed by the child.

Many boys who were physically abused by their fathers or surrogate figures become violent and harbor persistent feelings of vengeance. These sentiments are intensified if the children, in addition to their own victimization, have witnessed parental abuse against their mothers or siblings.

Reactivation of memories of abuse brings strong feelings of anger, for which these children have limited control. In working with both physically and sexually abused children, examiners need to respect children's reservations or fears of verbalizing these events, and they need to be cognizant of the risks of opening the gates of bad memories. Not being sensitive to these fears may destabilize a child, unleashing aggression and other acting-out behaviors. Furthermore, the reactivation of traumatic memories may stimulate the emergence of a severe regression, which complicates and extends emotional suffering and maladaptation. The examiner should make efforts to strengthen the child's adaptive behaviors and to deal with the traumatic past as it surfaces rather than dealing with the abusive past head on.

Most children in the custody of Child Protective Services agencies harbor deep resentments against the system or systems that promoted the family breakup. Most of these children blame Child Protective Services and the judges for the separation from their families. Despite clear prohibitions against contacts with the abusive parental figures, many children find ways of secretively talking or having in-person contact with their parents.

The psychiatrist needs to be attuned to the child's longing to be reunited with the original family and wish to recover his or her lost family. The psychiatrist should also be cognizant of the child's tenacious attachment to the original parents and realize that the child's ongoing difficulties with substitute parents may indicate a sign of loyalty to the biological parents.

Migrant Children

Migrant children spend a few weeks or months in one place and the next somewhere else. These children do not have a stable rearing or learning environment; those children who attend school must repeatedly readapt to various school environments. Also, these children have difficulty establishing long-lasting bonds to peers and to the local schools because they are on the move. Migrant families form strong, close nexuses among themselves, and for many of them, the opportunities for socialization become endogamic. Many migrant children have academic retardation and difficulties with English proficiency; others have a number of cognitive deficits or learning disorders that elude identification and remediation. Migrant families straddle the poverty line and lack basic medical services. As in working with children from poverty-level families, the examiner needs to pay closer attention to the migrant children's most basic needs and to medical and odontological care. If the child is from a family of undocumented immigrants, in addition to the disadvantages cited above is the ongoing fear of detection and extradition that frequently results in family separation (see section "Undocumented Immigrants").

Displaced and Refugee Children

Families sometimes are forced to leave familiar environments because of political reasons or natural disasters. During the middle of the second decade of the 21st century, the mobilization and displacement of millions of refugees from the Middle East and North Africa has required humanitarian relocation for thousands and thousands of people, children and adolescents included. Displaced families are removed from their supportive networks, and many family members become separated during the mobilization; worse yet, many children are separated from their parental figures. Displaced families are under extraordinary stress and in need of global supports. Displaced families need shelter and food, recreation, and other basic needs; these families are frequently housed in crowded dwellings that lack opportunities for privacy and intimacy. Many of the temporary camps lack amenities for distressed children. Refugee accommodations are not the most auspicious environments for the families to comfort and settle their anxious children.

Under such immense stress, many families break down. Then, secondary to the family malfunction, many children start to display maladaptive behaviors, including unlawful behaviors toward members of the host country, leading to a referral for a psychiatric evaluation and intervention. For children without prior maladaptive behaviors, adjustment reactions and acute stress disorders are common explanations.

For children with prior psychiatric history, who are already vulnerable to stress, the additional stress of displacement aggravates previous psychopathology or reactivates previous psychiatric disorders. These displaced children often show maladaptive behaviors in the school environment and in relating to unfamiliar peers and teachers. Areas the examiner needs to explore include the intactness of the family, the family's ability to cope with the precipitating stress, and the family's need to communicate with close friends and relatives. The examiner may ask the child questions such as the following: "Are you living with your parents now?" "Are your siblings with you?" "Where is the rest of the family?" "Tell me what happened that made your family move from where you were living before." "How did your family get out?" If family members are separated, the examiner should ask additional questions: "Where is your mom?" "Where is your dad?" "Where are your siblings?" "When was the last time you heard from them?" "How can you get in touch with them?" "How is everybody in the family doing now?" Other important questions relate to the child's general health, such as the ability and quality of a child's sleep.

Issues of Posttraumatic Stress Disorder Related to Terrorism

Armed conflicts provide an ecological shock or destabilization that creates a culture of violence that damages child protection and support at multiple interacting levels (Boothby 2008). Available evidence suggests a clear relationship between exposure to violence and the onset of traumatic symptoms; however, a number of children do not develop symptoms, likely because of protective factors that may buffer potentially harmful experiences. Findings are consistent with related research in traumatic stress. Variables such as the nature of the violent event, the availability of family and social supports, the meaning of the violent experiences, and the range of coping strategies and available resources all seem to play a role in the long-term impact of the violence on children's development. An additional factor is the extent to which acts of violence result in the loss or incapacitation of the children's parents or caretakers (Boothby 2008).

The importance of polyvictimization—that is, exposure to multiple adversities and multiple traumatic events—is something that the evaluator needs to keep in mind. Any type of child victimization increases future vulnerability for re-victimization. Polyvictimization is probably the norm for children who have been exposed to chronic situations such as war, child abuse, and domestic violence (Cohen 2008).

In working with refugee children and adolescents, the psychiatrist needs to consider the possibility of torture. The examiner needs to explore the exposure of the child and his or her family to war trauma or political persecution, and to keep in mind that the child may have had prior exposure to other kinds of trauma, including neglect and physical and/or sexual abuse. The psychiatrist should identify the diverse nature of the traumas and take measures to address each traumatic event comprehensively and in coordination with other complementary approaches.

The psychiatrist should keep in mind that social supports (family, schools, peer relationships, and religious supports) buffer the impact of terrorism (Henrich and Shahar 2008). These beneficial forces need to be explored, promoted, or strengthened.

Undocumented Immigrants

U.S. Immigration and Customs Enforcement had established a number of immigration detention facilities for undocumented immigrants who were caught attempting to enter the country illegally. Within the United States, more than 5,000 children annually were held in immigration detention facilities. The U.S. government had an ongoing commitment to keep detained family groups together; in 2006, a 512-bed facility was opened in Texas for family detention (Newman and Steel 2008). Some of these detention centers have been closed since then for allegations of mistreatment or/and abuse.

The number of unaccompanied minors crossing into the United States has grown considerably over recent years. According to the U.S. Customs and Border Protection, the number of apprehended unaccompanied minors in the southwest border region of United States increased from 10,105 in the first four months of fiscal year 2015 to 20,455 in the same time frame in fiscal year 2016 (U.S. Customs and Border Protection 2016). Some adolescents come without their families to the United States from Mexico and many Central American countries; they do not speak English, have low academic education, and come from low socioeconomic backgrounds; some of these youths come from neglectful and abusive/violent environments. Their backgrounds and the efforts they make to reach the United States are extraordinary. Leaving their homes and familiar lands, these children flee from appalling family circumstances and most go through incredible ordeals to reach the U.S. border. Many fall prey to "coyotes" and sexual predators; some female adolescents are sexually exploited and forced into prostitution. Not surprisingly, child asylum seekers arrive with a range of experiences that put them at high risk for psychological distress and for the development of a mental disorder (Newman and Steel 2008).

After being placed in the detention centers, these adolescents face reality, and their dreams of settling in the United States promptly vanish. Being in a foreign land, away from their supportive networks, in close quarters, unable to speak the language of their custodians, unable to make their needs understood, and facing a return to their country of origin, may—and in many cases does—cause a mental breakdown. Some of these adolescents become suicidal or psychotic. Under these conditions, the detention facilities request a psychiatric evaluation for these adolescents.

Non-Spanish-speaking psychiatrists require the assistance of a competent and fluent translator. Even Spanish-speaking psychiatrists may be challenged because these adolescents use slang and colloquialisms from their original cultures and usually have a low level of education.

Key Points

- Various medical conditions (e.g., neurodevelopmental disorders, cerebral palsy, neurogenetic disorders) and socioeconomic situations (e.g., poverty, migrant work) can pose a challenge to the diagnostician. These conditions create special needs that require timely identification in treatment
- The examiner needs to have broad familiarity with and sensitivity to these various circumstances to achieve an optimal diagnostic engagement with children and families from different backgrounds and medical-neurological-genetic circumstances.
- The evaluation of children with special needs should incorporate multiple disciplines to encompass the various areas of function and to facilitate the development of a comprehensive treatment plan.

Notes

1. Dissociation is considered a parasympathetically mediated response that occurs after exhaustion of sympathetically mediated defenses or coping mechanisms. Change in vagal tone, a well-documented parasympathetic marker, is associated with PTSD. Situations of extreme threat may lead to the parasympathetically mediated shutting down of emotions phenotypically observed as dissociative symptoms and prospectively related to PTSD (Saxe et al. 2005).

CHAPTER 7

Psychiatric Evaluation of Preschoolers and Very Young Children

Egger (2009) recommends that the psychiatric assessment of very young children, preschoolers, should be done in "multiples":

1. **Multiple sessions.** It is not possible to perform an adequate psychiatric assessment of a young child in a single session. In some centers, parents meet with the evaluating psychiatrist without the child to provide a detailed account of their emotional and behavioral concerns and for the psychiatrist to obtain developmental, marital, and family histories. A major goal during this meeting is to ascertain the functional status of each parent and to estimate the quality of the rearing environment parents are able to provide. Some examiners construct an organigram or a genogram to highlight the presence of family members, in the current or previous generation, who have been affected by emotional, substance abuse or other psychiatric problems, or members who have committed suicide.
2. **Multiple informants.** Multiple informants must contribute to the history and evaluation. Informants include biological parents, stepparents, and nonbiological parent figures, foster parents, day care providers, teachers, grandparents, nannies, baby sitters, and the child. (As Egger [2009] categorically states, "It is not possible to conduct a psychiatric assessment

of a young child based solely on adult report…every child is a critical informant" [p. 566].)

3. **Multiple experts.** A multidisciplinary approach is undertaken to ascertain the child's level of functioning in multiple domains. Psychiatrists, developmental pediatricians, developmental and clinical psychologists, school psychologists, pediatricians, neurologists, speech and language therapists, occupational therapists, social workers, caseworkers, early interventionists, and child welfare providers, among others, will contribute to the understanding of the child's strengths and difficulties. On the one hand, psychiatrists, psychologists, psychotherapists, substance abuse counselors, and marital and family counselors who work with the parents may assist in understanding parents' or caregivers' parental functioning, while siblings or even close friends may help contribute in the understanding of the family history or ongoing parenting difficulties. It is the responsibility of the child psychiatrist to assemble and to interpret all the different diagnostic assessments into a comprehensive and integrative diagnosis and treatment plan.

4. **Multiple modes of assessment.** Because of the challenges of gathering information about the emotions and experiences of very young children, different modes of assessment, including structured screening and diagnostic measures, psychological and developmental testing, observational assessments, direct interviewing, laboratory tests, and structured and unstructured play, are necessary to obtain multiple perspectives needed to understand the child and his or her symptoms within the context of the child's relationships and environment (Egger 2009, pp. 565–569).

5. **Multicultural perspective.** It is important to recognize that the evaluation of parenting and upbringing, as well as the evaluation of childhood behaviors, occurs within the context of specific cultural experiences, norms, and expectations of patients and clinicians. Clinicians should make a deliberate attempt to understand how culture shapes parents' understanding of their child's emotions, behavior, and needs, and how that affects the child's experience within the home environment and within the wider community. Clinicians must also be aware of how their own cultural values, beliefs, and assumptions affect their understanding and interpretation of the child's needs and experience.

6. **Multiaxial assessment.** DSM-5 (American Psychiatric Association 2013) dispensed with the multiaxial diagnostic system, but something has been lost with its omission. The DC: 0–3 and the DC: 0–3R had in Axis II "Relationship disorder classification" and "Relationship classification," respectively, that enabled the examiner to record information about the nature and quality of the child's relationship with his or her primary care givers (Egger 2009, p. 570). This lack of a multiaxial approach should be filled

by a narrative description of the quality of the child's relating to his or her care givers during the comprehensive formulation (see Chapter 13, "Comprehensive Psychiatric Formulation").

For the different areas or domains that need to be covered in the comprehensive assessment of very young children, see Table 7–1.

In general, the younger the child needing a psychiatric evaluation in the preschool years, the larger the odds that the child has a neurodevelopmental problem, that the psychiatric disorder has strong genetic loading, or that the child is being subjected to major adversities, formerly and aptly called "psychotoxic states" (i.e., neglect or abuse). Furthermore, the younger the child, the higher the likelihood that the parent(s) will suffer from a psychiatric disorder or a substance abuse condition.

Attachment and Bonding

What is the nature or quality of attachment is a question that frequently arises in the process of evaluating preschoolers. Attachment and bonding and their associated disturbances are described next.

Zeanah and Smyke (2015) define *attachment* as a tendency for human infants to seek comfort, support, nurturance, and protection preferentially from one or more caregivers. This is sometimes referred to as "focused," "preferred," "selective," or "discriminated" attachment between child and parent (Zeanah and Smyke 2015, p. 795). According to Marvin and Britner (2008), attachment and bonding are the mechanism by which "children and their caregiver organize protective proximity and contact, and how they [children] continue to use their caregivers as a secure base for exploration" (p. 270) (see Note 1 at the end of this chapter).

Attachment is classically assessed in infants and very young children by child responses elicited through the Strange Situation, which was developed by Mary Ainsworth and her colleagues. Ainsworth started her research on attachment in the early 1960s and consolidated her findings in the late 1970s. The Strange Situation utilizes a series of interactions that involve separations, reunions, and the introduction of a stranger (see Note 2 at the end of this chapter). The observations gathered during these events are used to assess not only the child's response to the scenarios but also the parental response to the child's emotional reactions (Solomon and George 2008) (see Note 3 at the end of this chapter).

Solomon and George (2008) describe the following attachment styles: the *secure* attachment style is characterized by the child's ability to explore, return to the parent for comfort or reassurance when upset, and explore again. The *avoidant* style involves minimal behaviors indicating a sense of a secure

Table 7–1.   Domains that need to be assessed in the comprehensive psychiatric evaluation of very young children

Current history of emotional and behavioral symptoms (frequency, duration, content, onset, relationship context, and triggers of symptoms)

Past history of emotional and behavioral symptoms (frequency, duration, content, onset, relationship context, and triggers of symptoms)

Developmental history (history of pregnancy, maternal prenatal care [use alcohol, drugs or tobacco during pregnancy], neonatal history, development of the milestones and history of developmental delays)

History and patterns of sleep, feeding (including history of breast feeding), eating, and toileting

Family composition; construction of a family genogram

Experiences in day care and preschool settings

Quality of the child's play (content, variety, enjoyment)

Quality of the parent-child relationship (nature of the affect when they interact, child's reaction to separations and reunions, level of conflict, coercion, or intrusiveness); history of participation of other caretakers in the rearing of the child and the reasoning for it

Current cognitive and developmental assessment of expressive and receptive language abilities, gross and fine motor capacities, and adaptive functioning

Medical history, including history of streptococcal infections, ear infections, hospitalizations, traumatic medical experiences; exposure to toxics (e.g., lead), central nervous system disorders, such as epilepsy, head injuries, and others

Recent physical examinations, including height, weight, BMI, and blood pressure; history of developmental growth

Medication history, including psychotropic medication exposure, other medications: antibiotics, anti-asthmatic medications (names, doses, length of treatment, side effects)

Laboratory tests including genetic testing when indicated

History of stressful life events, including major traumas (e.g., death in the families, abuse, witnessing violence), minor stressors (birth of a sibling, change of day care or schools), ongoing stressors (parental hardship, parental deployment, or parental illness); history of family relocations

Emotional resources of the family; details of how each family member is doing

Family structure and functioning (discipline practices [e.g., corporal punishment])

Relationship with siblings, peers, and other-age children

Table 7–1. Domains that need to be assessed in the comprehensive psychiatric evaluation of very young children *(continued)*

Child's family culture as well as the appreciation of the impact of cultural differences and conflicts between the child's culture and the culture of the wider community

Day care and school experiences, including type of setting, teacher/child ratios, length of time in the setting, relationship with teachers and child care providers, and relationship with peers

Three-generation family psychiatric and substance abuse history, ideally collected as a genogram with a record of symptoms, diagnoses, and events; age at onset; treatments, including inpatient and outpatient interventions, psychotherapy, and medications (name, doses, adverse side effects), including details about anxiety and depression

Current history of parental psychiatric symptoms, including symptoms of depression, anxiety, psychosis, or substance abuse; history of compliance and treatment

Current and past history of domestic violence between adults and between adults and child in child's home

History of Child Protective Services (CPS) intervention; reasons for CPS involvement

Assessment of the child's strengths and competencies

Impact of the child's symptoms on the family's functioning (e.g., unable to leave child with a sitter due to child's anxious distress or the child's violent behavior)

Assessment of how the child's problems interfere with parents' work

Degree of parental stress, both overall and in respect to the child's evaluation

Gathering information regarding the living conditions, parental employment, persons living in the household, socioeconomic status, quality of the neighborhood, and religious and cultural practices

Source. Modified from Egger 2009, p. 571.

base: little distress with separation and avoidance of parental comfort. The *ambivalent* attachment style is characterized by distress displayed in novel situations and separations, expressions of extreme responses to reunions, and lack of comfort from the parent. The *disorganized* or *disoriented* style reflects confusion and disorientation in the strategies utilized to cope with novel situations and separations and reunions (Solomon and George 2008, p. 387).

The attachment styles or their classification is not diagnostic. The secure attachment is considered a protective factor; the others are considered risk factors. Disorganized attachment has a prevalence of 14% in low-risk samples, but it is as high 70%–80% in maltreated or institutionalized samples. Disorganized attachment is associated with various disturbances of caregiving behavior, including frightening/frightened, antagonism, withdrawal, role confusion, and contradictory cues (Zeanah and Smyke 2015, p. 796). These attachment patterns of behavior seem to continue in a variety of maladaptive behaviors, such as overfamiliarity with strangers, lack of boundaries, intrusiveness, and inappropriate nonverbal social behavior (e.g., staring at people, inappropriate body contact). These behaviors are not perceived as sociable or friendly by those in the receiving end. Disorganized attachment tends to persist up to middle adolescence (Zeanah and Smyke 2015, p. 798). For the differential diagnosis of attachment and autism and other psychiatric disorders, see Table 7–2.

When children have formed a secure attachment, they are able to face novel situations with confidence and have acquired the knowledge (internalization) that the parent or caregiver will be reliably present to provide comfort and reassurance; the child develops confidence that upon separation, the parent will be there—will still be there (O'Connor et al. 1999; Oliveira et al. 2012; Stacks et al. 2014) (see Note 4 at the end of this chapter).

O'Connor, Bredenkamp, and Rutter, in their 1999 study of children in Romanian institutions who were subsequently adopted by families in the United Kingdom, demonstrated that neither cognitive impairments nor nutritional deprivation was correlated with the development of attachment disorders; instead, it is the lack of a consistent caregiver in the earliest stages of life with whom a child might form selective attachments (O'Connor et al. 1999). This lack may be the critical factor in the development of attachment disorders (see Joel's case in Chapter 3, "Special Interviewing Techniques," Case Example 15). Trauma may include physical or sexual abuse (see Case Example 1 later in this chapter), loss of a loved one (especially parent or caregiver), natural disasters, or displacement (such as by fire, war, or migration). Neglect or parental absences may have occurred because of physical or medical illnesses, imprisonment, family conflicts (such as custody disputes), or drug abuse or addiction.

Maternal Pathology and Attachment Subtypes

During the exploration of attachment patterns, the examiner should explore experiences that derail the development of healthy attachment between parent and child. Very early separations and lack of maternal emotional availability (due to depression, obsessive-compulsive disorder, psychosis, substance abuse, and other conditions, that interfere in the formation and organization of at-

Table 7–2. Differential diagnosis of attachment disorders and other psychiatric conditions

	Reactive attachment disorder	Disinhibited social engagement disorder	Autism spectrum disorder	Intellectual disability	Williams syndrome	Attention-deficit/ hyperactivity disorder	Callous unemotional traits	Posttraumatic stress disorder
Institutional rearing	+++	+++	+/?	+/?	?	+/++	+	+
Disturbance emotional regulation	+++	+++	+++	+	+	+	+	+
Disturbance of reciprocity	+++	+++	+++	+	+	+/-	+	+
Adverse caring	+++	+++	-/+	-/+	-/+	-/+	-/+	-/+
Indiscrimination social behavior	+++	+++	+/-	+/-	+++	+/-	+/-	+/-
Pretend play	+	+	-/+	+/-	+	+/-	+?/-	+/-
Repetitive behaviors	+/-	+/-	+++	+/-	+/-	-	-	-
Language disturbance	Delays	Delays	Delays Absence	Delays	Delays	+/-	-	-
Restlessness	+	+	+/-	+/-	+/-	+++	+/-	+/-
Inattention—inability to concentrate	+/-	+/++	+/-	+/-	+/++	+++	+/-	+/-

Source. Zeanah and Smyke 2015, p. 800.

tachment) are critical factors to explore (see Case Example 15 in Chapter 3, "Special Interviewing Techniques"). The examiner needs to determine the maternal figure's emotional disposition and her capacity and commitment to bond with her child and to be attuned to the baby's (infant, toddler, or preschooler) needs.

Examination of parental mental health and substance abuse offers insight into genetic loading for psychopathology and identification of risk factors for insecure attachment. Maternal perinatal depression appears to be associated with negative birth outcomes (obstetric complications, preterm delivery, decreased fetal growth and birth weight), impaired child function (overall health, cognitive, social and academic), and hostile or withdrawn parenting (Lefkovics et al. 2014). Increased levels of psychological distress in mothers are consistently associated with avoidant attachment styles (Mills-Koonce et al. 2011). Rosenblum et al. (1997) found that the manifestations of maternal depression influenced the development of the insecure attachment subtype. The children of mothers with more irritable and anxious depressive features tended to have an ambivalent attachment, whereas children with mothers experiencing anhedonia and psychomotor retardation presented with a more avoidant attachment. Children of substance-abusing mothers similarly demonstrate problematic pattern of interactions that manifest as insecure attachment (Flykt et al. 2012). (See Note 5 at the end of this chapter.)

It is very concerning that a study in the United Kingdom revealed that up to 20% of mothers indicated that talking to and cuddling their child were not important in the psychological development of a child. The author suggests that about a third of the social gradient (for people with longer life expectancy, their health is better) in linguistic development and about half of the social gradient in emotional development could be attributed to parental attitudes (Marmot 2016, p. 24).

Assessment of the Mother or Caretaker

An exploration of the mother figure's current and past environmental stressors is a vital component in the assessment of the infant or very young child. Maternal age at time of pregnancy, overall perceptions of the pregnancy (planned versus unplanned), and sense of preparedness for parenthood play significant roles in the development of functional versus dysfunctional parenting styles (Walsh et al. 2014). An inquiry regarding toxic exposures should include illnesses and surgeries as well as alcohol and drug use during pregnancy (prescription and illegal). The examiner should explore whether the mother experienced significant prenatal and postnatal stressors such as abuse, marital or financial problems, and other adversities or health issues. If the mother has a stable partner or spouse, is that relationship loving? Is it supportive? Does the partner share the obligations of child care? Is the extended family assisting the mother? Is the extended family involved? Are they supportive? Were there periods of insecurity, regarding health, financial resources, or housing or other burdens during the child's infancy? Homelessness not only compromises the physical well-being of the child but also affects the mother's ability to respond in a sensitive manner to a distressed infant (David et al. 2012). Was or is there adequate social support or a network to support the parent and child (i.e., family, friends, church or ethnic community)?

The psychological stability of the mother is of particular relevance in relation to the preschooler's welfare. Perry (2016) describes how the quality of the mother's defensive operations at birth has a bearing on the infant's mental health in toddlerhood. Specifically, mature or highly adaptive maternal defenses were subsequently associated with greater toddler attachment security and social/emotional competence and lower behavior problems.

Family organization is also a key factor in the assessment of a young child. In several studies, a paternal involvement may compensate for deficits in maternal parenting and, in fact, may provide opportunities to form secure attachment paradigms (Braungart-Rieker et al. 2014; Bureau et al. 2014; Galdiolo and Roskam 2016). Questions regarding the presence of a single-parent versus two-parent structure in the household should also include presence of other caregivers (grandparents, aunts or uncles, adult siblings of the parent or child, friends and nannies). An understanding of the level of involvement of the noncustodial parent should also incorporate inquiries regarding the relationship between parents and the degree to which there may be differing parenting philosophies. The examiner should also identify the presence of other children in the household, their biological relationship to one another, and their psychological relationships (e.g., contentious versus harmonious). The examiner needs to hear how the other children and other members of the family are doing. How big is the burden of caring for the mother? Are the offspring very near to each other in age? How many children demand the mother's attention?

Nowadays, almost 40% of new mothers are unmarried; one in five white children, one in four Hispanic children, and one in two black children live without a father at home (Porter 2016). Children living in single-parent households do worse than those living in two parent families; they tend to engage in risky behaviors and drop out of high school and are more likely to end in the criminal system. Selection plays a role: single mothers and their fathers are less educated; they tend to have lesser paying jobs and have more mental health issues. Single households tend to be poorer (Porter 2016). In 1970 10% of children lived in a single parent home; in 2015, it was 27%. On the other hand, in 1970, 86% of children lived in a two-parent home, in 2015, 69%. Six out of 10 births among mothers under the age of 30 are the result of unplanned pregnancies. The United States has one the highest percentages of children living without a father among advanced countries as well as one of the highest shares of children living in poverty (about 21%); among rich and industrialized nations, only three countries have as high a percentage as or higher percentages than the United States: Spain (21%), Mexico (22%), and Turkey (26%). Among industrialized nations, the United States has the highest rate of children living with a single parent (about 27%) (Porter 2016).

Observations of the Child

The examiner's observation of the child should begin in the waiting area. The behaviors of the child and the parent during this time should be noted. The examiner should note the location and relationship of parent to child and as well of child to parent. Is the child sitting quietly with the parent or running around without parental redirection? Does she interact with other children or adults? Is she attentive to parental directions? How does the parent respond to disruptive behaviors? When the examiner calls the child and parent to the examination area, does the child race ahead of the parent or cling to the parent? How does she respond to the examiner's greeting and introduction? These observations often provide the basis for an understanding of attachment and bonding between parent and child as well as indicators of social-pragmatic deficits that may assist in the elucidation of the presenting problem or problems.

When conducting the interview of a preschool-age child, the examiner should take special care when interviewing the child alone. Young children frequently resist or become distressed when informed that they are seeing a "doctor" because of the association of doctor's visits with "shots," vaccinations, or invasive testing. If a child resists the parent leaving the interview room, it is advisable to support the child's level of comfort. The parent's presence during the interview may provide helpful information regarding difficult to understand speech, parent/child relatedness, and parenting style.

A child's response to the examiner during the evaluation may also provide useful information regarding development and potential deficits. The presence or absence of understandable speech as well as age appropriate vocabulary and syntax should be noted and provides a basis for identifying problems in speech production. The examiner should inquire about the presence of birth defects (such as cleft palate) and conduct a visual survey of the oropharynx for any obvious physical barriers to the development of understandable speech (such as ankyloglossia, enlarged tonsils or poor dentition). The child's ability to answer questions appropriately provides insight into receptive language as well as expressive language. When a child does not appear to answer questions appropriately but does follow directions accurately, this suggests that receptive language may be intact, but expressive language deficits may exist. Difficulties in both answering questions and in following directions may indicate problems with receptive or receptive and expressive language. When speech and language are evidently poor, the examiner may also utilize pictures (especially faces expressing different emotions) to assist the child in communicating feelings or difficulties. No conclusions about speech development should be made without a prior audiological evaluation.

During the evaluation of a preschool-age child, the examiner may also incorporate the use of toys and art materials into the interview. Observations of playfulness and attempts to engage the examiner, the parent, or other adults present in the interview provide information regarding level of social reciprocity as well as temperament. For instance, children who display poor eye contact, lack of imaginary play, or unusual behaviors (such as preoccupation with lining up objects or with parts of objects) may have an underlying autism spectrum disorder. Responses to redirection, taking turns, and limit setting by the examiner—and by the parent—should also be noted.

Common Psychopathology in Preschool-Age Children

The estimated prevalence rates of psychiatric problems in preschool-age children reported by McDonnell and Glod (2003; quoted in Zuckerman et al. 2009, p. 3) are as follows: oppositional defiant disorder, 0.7%–26.5%; anxiety disorder, 0.3%–11.5%; attention-deficit/hyperactivity disorder (ADHD), 0.5%–6.5%; conduct disorder, (0.8%–4.6%); major depressive disorder, 0.9%–1.1%; and posttraumatic stress disorder, 0.1%–0.4%.

The following vignette is an extreme example of attachment disorder and severe psychopathology due to neglect and physical or sexual abuse.

Case Example 1

Elliott, a 4-year-old Hispanic male, was admitted to a preschool inpatient unit for command auditory hallucinations, visual hallucinations, and severe aggression toward his 6-year-old brother and school peers. His mother and stepfather reported that prior to the hospitalization Elliott had been sleeping only 2–3 hours a night. He reported seeing monsters all around his bedroom and expressed that a large bug was occupying his bed and had instructed him to get a knife to kill his brother.

Information from the parents revealed that Elliott was born at 34 weeks because of his mother's preeclampsia. He spent 1 month in the neonatal intensive care unit. Shortly after his birth, his mother developed a postpartum depression. Elliott's mother, as a child and also as an adult, had been diagnosed and treated for ADHD, depression, and hallucinations. During her pregnancy she needed to continue her psychotropic medications for depression and hallucinations. Elliott's mother reported that during the child's infancy, she was able to provide for his daily needs but that she did not bond with him; it was difficult for her to hold and cuddle him. In his first year of life, Elliott displayed hearing difficulties and feeding difficulties and had problems digesting solid foods. He later required a foot brace and glasses to address his strabismus.

Elliott's biological father was physically abusive, and when Elliott was 18 months old his father was arrested for domestic violence. At the age of 2, Elliott's 4-month-old brother died of sudden infant death syndrome. Elliott reportedly stopped talking at that time for several months and displayed other signs of depression: emotional withdrawal, lack of play, and decreased eating—all signs of a very severe developmental regression. During this time, he also began to exhibit self-harm behaviors that included banging his head, pinching himself, and stabbing himself with sharp objects. Despite previous medication and behavior therapy, the self-harm behaviors persisted, and Elliott's aggression began to turn outward when he began preschool. He struggled to make friends, displayed poor social skills, and appeared to interact only with his brother and parents.

During the diagnostic meeting with the examiner, Elliott, a small-for-his-age child with coke-bottle glasses, accompanied the examiner without hesitation and was initially cooperative in speaking with the examiner. While his speech was comprehensible, he spoke with short phrases or single words. The overall story of the incidents leading to the child's admission was disjointed and difficult to piece together. He was able to sit in his chair but would swing his legs back and forth. After answering questions about his family, he got up and began to walk around the room and attempted to open the door to exit. When he was unable to open the door, he asked the examiner for assistance and left the room.

Of note, several months after this acute admission, Elliott reported rectal pain. An emergency room evaluation confirmed the presence of rectal trauma. Elliott disclosed to his parents that over a period of several months, his stepfather's 13-year-old nephew had repeatedly assaulted Elliott with a variety of kitchen utensils when the nephew's mother had been babysitting Elliott.

There were multiple developmental interferences with the attachment process in Elliott's vignette. In the first place, he was born prematurely and was exposed to psychotropics during pregnancy; there was a prolong separation from mother due to his prematurity; then, mother became emotionally unavailable to Elliott due to postpartum depression. The early developmental environment was tense and violent, and in addition to all the previous adversities, Elliott had been severely sexually traumatized by his adolescent cousin.

For other examples of interviewing preschool children, see the cases involving Rudd (Case Example 2), Pedro (Case Example 10), and Chad (Case Example 16) in Chapter 3.

In the assessment of very young children, the examiner should be attentive to early experiences of trauma or neglect (see Table 7–1 for the elements or domains of the evaluation of preschool-age children).

Attention-Deficit/Hyperactivity Disorder

ADHD frequently begins between 2 and 4 years of age and is often associated with significant impairment in terms of emotional distress for the preschool child and the caregivers due to expulsion from day care and early education settings; ADHD puts significant demands on caregivers' time and often causes exclusion from family events secondary to accident proneness and safety concerns. Children with ADHD have comorbid mental health and chronic health problems and are frequent users of health care services. Behavior problems in preschool children persist to school-age years and cause and continue to be associated with significant impairment; 79.2% of children with symptoms meeting full diagnostic criteria for ADHD, and 34.5% of those with symptoms meeting criteria for one situation only at initial assessment, continue to have symptoms that meet the full ADHD diagnostic criteria and to exhibit global academic and social impairments 3 years later (Ghuman et al. 2009, pp. 221–222). The rates of depression are increased in patients with ADHD and their parents (Brent and Maalouf 2015, p. 877).

Oppositional Defiant Disorder and Conduct Disorder

Unfortunately, oppositional defiant disorder (ODD) and conduct disorder (CD) are still viewed by some not as "true" psychiatric disorders but more as character flaws, with children being seen as nasty and bad. In recent years there have been important discoveries about what contributes to the development of ODD/CD, with a substantial biological component involving genetic and brain differences becoming evident. In many cases the problems are not due to just poor socialization. There are very different trajectories for children who exhibit early versus later onset of ODD/CD and for those with unemotional callous traits. Although at one time effective treatments for these disorders were not available, this is not the case anymore (Scott 2015, p. 913). ODD is more common in preadolescents and in males. CD is more common in adolescence and far more common in males than in females, and in low socioeconomic status (Scott 2015, p. 915). Among the CD subtypes, the early onset–lifetime persistent subgroup (8%) is associated with low IQ, hyperactivity and inattention, poor memory, peer difficulties, and severe family and psychosocial circumstances. This group has the worst prognosis. The adolescent-limited subgroup (15%) continues a pattern of offending at moderately high levels until the 30s. In the childhood-limited subgroup (7%), antisocial behavior emerges earlier than age 5 years but decreases in intensity, with a major deescalation of antisocial behavior from ages 5 to 10 years, and a progressive decrease in antisociality up to age 20. Most of the ODD and CD children (≥70%) do not display antisocial behavior (Scott 2015, pp. 915–916). Dividing children with ODD into irritable, headstrong, and hurtful has a predictive longitudinal outcome: individuals with irritable traits (angry outbursts, temper tantrums) are likely to develop anxiety and depression but not fears. Headstrong individuals (defiant and disobedient) are likely to develop conduct disorder, and hurtful individuals (those with callous unemotional traits) are likely to develop aggressive conduct disorders (Scott 2015). Harsh, inconsistent, and frightening parenting could cause or worsen antisocial behaviors (Scott 2015, p. 919).

Children with conduct problems are rejected by normal peers; at as young as 5 years, aggressive- antisocial children tend to associate with other deviant children (Scott 2015, p. 921).

The examining physician needs to obtain a very detailed and truthful picture of the disciplinary practices in the household. It is important to find out if the parents and the child have good times together. Is the child able to find comfort in the parents? Does the child feel close to the parents? In younger children, the examiner will strive to determine the quality of attachment, what the child enjoys doing, and what his or her future plans are.

Mood Disorders

It was long believed that depression exhibited a marked developmental discontinuity such that depression was not possible in children because they lacked the necessary intrapsychic structures. "It is now clear that depression occurs across the life span, even in infants, although the symptoms naturally vary somewhat as a function of the patient's developmental level" (Pennington 2002, p. 103).

The examiner needs to remember that irritability is a prominent symptom of ODD and CD and that in the absence of other mood symptoms, irritability is more likely to be secondary to a behavioral disorder than to depression. The Preschool Feelings Checklist, a one-parent report instrument validated for preschool depression, can be used as an aid in the differential diagnosis (Brent and Maalouf 2015, p. 875).

Depression has genetic and environmental influences. The influence of common environmental factors shared by twins of the same family on the stability of Anxious/Depression (A/D) is highest in early childhood (around 50% for the preschool children) and is reduced after age 7 years. Across ages, the same common environmental factors were suggested because a single C (common environmental) factor could explain the covariance pattern across ages. Family variables such as parental conflict, negative family environment, and separation are likely candidates for these shared environmental influences. Future genetic research should include such environmental variables (e.g., parental divorce) to specify the role of these environmental experiences (Boomsma et al. 2008, p. 184). It appears that the expression of A/D is influenced significantly by genetic factors. These data are consistent with a wide literature on infant anxiety, behavioral inhibition, and temperament. Life experiences can both positively and negatively affect the child, adolescent, and adult outcomes of anxious children. With the knowledge that shared environmental influences increase with age comes the possibility that children at risk for anxiety can be influenced away from the expression of A/D or, sadly, that this factor may contribute to the expression of the same phenotype. Recent remarkable findings from association studies of the serotonin transporter gene and tryptophan hydroxylase provide evidence that children with different genotypes have variable responses to different environmental stimuli and are at a highly variant risk for negative outcomes (Boomsma et al. 2008, p. 185).

The prevalence of depressive disorders is 1%–2% in preschool-age children and 3%–8% in older prepubertal children, with a lifetime prevalence by the end of adolescence of 20% (Brent and Maalouf 2015, p. 876). Adolescent-onset depression has higher heritability than prepubertal depression. A less functional allelic variant of the serotonin transporter gene *5HTTLPR* is associated with early-onset depression, in the presence of stressful life events, a history of abuse, or peer victimization. This finding has not been consistently replicated. Difficulties with emotion regulation (i.e., the ability to achieve emotional equilibrium in the face of perturbation) are considered a core deficit predisposing to depression (Brent and Maalouf 2015, p. 877).

Physical or sexual abuse, neglect, and exposure to domestic violence are potent risk factors for the onset and recurrence of depression. Peer victimization may have a long-lasting effect on increasing depression symptomatology, and parental or peer bereavement is associated with a threefold increased risk of depression even after preexisting risk factors are taken into account (Brent and Maalouf 2015, p. 878).

Sleeping Disorders

The most common sleep disorders in preschool years are disorders of initiating and maintaining sleep, night terrors and nightmares, and parasomnias. Sheldon (2005b) notes that the diagnosis and management of sleep disorders in children may hold a unique significance in at least three important ways: 1) primary sleep-related pathology may cause daytime symptoms, 2) sleep-related pathology may be a comorbid condition contributing to day time symptomatology, and 3) a child's sleep difficulties may have a greater impact on other family members than on the affected child, causing the caregiver, for example, to be sleep deprived, with medical and emotional consequences, including an impaired ability to take care of the child. Sleep disorders in infants and children reflect an interplay among many factors, including central nervous function, parent-child interaction, social stress, patient needs, and other medical conditions. Comprehensive knowledge of these interactions is essential for all child care professionals who want to deliver optimal management (Sheldon 2005b, p. vii). Non–rapid eye movements (NREM) are considered to be restorative to the body, and rapid eye movement (REM) is considered to be restorative to the brain. (For the physiological role of REM and NREM sleep, see Note 6 at the end of this chapter.)

Among the sleep disorders described in DSM-5, the following are particularly relevant for preschool psychiatry: insomnia disorder, breathing-related sleep disorders (obstructive sleep apnea hypopnea), and parasomnias: non–rapid eye movement sleep arousal disorders (sleepwalking and sleep terrors) and nightmare disorder. The examiner needs to differentiate night terrors from nightmares.

Night terrors arise during the first third of a major sleep period; The episodes last from 1 to 10 minutes, or longer in small children. The episodes are accompanied by impressive autonomic arousal and behavior manifestations of a great fear. The child does not respond to comfort and is difficult to awaken. Usually, there is no recollection of any dream content. During a typical episode, the child abruptly sits up in bed screaming or crying with a very frightened expression and displays signs of autonomic arousal (tachycardia, rapid breathing, sweating, and dilation of pupils). The child may be inconsolable and difficult to awake (American Psychiatric Association 2013, p. 400).

DSM-5 now recognizes the diagnosis of *nightmare disorder* (American Psychiatric Association 2013, p. 404). The diagnostic criteria are as follows:

A. Repeated occurrences of extended, extremely dysphoric, and well-remembered dreams that usually involve efforts to avoid threats to survival, security, or physical integrity, [and that relive or is closely associated with past traumas,] and generally occur during the second half of the major sleep episode.
B. On awakening from the dysphoric dream, the subject becomes readily oriented and alert.
C. The sleep disturbance causes clinically significant distress or impairment in social occupational or in other important areas of functioning.
D. The nightmares are not related to the physiological effect of a medication or a substance of abuse.
E. Coexisting medical or mental disorders do not adequately explain the dysphoric dreams.

Sleepwalking represents a repeated complex motor behavior initiated during sleep, including rising from bed and walking about. Sleepwalking can arise from any NREM stage. These episodes are more common during slow wave sleep, and therefore sleepwalking occurs most frequently during the first third of the night. During episodes, children have reduced alertness and responsiveness and a blank stare and display relative unresponsiveness to communication with others or to efforts by others to awaken them. As a rule, children do not have recollection of the episodes. After the episode, there may initially be a brief period of confusion or difficulty orienting, followed by a full recovery of cognitive function and appropriate behavior (American Psychiatric Association 2013, p. 400).

Virtually all psychiatric disorders in children may be associated with sleep disruption. A psychiatric disorder is the most common cause of insomnia and can also be the cause of daytime sleepiness, fatigue, abnormal circadian sleep patterns, and disturbing dreams and nightmares. Growing evidence indicates that primary insomnia (insomnia with no concurrent psychiatric disorder) is a risk factor for depressive and anxiety disorders (Owens 2005, p. 31). Sleep disturbances in the pediatric special needs population are extremely common. Significant sleep problems occur in 30%–80% of children with severe intellectual disability and in at least half of children with less severe intellectual impairment. Children with autism spectrum disorder are in the range of 50%–70%. A variety of sleep disorders have been reported in children with neurodevelopmental disorders (Asperger, Angelman, Rett, Smith-Magenis, and Williams syndromes). Similar findings have been reported in children with blindness (Owens 2005).

In children with obesity, the examiner needs to explore the presence of snoring or, worse, the presence of sleep apnea. A sleep study may provide good diagnostic help.

Psychosis

The examiner needs to rule out the presence of psychosis as a cause for difficulties of initiating or maintaining sleep. Psychosis in preschool years is not common but is not rare either; it does exist. The inquiry, as elaborated in the evaluation of psychosis in Chapter 9 ("Evaluation of Internalizing Symptoms"), may start with the examiner asking the child if he has any fears at night. The examiner wonders if the child hears creepy or scary noises; if so, the examiner explores the nature of the noises. At this point the examiner may ask the child if he has ever heard any voices talking to him when nobody is around. Depending on the response the evaluation proceeds in the pertinent line of questioning. The same is done with visual hallucinations. "Have you ever seen monsters, ghosts, people, shadows?" The examiner equally follows the pertinent exploration in case of positive responses. Some children are afraid that someone may come in the middle of the night to snatch them away from the family or to harm or kill them. Children ought to be asked if they are afraid of the closet, where monsters or ghosts or scary people may hide, or of the windows and under the bed for related reasons. No evaluation of psychosis in children is complete without asking questions pertaining to paranoia: "Do you feel people say bad things about you?" "Do you feel people watch you?" "Do you feel followed?" "Do you need to check your back to see if somebody is behind you?" "Do you feel somebody is after you? How come?" Trauma (physical and sexual abuse) needs to be ruled out in psychosis in preschool.

For vignettes of preschoolers with psychosis, see cases of Fabio (Case Example 4) and Blond (Case Example 5) in Chapter 8, "Documenting the Examination."

Developmental Scales

Developmental scales may play an important role in the assessment of a young child's functioning (see Note 7 at the end of this chapter). The Child Behavior Checklist 1.5–5 is a symptom checklist for children 18 months or older and younger than 5 years. The Autism Diagnostic Observation Scale is considered the gold standard for the diagnosis of autism spectrum disorder. The Preschool Age Psychiatric Assessment is a comprehensive parent psychiatric interview for assessing symptoms and disorders in children between 2 and 5 years of age. The Denver Developmental Screening Test II (DDST II) provides a general developmental screening for children from birth to age 6½ years (Rush et al. 2007). Administered by a trained clinician, the DDST II examines a child's skills in four areas: personal and social, fine motor–adaptive, language, and gross motor. This scale also aids in the assessment of speech intelligibility, ability to comply with requests, alertness, fearfulness, and attention span. The use of this screening tool assists the clinician in identifying possible delays that may warrant referral for additional evaluations and interventions.

The Infant-Toddler Social and Emotional Assessment (ITSEA) is a questionnaire that elicits parent or caregiver information regarding social-emotional problems and strengths in children age 12–36 months; it provides a more comprehensive view of a child's social development with the intent of identifying strengths and areas of risk (Rush et al. 2007). The ITSEA consists of 166 items that examine three problem domains (internalizing symptoms, externalizing symptoms, and dysregulation areas) and the domain of competence (examining a child's aptitude to function and perform socially) (see Note 8 at the end of this chapter). The Brief ITSEA (BITSEA) is a shorter form of the ITSEA that allows for screening of the same general areas but in a much more time and cost-efficient manner (Rush et al. 2007). The Bayley Scales of Infant Development, 2nd Edition (BSID-II) assesses the language, social, cognitive, and motor skills of children ages 1–42 months (Rush et al. 2007). Although the BSID-II is not a diagnostic tool, the clinician may administer the examination to assess for the presence of low function or developmental delays in infants and toddlers.

Key Points

- History, collateral information, observation, and developmental assessment with standardized developmental scales or protocols are the main tools used in the psychiatric assessment of preschool-age children.
- Familiarity with normal and abnormal childhood development is critical in the assessment of young children.
- Gaps in data gathering created by deficits of communication (language and speech) are filled with keen observations of the child and the mother (or caretaker) and of the interaction between mother and child.
- Observations of the interaction between the child and parent provide the foundation for an understanding of the child and caretaker relationship—that is, the quality of the child's attachment and the parental bond. The ways in which a child relates to a parent (attachment) and a parent relates to a child (bonding) provide a framework for exploring the etiology of behavioral disturbances present in young and very young children.

Notes

1. The concept of the development and implications of attachment are based on the foundational works of John Bowlby and Mary Ainsworth. Marvin and Britner (2008) provide a history of the development of attachment theory.
2. The components of the Strange Situation include the introduction of the parent and child to a room that the child explores with parental assistance as necessary. A stranger is then introduced into the room and plays or interacts with the child. The parent leaves the infant with the stranger but eventually returns and the stranger exits. The parent then leaves the

child alone in the room. The stranger reenters the room and interacts with the child as needed. In the final phase, the parent returns and the stranger again exits (Solomon and George 2008).

3. As children develop additional language and cognitive skills, other assessment tools utilize the rubric of the secure/insecure subcategories but take maturation into consideration in expanding those subcategories. The Cassidy-Marvin Assessment of Attachment in Preschoolers utilizes the child's responses to reunions with the mother but expands the description of "controlling/disorganized" and "insecure/other" (Solomon and George 2008, p. 394). The Preschool Assessment of Attachment "emphasizes dynamic changes in the quality of attachment that arise from the interaction between maturity and current experience…[and] emphasizes… the possibilities for changes in quality of the attachment relationship over time" (Solomon and George 2008, p. 393). Other attachment assessment protocols utilize symbolic representations of attachment such as the interpretation of projective photographs from the Separation Anxiety Test or the observations of doll play with a focus on attachment-related themes as in the Attachment Story Completion Task or the Attachment Doll Play Assessment (Solomon and George 2008).

4. As a result of impaired parental responses, children develop insecure attachments and display dysfunctional behaviors upon reunion (O'Connor et al. 1999; Oliveira et al. 2012; Stacks et al. 2014).

5. Multiple factors may greatly affect the development of attachment and subsequent child dysfunction. Multiple studies indicate that the effects of stressors on the parent (most often the mother) affect the *quality* of parenting behaviors with a particular emphasis on parental management of expressed emotion (Borelli et al. 2012; Parfitt and Ayers 2012). Substance-abusing mothers demonstrate "emotionally avoidant language… [that] is associated with risk for parenting self-dysregulation" (Borelli et al. 2012, p. 516). Parents with anger issues express greater frustration and lack of understanding of their infants which compromises the quality of interactions and subsequent development of attachment in their children (Parfitt and Ayers 2012). Mothers with histories of childhood trauma and domestic violence may be at greater risk for dysfunctional parenting styles and the development of insecure attachment in their infants as a result of distorted or negative representations of the parent/child relationship (Malone et al. 2010) and an inability to conceptualize the mental states and motivations of themselves and others especially in regard to their past trauma (Berthelot et al. 2015). Because of narcissistic injuries, some mothers who may have had attachment disturbances themselves cannot empathize with their infants' needs and sense of helplessness; they are bothered by the infants' demands and attempt to promote precocious self-reliance. How-

ever, the effects of trauma on parental caregiving may be mitigated by the presence of a parent's own history of positive caregiving experiences in development (Burrous et al. 2009; Huth-Bocks et al. 2014; Lieberman et al. 2005; Shlafer et al. 2015; Stacks et al. 2014). Therefore, inquiries into parents' own attachment history with their caregivers should accompany an exploration of parental trauma experiences.

6. The NREM restorative function to the body comes from research that has demonstrated the following (Sheldon 2005a, pp. 1–2):

   a. Slow-wave sleep (SWS) increases following sleep deprivation.
   b. SWS percentage increases during the developmental years.
   c. Total sleep duration increases with body mass.
   d. Growth hormone release occurs at sleep onset, and peak levels occur during SWS, in prepubertal children.
   e. Release of endogenous anabolic steroids (prolactin, testosterone, and luteinizing hormone) occurs in relation to a sleep-dependent cycle.
   f. The nadir of catabolic steroid release, such as corticosteroids, occurs during the first hours of sleep, coincident with the largest percentage of SWS.
   g. Increased mitosis of lymphocytes and increased bone growth occur during sleep.
   h. There is a gradual increase in SWS percentage of total sleep in response to an increase in physical exercise. However, in adolescents and adults, somatomedin levels are the highest during wakefulness, not during sleep as they are in preadolescent children.

REM sleep, characterized by intense central nervous system (CNS) activation, has been thought to restore CNS function. It may have evolved to "reprogram" innate behaviors and to incorporate learned behaviors and knowledge acquire during wakefulness. The synthesis of CNS proteins is increased during REM sleep. This sleep state is present in a higher proportion during the fetal and newborn periods and decreases progressively over the first few years of life (Sheldon 2005a, p. 2). REM sleep is deeply involved in the reprocessing and optimization of high-order information contained in the material to be learned, suggesting that cerebral reactivation is modulated by the strength of the memory traces developed during the learning episode (Sheldon 2005a, p. 3). NREM sleep is necessary for declarative memory consolidation; spindle density correlates with recall performance before and after sleep, and spindle activity during NREM sleep is very sensitive to previous learning experiences. REM sleep is associated with creative processes and abstract reasoning, with an increased strength of weak associations in cognitive networks (Sheldon 2005a, p. 4). Research has demonstrated support for the neuronal activity correlation theory by Emmons and Simon: REM sleep actively consolidates and/or integrates complex associative information, and NREM sleep passively prevents retroactive interference of recently acquired complex associate information (Sheldon 2005a, p. 6).

7. Tables of developmental milestones are available in most textbooks of child and adolescent psychiatry. One detailed reference book is *From Birth to Five Years: Children's Developmental Progress* by Mary D. Sheridan and revised and updated by Marion Frost and Ajay Sharma (Sheridan 1997).

8. Internalizing scales in the ITSEA include those for depression/withdrawal, anxiety, separation distress and an examination of inhibition to novelty. The externalizing scales assess activity/impulsivity, aggression/defiance, and peer aggression. The dysregulation scales examine constitutional areas such as sleep and eating as well negative emotionality, and sensory issues (Rush et al. 2007).

CHAPTER 8

Documenting the Examination

Using AMSIT

In every diagnostic interview, the examiner must document the patient's mental status examination. AMSIT is an acronym representing the components of the mental status examination: A (appearance, behavior, and speech); M (mood and affect); S (sensorium); I (intelligence); and T (thought). AMSIT is a documentation protocol that was developed in the Department of Psychiatry at the University of Texas at San Antonio for the systematic documentation of psychiatry examinations in adults. It was originated in the early 1970s by David Fuller, M.D. (Fuller 1998). The documentation in AMSIT should mainly include observations and clinical evidence gathered during the psychiatric evaluation. Over the years, AMSIT has undergone a number of improvements. Medical students, interns, general psychiatric residents, and fellows in child and adolescent psychiatry are expected to be proficient in the use of AMSIT. The present chapter represents a modification of the original protocol for documenting the mental status examination of children and adolescents.

The psychiatric examination provides the data needed to establish a psychiatric diagnosis and to develop a comprehensive treatment plan. A comprehensive psychiatric evaluation of a child includes an inquiry into the child's presenting problems, his or her developmental course, and the nature of the family context or rearing environment. The developmental progression (which refers to the acquisition of abilities or skills at a given age) and the developmental context (which refers to psychosocial factors and the nature of the rearing environment) are fundamental concepts in the field of child and adolescent psychiatry.

Although the psychiatric examination of the child is a valuable component of the diagnostic process, it is only part of the process. The examiner must remember that the examination removes the child from his or her natural environment context; therefore, the child's family and other aspects of the child's psychosocial environment also need to be evaluated.

A child's mental status is an active, dynamic process, and it changes from one moment to the next. For example, a child who is withdrawn one moment may be active and engaging a moment later, and vice versa. In general, children and adolescents are environmentally reactive; whatever is going on around them influences their mood and other psychological processes. This reactivity may mislead the examiner who is determining the existence or severity of a given disorder. AMSIT is a valuable tool for documenting the psychiatric examination. In the remainder of this chapter, we describe the components of AMSIT as it pertains to child and adolescent psychiatry. (See the appendix to this volume for an example of a protocol used at ClarityCGC, San Antonio, for the documentation of the psychiatric evaluation of children and adolescents.)

Appearance, Behavior, and Speech

Table 8–1 summarizes the specific areas of AMSIT that are related to appearance, behavior, and speech in children and adolescents. Keen, disciplined, and systematic observations must be made during this part of the examination. Methodical inspection and careful observation probably account for up to 75% of the work involved in arriving at a diagnosis. A "clinical eye" and expertise give examiners an advantage in this area.

First impressions are significant. The examiner should consider the following questions: What is my first impression of the child (or the family)? Is the child likable? What is likable about this child? Is anything odd about the child? Is there any sense of detachment, apprehension, or even danger? The answers to these questions are important in the overall assessment of the child and family. The examiner also needs to keep in mind that while he or she is assessing the child and the family, they are also assessing the examiner, too: Is the doctor likable? Does the doctor come across as reassuring or as critical and severe? Does the doctor appear to be comforting? Does the doctor seem willing to help?

Table 8–1. **Elements of the appearance, behavior, and speech section of AMSIT for children and adolescents**

Appearance

Physical appearance

Gait and posture[a]

Behaviors

Exploratory behavior[a]

Playfulness[a]

Relatedness

Eye contact[a]

Behavioral organization[a]

Cooperative behavior[a]

Psychomotor activity[a]

Involuntary movements[a]

Behavioral evidence of emotion

Repetitive activities

Disturbances of attention

Speech

Disturbance of speech melody (dysprosody)[a]

[a]Section not included in the AMSIT original protocol, which was created to document adult psychiatric evaluation.
Source. Modified from Cepeda 2010, p. 169.

Appearance

Physical Appearance

The examiner should note whether the child appears his or her chronological age or looks younger or older than the stated age. The examiner should observe the child's nutritional state, his or her sense of vitality, and the presence or absence of secondary sexual characteristics. Marked slimness, cachexia, heaviness, and obesity are readily apparent. In children showing such characteristics, issues related to eating disorders need to be explored, no matter what the presenting problem may be.

The examiner should note the presence of dysmorphic features in any of the following areas: facial complexion, shape and configuration of the eyes (e.g., separation of the eyes [hypertelorism], slanted or mongoloid; different-colored irises), breadth or shape of the forehead, setting or configuration of the ears, and texture and docility of the hair (e.g., "electric" hair). The shape and configuration of the head should be noted. The examiner should also note any other unusual facial or cranial features.

The examiner should pay attention to the child's attire and physical presentation. Children with deviant social behavior often wear striking and unconventional attire. The examiner should note the child's footwear, hairstyle, and hair color. With female patients, the examiner also should note the use of nail polish and the quality of any makeup. Revealing or see-through garments may indicate a defiance of norms and the transgression of social conventions. Children who wear such garments may also demonstrate precociousness, sexualization, or evidence of antisocial behavior. Rings and perforations are in style among some youths and young adults. If the child has nose, eyebrow, or tongue piercings, the examiner might also inquire about perforations elsewhere on the body, including the navel, nipples, or genitals. Children with sexual identity conflicts often present with ambiguous attire or with makeup that is more appropriate to the opposite sex. Masculine females frequently present without makeup, and their attire and demeanor betray their intentions of wanting to be male.

The examiner should observe any visible skin for the presence of tattoos, for signs of recent injuries or self-abusive or suicidal behaviors, or for evidence of old injuries, such as multiple scarring of the knuckles, wrists, or forearms. These marks may be indicative of chronic self-abusive behavior or impulsive aggressive tendencies. If the patient's upper limbs show evidence of self-abusive behavior, the examiner should explore whether the patient abuses other parts of the body (e.g., legs, chest, breasts, genitals). The examiner should ask the child about all visible scars: each scar has a history to tell. The possibility of nonvisible scars needs to be kept in mind, even if no scars associated with self-abusive behavior are visible.

Alert examiners may detect vein tracks or other signs of drug abuse. An attentive interviewer will detect evidence of hair pulling (trichotillomania) of the scalp or of the eyebrows, as well as signs of nail biting, nose picking, skin picking, and other compulsive traits. If the patient has an obvious disability, the examiner should note it and observe the limitations that it imposes on the patient and how the patient copes with it.

Gait and Posture

As the examiner enters the waiting room and guides the child to the interviewing room, he or she should note the child's gait, including the child's grace, smoothness of movements, and coordination. Does the child waddle, shuffle, or tiptoe? Does he or she move with agility? Are any unusual movements associated with the child's gait? For these and related observations, see Chapter 12, "Neuropsychiatric Interview and Examination."

Does the child sit or stand erect, or does the child slouch? Some children are unable to keep an erect posture while sitting or standing. Does the child lean on the chair, the table, or other available support? Some children look hypotonic, or sluggish. Children with a background of early deprivation display unusual and ungraceful postures and may seem hypoactive or even apathetic. Children with chronic regressive states are likely to lean on the chair or to lie down on the couch or the floor, even though they exhibit no neuromotor impairment. The same is true for children with severe melancholic features. In severe psychomotor retardation, the child's inactivity may reach a catatonic state.

If the child is catatonic, the examiner should evaluate the degree of akinesia, including lack of blinking, persistence of unusual postures, vacant staring, or flatness of emotional display. The examiner may observe echopraxia (imitates the examiner's behavior), echolalia (imitates the examiner's speech), and other automatic imitative behaviors. The examiner may test the patient for *cerea flexibilitas* (child maintains whatever body position he is placed in).

Some children come across as weak, anergic, or temperamentally hypoactive or hyporeactive. These children lack enthusiasm, and it is difficult to keep them motivated about anything.

Behavior

Exploratory Behavior

Some children demonstrate no reticence when entering the examiner's office. Some children appear fearless in new circumstances and do not show any restraint in unfamiliar settings. These children often show a sense of familiarity with the examiner, even though this is the first time they have met him or her. Some children look around first but seem comfortable, even though they are in a new environment. Others are apprehensive about entering the office and need the active encouragement or assistance of a parent or other caregiver. These children show evidence of behavioral inhibition (Kagan 1994); they hide behind their mothers and stay near them, or they hide their faces with their hands to avoid eye contact. Other children fret or show wariness and need reassurance before any diagnostic engagement.

Playfulness

Playfulness is a quintessential characteristic of childhood. It should be present in well-adapted, so-called normal children. If the examiner encounters an overtly serious child, he or she needs to seek explanations for this demeanor. If the child lacks the quality of playfulness, the examiner will probably observe other evidence of developmental deviations, such as lack of behavioral organization and exploratory behavior or other atypical behaviors. The examiner may also observe inhibition, passivity, and separation problems.

Once the child engages in play, the examiner should attend to the content and process of the child's play. The examiner should note the nature of the child's enactments (see Chapter 2, "General Principles of Interviewing"), the degree of the child's affective involvement (i.e., the child's emotional involvement with the examiner and the child's overt affective display), and the manner in which the child involves the examiner in the play. Frequently, children enact themes related to the major psychological issues that preoccupy or surround them (e.g., major anxieties or conflicts going on in their families).

Relatedness

Relatedness refers to the child's manner of relating to the examiner and to his or her significant others: parents, siblings, extended family, peers, friends, and others. Normal preschool and preadolescent children are reserved when they meet strangers. After they get a "feeling" for the situation and become reassured, they relate more warmly. Adolescents may be expectant and hesitant. Once they feel comfortable, they become more spontaneous and engaging. Anxious children need more time and more reassurance to feel at ease and to develop rapport. Children with schizoid personality disorder appear distant and uninvolved. These children will not warm up to the interviewer, no matter how much effort is made to engage and comfort them. Children with psychotic disorders show oddness and inappropriateness in relating, or they may display signs of self-absorption, evidence of response to internal stimuli, or inappropriate affect.

Some children show immediate familiarity with the examiner and, for that matter, with any stranger. Such children demonstrate boundary problems and require ongoing structure to behave adaptively. Children who demonstrate promiscuous relating may also show evidence of seductive or even overt sexual behavior (see section "Reverse Engagement" in Chapter 1, "Diagnostic and Therapeutic Engagement"). Management of these behaviors requires active limit setting throughout the diagnostic interview (see Chapter 3, "Special Interviewing Techniques"). Other children behave in a hostile and aggressive manner or even in a paranoid fashion. These children are hyperalert and suspicious.

Eye Contact

Eye contact is a fundamental interactive behavior. It is a universal nonverbal behavior that increases attachment and rapport. Warm eye contact is a basic element of interpersonal engagement, and its absence indicates a significant relational problem. Children who display poor eye contact also display problems in interpersonal social behavior. Some children avoid eye contact when they are anxious or when attachment or neuropsychiatric difficulties are present.

The more deviant the nature of the eye contact, the more serious the likelihood of profound developmental psychopathology in the social-relational area. Examples of deviant eye contact include the "see-through" eye contact observed in children with autism and the "staring" eye contact observed in children with paranoid personality or psychotic disorders. Seizure disorders and dissociative states must be considered in the differential diagnosis when staring is observed.

Behavioral Organization

The examiner should note the patient's degree of adaptability and organizational behavior. Some children, no matter what is happening around them, are able to initiate or create adaptive activities or to immerse themselves in generative endeavors (e.g., play). Other children, even in the most propitious circumstances, are unable to generate constructive or productive activities and depend on the alter-ego functions of responsible adults in order to organize and display adaptive behavior. Children who lack behavioral organization also show other deficits, such as the inability to focus, the absence of an organized approach to problem solving, or a lack of self-soothing functions.

Some children exhibit behavioral disturbance as soon as they enter the psychiatrist's office. They are fidgety, restless, and hyperactive. These children need active structuring throughout the evaluation. The structuring may include verbal redirection, limit setting, or even physical redirection or restraint.

Cooperative Behavior

The examiner should note the child's active and cooperative participation during the psychiatric examination. This quality is associated with the child's understanding of the presenting problems, the dystonicity of the symptoms, and his or her motivation to change.

Problems with compliance or with following directions are common and challenging complaints in the field of child and adolescent psychiatry. When faced with a child's oppositional behavior, the examiner should attempt to determine whether the behavior stems from a need to control, a power struggle motivation, or a sense of personal incompetence. Children who are aware of their real or perceived incompetence (or mastery limitations) are reluctant to try a given task because they know, or believe, they cannot do it. Many so-called oppositional children have significant unidentified language disorders. These children often have major receptive language problems and cannot understand expectations or given commands. They may also have neuropsychological deficits that interfere with their ability to understand a task or its solution. The examiner should also determine whether these patients have any hearing problems.

Psychomotor Activity

Disturbances of psychomotor activity are probably the most commonly encountered disruptive behaviors in clinical settings. Psychomotor disturbances are caused by a multiplicity of medical, neurological, and psychiatric conditions. Attention-deficit/hyperactivity disorder (ADHD) is one of the most prevalent psychiatric diagnoses, and some of its features are among the most common behavior problems cited by schoolteachers (see subsection "Attention and Concentration Deficits" in Chapter 12, "Neuropsychiatric Interview and Examination"). The triad of hyperactivity, distractibility (inattentiveness), and impulsivity may occur as a primary disorder, as a complicating comorbidity, or as a secondary manifestation. When the examiner observes signs of ADHD, he or she should search for evidence of medical, neurological, and common comorbid disorders that are associated with this condition—for example, oppositional defiant disorder, conduct disorder, depressive disorders, anxiety disorders, developmental language and learning disorders).

The examiner should distinguish between a child who exhibits hyperactive behavior (e.g., fidgetiness, aimless behavior) and a child who is driven by goal-directed behavior. The examiner should test the child's response to redirection or structure to determine whether the hyperkinesis is responsive to or impervious to structuring or limit setting. The examiner also should attempt to determine whether the child's impairments are secondary to ADHD, one of the associated conditions (comorbidity), or both.

Agitation and sensorium disturbances should alert the examiner to the possibility of delirium. Because delirium is a potentially life-threatening process needing urgent medical attention, it should be considered in the differential diagnosis of hyperactivity, agitation, and restlessness in children.

Mania and akathisia should be considered in the differential diagnosis of agitation and restlessness. Manic patients are frequently hyperactive. The examiner should pay attention to other manic manifestations, such as pressured speech, loose associations, hypersexuality, and grandiosity. If akathisia is suspected, the examiner should determine whether the patient uses neuroleptics or selective serotonin reuptake inhibitor (SSRI) antidepressants (see below) and should look for other extrapyramidal symptoms or other evidence of a neurological disorder.

Involuntary Movements

The examiner should observe whether the child displays tics of the face or limbs, or muscle twitching or jerking. These signs should immediately raise the examiner's suspicion that the child may have an involuntary movement disorder or Tourette's syndrome. Other involuntary movements (e.g., choreic or dyskinetic movements) may indicate a movement disorder, cerebral palsy, or other neurological condition (e.g., Sydenham's chorea, Huntington's disease, Wilson's disease). The examiner should also be attentive to the child's production of vocal tics or guttural noises such as grunting, throat clearing, involuntary noises (including shrilly noises), or barking.

With children who are taking neuroleptic medications, the examiner should be alert to the presence of involuntary movements associated with acute dyskinesia and the orolingual and choreiform movements associated with acute or tardive dyskinesia. Any of these findings require full neurological clarification. SSRI antidepressants can also induce extrapyramidal symptoms (Pies 1997).

Behavioral Evidence of Emotion

The examiner should observe any affective or emotional manifestations and pay special attention to the flow and vicissitudes of the child's emotional display. The examiner should note whether the child's emotional display is enduring or whether it is variable and unstable.

Anxiety disorders and depressive disorders are common afflictions in child psychiatric practice. Common signs or features of anxiety disorders include the presence of specific and unspecific fears, thumb sucking, nail biting, hair pulling, frequent scratching, skin picking, skin flushing, and bowel sounds. Cracking of the knuckles or the back is common in anxious adolescents. Preadolescents may exhibit manifestations of primitive anxiety and fear (e.g., urinating, passing gas, defecating) during the interview.

Separation anxiety complaints are common. Children with this disorder refuse to separate from their mothers, stay close to their caregivers, and display limited curiosity and exploratory behavior. Equally common in anxious children are inhibitions in social settings, "freezing" in social situations, and elective mutism.

Common features of melancholia include a sad face, a downcast demeanor, crying, and a limited level of activity. Melancholic signs are commonly accompanied by negative cognitions such as helplessness, hopelessness, and worthlessness and by suicidal thoughts or behavior. Tiredness, sleep and appetite disturbances, and anhedonia are other components of melancholia. In contrast, euphoric mood coupled with restlessness, distractibility, a sense of grandiosity, hypersexuality, and pressured speech should make the examiner suspect mania or hypomania. In general, mania and melancholia are infectious moods, meaning that the examiner is "contaminated" by the patient's prevailing mood. Often the examiner evolves a countertransference that is concordant with the child's prevailing mood (Racker 1968). In addition, the examiner needs to recognize signs of fear, confusion, perplexity, hostility, seductiveness, and many other emotional states.

Repetitive Activities

The examiner should pay attention to the presence of repetitive motoric activities. On the most benign end of the spectrum are continuous hand rubbing, frequent preening, and other behaviors associated with anxiety and tension. In the middle of the spectrum are behaviors such as thumb sucking, nail biting, and knuckle or spine cracking. At the most pathological end of the spectrum are behaviors such as rocking, arm flipping, and other autistic behaviors. When careful inspection does not reveal the presence of overt repetitious activities, the examiner should proceed with sensitive probing to rule out the presence of less obvious compulsive activities (see Chapter 9, "Evaluation of Internalizing Symptoms").

Disturbances of Attention

Although hyperactivity is commonly associated with inattentiveness and impulsivity, disturbance of the attentional processes sometimes occurs without hyperactivity or impulsivity. In general, disturbances of attention reflect *distractibility* (i.e., a lack of a capacity for selective and sustained attention). Distractible children move from one activity to the next without finishing any of them.

Attention comprises many functions, including selective attention, sustained attention, intensity of attention, inhibitory control, and attentional shifts. The selection and organization of responses to stimuli depend on high-level executive functions. Attention is a fundamental function in information processing and cognitive and language functioning. Attention disturbances are implicated in the etiology of schizophrenia.

Speech

The speech component of the mental status examination is rich in findings and rewarding in the overall diagnostic process. The findings in this area range from overt aphasias with associated neurological findings to the less specific developmental language disorders. If a child does not seem to understand what the examiner is attempting to convey, or if the child's responses seem to miss the point (e.g., non sequitur responses), the examiner should suspect a receptive language disorder. The examiner must ascertain whether a hearing loss is present in these cases.

Children with receptive language difficulties look lost and confused. The examiner should consider the following questions: Is the child attempting to communicate at all? Is the child gesturing or attempting to use other nonverbal behavior? Is the child capable of developing rapport? Is the child attempting to connect with the examiner? The answers to these questions will assist the examiner in differentiating autism from other communication disorders.

As the child speaks and responds to the examiner's questions, the examiner should pay special attention to the spontaneity and flow of the child's speech, the richness of the vocabulary, the child's capacity for abstraction, the quality of the grammar, the child's ability to communicate emotion and meaning, and the melody of the speech.

Limited lexicon, grammatical mistakes, inappropriate use of prepositions, and problems with syntax are common in children with expressive language delays. Their speech and language are usually immature. Expressive language disorders may be associated with psychosocial developmental immaturity.

The examiner should also note the naturalness of the patient's speech and the quality of the communication process. Odd speech, affectation in the communication (i.e., pedantic talk), or unusual features of the communication process or of its contents, such as echolalia, neologisms, or bizarre productions, should raise the suspicion of a thought disorder (e.g., schizophrenia).

The examiner must attend to the volume and rate of the child's speech, as well as to the quality of its articulation. The examiner should note whether the child's speech is loud, pressured, or slurred and whether evidence of mispronunciations, stuttering, or other unusual speech qualities is present.

The examiner should note the response latency—that is, the amount of time that elapses before the child initiates a verbal response. Some children take a rather long time before beginning any response, whereas others blurt out responses impulsively before the examiner finishes the question or completes a thought.

Disturbances of Speech Melody

Disturbances of speech melody (dysprosodies) are prevalent in severe aphasias and developmental language disorders. The examiner should pay attention to these speech qualities because they are revealing. Disturbances of the musicality and rhythm of speech indicate that an injurious event affected the child's neurolinguistic development in early periods of language and speech formation. Instead of the soft, childlike, sweet, and melodious quality of the typical child's speech, the examiner may hear a grave, hoarse voice that resembles an adult's or elderly person's voice. The child's voice may have a high-pitched tone, or a male child's speech may have an effeminate quality.

Children who have neurodevelopmental disorders also exhibit problems with voice melody and voice inflection. For instance, when they attempt to make a statement, they may raise their voice as if asking a question.

Mood and Affect

Cummings's (1995b) definitions of mood and affect are clear and succinct: "Mood is an internally experienced pervasive emotion. Affect is the outward emotional display" (p. 168). During the mental status examination, the examiner notes the child's prevailing mood and predominant affect and the subjective states that accompany it. He or she may also observe the quality and intensity of affective expression.

Among the most valuable and clinically relevant aspects of AMSIT is the expectation that the examiner will consider the presence of depression or mania in every individual's psychiatric evaluation. The examiner is expected to rate the patient's depressive or elated affect on a seven-point numerical scale. The scale includes depression at one extreme, euthymia at the center, and mania at the other extreme. Every examiner completing AMSIT should assess the patient's degree of mood disturbance or affective expression.

Loved and well-cared-for children are, by nature, bubbly and expansive. The examiner should describe any deviation from this state. A serious child may already be demonstrating emotional disturbance. A serious countenance may be part of a restrained, euthymic state in an adult; but this is not necessarily the case in children.

Reactivity to environmental factors complicates both the identification of affective disturbance and the determination of its severity. Many depressed children react positively to reassurance and may even engage in playful interactions. These behaviors mislead the diagnostician.

The examiner should note the child's spontaneous affective display and any changes of affect that occur during the interview. The examiner should describe the intensity and the range of the child's affective expression. It is equally important to observe if the affect is appropriate to the thought content or if it is inappropriate either to the thought content or to the interviewing context.

Silliness and inappropriateness of affect are common in immature and regressed children. These affective states may represent early forms of hypomania, immaturity or regression. Some children are openly silly, whereas others display overt euphoria. Affect disturbance is common in so-called borderline disorder, in autism spectrum disorders, and in schizophrenia.

Other mood and emotional states may be as prominent and as important as those associated with depression and mania. Anger, anxiety, fear, and other states of emotional arousal are common phenomena observed in clinical practice.

The examiner should differentiate depression related to a psychiatric disorder from depression related to neuropsychiatric dysfunction. As Harris (1995a) warned,

> In the assessment of affect, apathy must be distinguished from depression. Moreover, the experience of emotion must be clarified because in some conditions, such as certain right-hemispheric dysfunction presentations or in pseudobulbar palsy, the physical expression of affect (e.g., facial expression, voice tone) may be impaired although inner experience may remain intact. Finally, with some frontal lobe lesions and in some metabolic encephalopathies, severe apathy may be noted in the absence of depression. (p. 31)

Sensorium

This section of AMSIT tests the orientation of the patient to the real world and the capacity to track time.

Orientation

Children of normal intelligence, even early preadolescents, frequently know the day of the week, the month, and the year of the evaluation. In late preschoolers and early preadolescents, less precision should be expected with the date, but even so, alert and bright children typically give very close to the correct date. It is telling when the examiner asks the child questions regarding orientation, and the child turns to the mother for assistance or expects her to give the response. The examiner needs to look beyond the overt dependency and explore cognitive problems or generalized difficulties with orientation in time and space. Significant deviations from orientation to time or place are common in children who have cognitive impairments and in children who have neurodevelopmental disorders such as learning disorders and right-hemispheric dysfunctions.

Memory

Disorders of memory result from problems with encoding (i.e., registration secondary to attentional disturbances) or from difficulties with decoding or retrieval (see Chapter 12, "Neuropsychiatric Interview and Examination"). "The impairment of new learning, or anterograde amnesia, is a defining attribute of organic amnesia" (Zola 1997, p. 448). *Retrograde amnesia* refers to impairment for memories acquired before brain damage (Zola 1997). The examiner should notice the accuracy of the child's recall and the coherence and the relevance of details included in the child's narrative. Memory problems should be suspected when, in response to the questions posed by the examiner, the child looks confused or uncertain or seeks support for his or her answers from significant others.

A child of normal intelligence can talk about important recent events. For example, if the child is a sports enthusiast, the examiner may test the child's tracking of recent sporting events and the accuracy of the recall.

The task of remembering three different words is a classic and practical short-term memory test. The examiner should select unrelated words. This challenge becomes more demanding if one of the words is abstract (e.g., honesty, fairness).

Concentration

Concentration reflects the patient's ability to focus and sustain attention during cognitive tasks. An adolescent with normal intelligence and without specific learning disabilities in arithmetic should be able to demonstrate proficiency with the serial sevens test (e.g., "Take 7 away from 100, and keep taking 7 away from the result"). The response to this challenge is considered satisfactory when the adolescent gives four or five accurate responses. For an early-latency-age child, this task may be a formidable challenge, in which case the examiner may choose a less difficult task, such as the serial threes test (e.g., "Take 3 away from 20, and keep doing so from each answer you get").

The repetition of digits forward and digits backward is a traditional test of concentration and immediate memory. After the examiner says a series of numbers, adolescents with good concentration and good immediate recall should be able to repeat five or six of the numbers forward and up to four or five of the digits in reverse order. Younger children should be expected to be proficient with fewer digits.

Another simple test of concentration is to ask the child to spell his or her last name forward and backwards; the backward spelling being a bigger challenge.

Calculating Ability

If the examiner is using the serial sevens test to assess the child's calculating ability simultaneously with concentration, and the child finds the task too difficult, the examiner could try easier challenges such as serial threes (as described in the preceding section, "Concentration") or present simple calculation problems, such as $6+7=?$ or $9+4-3=?$ Even these simple tests may be trying for children who have cognitive limitations or for those with specific developmental learning disorders.

Overall Conclusion

The AMSIT approach requires the clinician to make an overall assessment of the patient's sensorium based on the entire examination or specific findings.

A significant impairment of the sensorium should raise the suspicion of delirium, which requires diligent exploration of the central nervous system needing urgent medical attention. Because delirium can be fatal, its elucidation and treatment are medical and neurological emergencies.

Intelligence

Even experienced clinicians err in their estimation of a patient's intelligence level. Children may appear to have an intellectual disability although they do not, or they may come across as being brighter than they are. Factors that may mislead clinicians in this assessment include the presence of comorbid conditions and the presence of language or learning disorders.

In ascertaining intellectual functioning, a detailed developmental history is required. A record of the child's achievement of milestones and the time at which the child began to produce speech is of particular importance. The child's history of academic progress or academic retention is also relevant. The fact that the child has a history of grade retention does not mean the child is intellectually impaired. Similarly, the fact that a child is promoted year after year does not mean he or she is devoid of cognitive or learning problems.

Sometimes teachers may perceive bright students as having an intellectual disability. For example, a child was referred for an evaluation because his teacher believed he was too "slow." The child came across to the examiners as extremely bright, creative, and imaginative; his IQ score was found to be about 142. Comprehensive psychometric testing, complemented, when indicated, with neuropsychological testing, will assist in the clarification of intellectual capacity and language or learning disabilities.

Thought

The basic caveat in the identification of thought disorders is that the presence of severe language disorders can confuse the clinical picture. Developmental and academic histories are very helpful in preventing this confusion, as are the child's affective expression and his efforts to communicate. Table 8–2 lists the topics covered in the thought section of AMSIT.

No typical symptoms make the diagnosis of schizophrenia unequivocal. Although first-rank symptoms were formerly thought to be associated only with schizophrenia, Akiskal and Puzantian (1979) demonstrated the presence of first-rank symptoms in affective disorders with psychotic features.

Some clinicians still confuse the concepts of psychosis and thought disorder. *Psychosis* refers to problems with reality testing and especially the presence of hallucinations or delusions; *thought disorder* refers to impairments of the process of thought production, thought concatenation, and thought organization.

Table 8–2.   Elements of the thought section of AMSIT for children and adolescents

Coherence	Perceptions
Logic	Delusions
Metaphorical thinking[a]	Thought content
Goal directedness	Judgment
Reality testing	Abstracting ability
Associations	Insight

[a]Not in AMSIT for adults.
Source.   Modified from Cepeda 2010, p. 184.

Coherence

The examiner should note the threading and convergence of the patient's thinking. The examiner should consider the following relevant questions: Are the child's thoughts threaded together to express the intended idea? Does the narrative make sense? Is the narrative clear? Are the topics or themes connected to one another? When the child speaks, can his or her train of thought be followed?

Logic

In assessing the child's logic, the examiner should consider the following questions: Does the child respect the laws of reasoning, of time and space, and of the contradiction of opposites (i.e., if you state something, you rule out or exclude the opposite; see Troy's case [Case Example 9] and Note 7 in Chapter 9, "Evaluation of Internalizing Symptoms")? Do the child's conclusions derive from established premises? Are cause-effect relationships respected in the child's arguments? According to Caplan (1994), illogical thinking is based on a defective control of cognitive processing and represents a negative sign of childhood-onset schizophrenia. This defect appears to reflect frontal lobe impairment (Caplan 1994; see also Chapter 9, "Evaluation of Internalizing Symptoms").

Metaphorical Thinking

Adolescents sometimes use metaphors to describe their conflicts or concerns. The examiner should attempt to stay within the metaphor and to make interventions that use the patient's metaphoric language. This approach parallels the process of interviewing in displacement (see Chapter 3, "Special Interviewing Techniques"). The following case examples illustrate the use of metaphors by adolescents.

Case Example 1

Tim, a 15-year-old Caucasian male, was evaluated for rebellious, aggressive behavior and anger dyscontrol. He said to the interviewer that he "felt like a bull." This metaphor was helpful in understanding the patient's sense of being untamable and out of control; it also clarified the child's narcissism and his concerns about losing control. When the interviewer stressed that the patient was behaving like a bull, the adolescent responded with satisfaction. This approach improved the therapeutic alliance and made the patient more receptive to the examiner's recommendations.

Case Example 2

Sharon, a 15-year-old Caucasian female, was referred for an evaluation because of her bulimic behavior, which had continued for more than a year. She was preoccupied with her looks and compared herself unfavorably to her more attractive mother, who had been a beauty pageant queen in her younger years. She was also very preoccupied with boys and sex. She said, "When I was younger, I could handle the 'small hormones,' but now that I'm becoming older, I feel I can't handle the 'big hormones.'" Sharon was terrified of the idea of turning 18 and being on her own. Her concerns with the "big hormones" clearly indicated her difficulties with her emerging sexuality and with the separation process involved in turning 18.

Goal Directedness

When observing goal directedness, the examiner should observe whether the child's narrative includes details that are relevant to the idea the child wants to communicate. Does the child branch off into unimportant details? Does the child deviate from the point that he or she initially wanted to make? The examiner should listen for irrelevant or unnecessary details. While listening to the child's narrative, the examiner should consider the following questions: Does the child go into the substantive matter of the idea he or she wants to communicate? Does the child get lost in minutia unrelated to the core idea?

The most common disturbances in goal directedness are circumstantiality and tangentiality. In *circumstantiality*, the child's train of thought branches off into irrelevant details, but the child eventually gets back to the main idea. In *tangentiality*, the child's main idea is lost, and he or she goes off into extraneous ideas. The following example illustrates a thought disorder involving goal directedness.

Case Example 3

Jennifer, an 11-year-old Caucasian female, underwent a psychiatric evaluation for explosive and assaultive behavior that resulted in her biting and punching a teacher. In less than 6 weeks, she had three episodes of dyscontrol at school, all involving fights with peers. School administrators felt that they no longer could provide a psychoeducational program for Jennifer on school grounds because she posed a serious risk to other students and the faculty. Jennifer had attended a day hospital program the previous year for similar reasons. She was described as moody and grandiose. She was her mother's only source of emotional support, and the mother and child were entangled in a dependent, symbiotic relationship.

During the mental status examination, Jennifer showed a mildly expansive mood and a clear thought disorder, exemplified by ever-present circumstantiality, tangential thinking, and loose associations. During the interview, the examiner asked Jennifer, an obese child, "What do you think of your weight?" She responded, "OK. My belly is good for many things. The belly floats in the water…I can bob other kids with my belly, it doesn't bother me…I've seen 500-pound guys. They are huge…in Sumo wrestling in Japan…Yokosama… It doesn't matter…This big guy…"

According to Caplan (1994), "Certain aspects of thought disorder, such as illogical thinking, are found in childhood psychiatric disorders other than schizophrenia. Looseness of the associations, however, seems to occur specifically in childhood schizophrenia" (p. 608). Caplan also asserted that loose associations are secondary to distractibility and represent a positive sign of childhood-onset schizophrenia. She postulated that this defect is secondary to a disconnection between the prefrontal cortex and the subcortical regions (i.e., basal ganglia and thalamus).

Reality Testing

By mid-latency age, a child's reality testing (i.e., ability to differentiate reality from fantasy) should be established solidly; however, reliable reality testing can be demonstrated even earlier. This issue relates to how old the child is before he or she can distinguish fantasy from reality and how old he or she is before hallucinations or delusions can be observed. The examiner will remember that girls are cognitively and language-based ahead of boys during preadolescence and early and middle adolescence. The following is an example of reality testing disturbance in a preschooler, one of the youngest children with overt psychotic features (i.e., visual and auditory hallucinations) that we had ever encountered.

Case Example 4

Fabio, a 4-year-old Hispanic male, was referred for evaluation of aggressive behavior. He demonstrated murderous behavior toward his baby brother. He spontaneously verbalized that the "jingle," a monster-like figure, was coming to kill him, and he added that the jingle was going to kill his family, too. To protect himself against the jingle, Fabio would take a knife to bed with him. He saw the jingle and heard it. He said that he heard the jingle telling him that it was coming to hurt him.

Cepeda (2007, pp. 15–16) described a 3-year-old Caucasian male with psychosis. (Notice that the child is using a neologism.)

Case Example 5

Blond, a 3-year-old Caucasian male, was evaluated for aggressive behavior toward his mother and 2-month-old baby brother. He threatened to kill his mother and other people. He claimed that monsters bothered him and that they hid in the closet. He stated that the monsters tried to "poke" him.

By early mid-latency age, children can clearly differentiate between thoughts coming from inside their heads and voices coming from outside their heads, as demonstrated in the following case example.

Case Example 6

Dionne, a 9-year-old African American female who was referred for suicidal behavior, complained of hearing voices. When the examiner asked Dionne if she was hearing her own thoughts, she said, "A thought and a voice are different. A thought comes from inside of my head; a voice comes from outside of my head."

The following case example illustrates confusion of reality with fantasy and gross impairment of reality testing in a late preadolescent child.

Case Example 7

Dwayne, an 11-year-old African American male, was evaluated for explosive and assaultive behaviors. He had hit his female teacher and bitten her nose. The school was no longer willing to put other students at risk because Dwayne had lost control around his peers several times before. Dwayne had been seeing a child psychiatrist for over a year, had been in acute inpatient programs, and had taken various psychotropic medications without any significant effect. He lived with his father at the time of the evaluation. Before that, he lived with his mother in another state. His father took custody of the child when he learned that Dwayne was being physically abused at his mother's house. Dwayne's stepbrother allegedly would encourage the family dogs to attack Dwayne. Dwayne had extensive scars on his back.

The mental status examination revealed a handsome child who was extremely dysphoric; he also displayed an apathetic demeanor. He was not spontaneous and did not respond verbally to any questions. He exhibited a disgruntled countenance and an ongoing sense of irritation. The omega sign (a persistent frown) was prominent. He appeared to be very depressed. Because his internal world was inaccessible to exploration, his thought processes could not be assessed. The dosage of his antidepressant medication was increased, and he was asked to return the following week for another diagnostic appointment.

When Dwayne came with his father to the second appointment, he brought several pieces of chewing gum. Upon entering the office, he put a piece of gum in his mouth. This time he was talkative. He began narrating a fantasy story, and his father pointed out that the theme of the story was related to a movie he and Dwayne had watched a couple of days earlier. Shortly after this, Dwayne opened his mouth and showed the examiner that the gum was stuck on his lower molars. He didn't seem to know what to do. The examiner suggested that Dwayne could dislodge the gum with his finger.

At this point, Dwayne said that he had fought with Mike Tyson the night before. His father promptly explained that Dwayne had played a Mike Tyson boxing video game the night before. Dwayne went on, saying that he had "blown out Tyson's teeth" and so on. Suddenly, Dwayne opened his mouth and indicated that the place where the gum had stuck was the place where Tyson had hit him the previous night. This was followed almost immediately by the revelation that he had bad dreams that night. Dwayne reported dreams of monsters eating his hands. He then showed the examiner his fingers and said, "I had some funny feelings where the monsters were eating my fingers." The nature and extent of this child's psychotic thinking had not been appreciated earlier. Dwayne received neuroleptics with positive results.

Associations

Associations refer to the manner in which the child's thoughts are connected among themselves. As the child speaks, the examiner should follow the sequence of the child's thinking and the links between each of the child's thoughts. The examiner should note whether the child's thoughts flow smoothly. The examiner should also observe the transitions between thoughts and note whether the child returns to the original thought after digressing into other topics. Does he or she jump from one idea to the next without a clear thread linking the two ideas? The examiner should note the affective prosody (i.e., the emotional coherence of the thought content). *Ideo-affective dissociation* means that the expressed thoughts and the associated emotions are incongruent. This concept is similar to isolation of affect.

The main disturbances of association are blocking, loose associations, and flight of ideas. In general, patients are unaware of disturbances in their thought processes. *Blocking* refers to the interruption of a train of thought. It is demonstrated when the child stops presenting the main idea and either becomes silent (i.e., making a prolonged pause) or, after a short pause, goes onto another thought that is not connected to the unfinished thought. When the examiner calls attention to this disturbance, the child has significant difficulty returning to the interrupted idea. When a child's ideas are weakly connected to one another, the disturbance is called *loose associations*. In flight of ideas, the ideas presented in a chain of thoughts are not connected to one another. In the most extreme case, the ideas are so disconnected from one another that no sense can be made of them. This condition is often described as *word salad*. In *flight of ideas*, the child presents his or her thoughts at a fast pace. The child's speech frequently is increased in rate, if not pressured. Sometimes, the patient is able to acknowledge that her thinking is rushing or going very fast. In other words, the patient cannot control his or her thinking. This symptom helps to explain the impulsivity or lack of judgment exhibited by hypomanic and manic patients.

Perceptions

Normal perceptions are those that have consensual validation within a given culture. *Consensual validation* means that what a person sees, hears, or touches is similar to what another person from the same milieu sees, hears, or touches. Disturbances of perception occur when the objects of the perception do not exist, do not have consensual validation, or both. This process is called *hallucinating*, and the experience itself is a *hallucination*. When the object of experience is present but is distorted in its nature or relation to the person, or when it is misidentified, the experience is called an *illusion*.

Hallucinations may occur in any of the sensory modalities—visual, auditory, gustatory, olfactory, or tactual—or they may be visceral (i.e., other body sensations) or experiential. Complex partial seizures represent a neuropsychiatric condition that must be considered in the differential diagnosis of perceptual disturbances and other psychotic disorders. (For a discussion of the evaluation of positive and negative psychotic symptoms, see Cepeda 2007, Chapter 2.) In the following case example, the examiner uses systematic questioning to ascertain the unsuspected diagnosis of complex partial seizures.

Case Example 8

Ralph, a 14-year-old mixed-race male, was admitted to an acute psychiatric care program for unrelenting suicidal ideation and serious conflicts with his mother. He had a background of gang involvement and other conduct disorder problems. Ralph lost his most important source of emotional support when his maternal grandfather died a short time before the admission. Ralph had been quite attached to his grandfather. Although his parents were divorced, they still continued a bitter relationship. Ralph was caught in a painful loyalty conflict because each parent was pressuring him to live with him or her. Ralph had witnessed his father abusing his mother physically and hated him for that. Ralph's medical background was positive for an episode of meningitis at age 15 months. He also had complained of "panic dreams" 2 years earlier, but a magnetic resonance imaging scan taken at the time was normal.

Ralph, who weighed 280 pounds, looked older than his stated age and appeared depressed. During the mental status examination, he denied hearing voices and denied visual hallucinations. When asked if he smelled any unusual smells, he readily reported olfactory and gustatory hallucinations: "An ugly smell, like a cadaver…a pretty bad taste, like rotten meat." While experiencing those hallucinations, he heard screeching, yelling, and beeping noises, and all of this was accompanied by a disturbance of consciousness and a sense of confusion for about 2 minutes. When this happened, he did not know what was going on. At times he felt like he was going to faint and his legs would get weak. During the previous summer, while playing basketball, Ralph's legs gave way after he experienced the olfactory hallucinations. He had a feeling of "strangeness" and experienced profuse sweating, even during the winter.

Additional exploration revealed that he had experienced déjà vu phenomena, dreams that foretold the future, and an urgency to urinate during these episodes. The diagnosis of complex partial seizures was substantiated; it had not been suspected initially.

Commanding auditory hallucinations are of particular clinical importance. The examiner should explore how strong the hallucinations are and what the child does when he or she hears the voices. Is the child able to fight them and resist their commands? Invariably, parents are skeptical about the validity of preadolescents' perceptual symptoms and need to be educated about them (see Note 1 at the end of this chapter).

A disturbance of perception may be centered in the sense of self, in the body image, or in aspects of the self-image. *Depersonalization* denotes a sense of strangeness in the sense of self; that is, the patient feels he or she is not the same as before or the child feels strange. This experience may be accompanied by a sense of confusion or bewilderment. This phenomenon occurs in affective disorders and dissociative states and is commonly observed in children with psychotic disorder.

When a girl with anorexia nervosa looks at the mirror and sees a fat person, she suffers from a *disturbance of perception of body image*, among other things. Disturbance of body image may be localized, as in the case of body dysmorphic disorder (when the patient thinks something is wrong with a specific body part). When the patient has a sense of internal body damage, uncorroborated by medical evidence and impervious to reassurance, the distortion is called *hypochondria*.

Out-of-body experiences are reported with some frequency. *Autoscopic hallucinations* are an uncommon experience in the field of child and adolescent psychiatry. A sense of the presence of a dead person, or even experiences such as talking to or hearing from dead people, are common for children during bereavement.

Delusions

Delusional thinking refers to a belief or system of beliefs without consensual validation in a given culture. *Ideas of reference* refer to the beliefs that everything the child perceives is related directly to himself or herself. The most common problems in this area relate to the belief that when people are talking or laughing, they are talking about or laughing at the patient. Some patients feel that people watch, spy on, or follow them. Others harbor persecutory delusions; these patients think that others are plotting to kill or harm them or their families. Patients may see signs in the environment that somehow convey a secret or special message to them. Delusions of guilt are described in Chapter 9, "Evaluation of Internalizing Symptoms" (see the cases of Salim and Fred [Case Examples 1 and 2, respectively]).

Children's concerns can sometimes be quite bizarre, as the following case examples show.

Case Example 9

Ted, an 8-year-old Caucasian male, reported that monsters were coming at night to exchange his blood for a green liquid. He was so terrified that he asked his father to cover the opening under his bed with a board. Ted believed that the monsters lived under the bed and that nailing the board there would keep the monsters from coming out.

Case Example 10

Mat, a 10-year-old Caucasian male, frequently worried that scorpions would come out from the shower head or climb into his bed while he slept. This child was ostracized, ridiculed, and rejected by his peers.

Extreme forms of disturbances of body image or body functions occur when the child complains that his or her body or body parts are damaged, or worse, that his or her insides may be "rotting." The following case examples illustrate the presence of such somatic delusions.

Case Example 11

Donna, a sophisticated and talented 16-year-old Caucasian female, was evaluated for intense and unremitting suicidal ideation. She had a long history of depression, dating back to when she was 7 years old. She had been a patient in a number of psychiatric hospitals. In explaining her sense of hopelessness, she reported that her "insides were rotten," that her "parts were dead inside." She acknowledged that 90% of her suicidal intent stemmed from that belief.

Case Example 12

Ming, a 16-year-old Asian American female and the mother of a 13-month-old infant, exhibited a severe major depressive episode with psychotic features. Besides commanding auditory hallucinations ordering her to kill herself, she had a deep-seated belief that she had cancer. No amount of reassurance or medical evidence could persuade her to the contrary.

In clinical practice, after the examiner observes the patient's thought processes, the following chain inquiry is useful: 1) systematic questioning regarding the presence of auditory, visual, olfactory, gustatory, tactual, and other atypical perceptions, such as depersonalization and out-of-body experiences;

2) systematic questioning about referential and persecutory ideation; and 3) systematic questioning regarding beliefs of thought intrusion or thought withdrawal. This line of inquiry may be completed with a full exploration of obsessive-compulsive symptomatology.

Thought Content

In addition to the concerns that the patient expresses, the examiner should note the presence of the following: 1) suicidal and homicidal ideation, 2) obsessional thinking, 3) compulsive activities, 4) alcohol and substance abuse, 5) gang involvement, and 6) other significant content not included elsewhere.

Judgment

The assessment of the patient's judgment should be based on observations and on the patient's response to specific situations presented during the psychiatric examination. A child is assumed to have good judgment if he or she gives a satisfactory answer to questions such as "What do you do if you are in a theater and you see smoke?" or "What do you do if you find a stamped envelope?" The determination regarding impairment of judgment needs to take into account the patient's history of chronic impulsivity and the patient's lack of forethought before carrying out impulsive actions. The patient's history tells far more about the patient's judgment than do his or her responses to standard questions. A clever and manipulative child may be able to give the right answers to hypothetical questions posed by the examiner, even though the child displays poor judgment in the real world.

Abstracting Ability

The assessment of the child's abstracting ability (i.e., capacity for categorical thinking) needs to take into account the child's cognitive development. A common but incorrect assumption is that when a person reaches late adolescence or adulthood, he or she has reached the cognitive developmental stage of formal operations. As such, this person should be capable of abstract thinking, as tested by similarities and interpretation of proverbs. Not everyone reaches this state of cognitive development. When they reach adulthood, children who are in the process of acquiring this cognitive sophistication should not be expected to perform well in this area, although some bright children do. In general, preadolescents and some adolescents tend to be concrete.

To assess abstracting ability, the examiner pays close attention to the patient's language and the sophistication of his or her responses. The examiner should also note the richness of the child's vocabulary and the manner with which the child discusses problems. For example, does the child use rich, complex, and metaphorical language?

Insight

Making judgments about a child's insight is difficult. Preadolescents begrudgingly acknowledge their problems, and adolescents more often than not only pay lip service to recognition of personal problems and express no willingness to change. Judgments about the presence of insight are based on the degree of the patient's dystonicity over the symptoms and his or her explicit desire to change.

Key Points

- Psychiatric examinations of children and adolescents are more nuanced than that of the adult. At all times, findings need to be correlated and developmental norms and expectations need to be documented systematically.
- The mental status examination of children and adolescents has many components that need to be considered in establishing a psychiatric diagnosis and creating a comprehensive treatment plan.
- Psychotic symptoms are not rare in child and adolescent practice.
- Psychotic symptoms should be explored systematically in every child and adolescent interview.
- Psychotic symptoms are rarely benign. They indicate severity of the psychiatric condition.
- Psychotic symptoms are associated with many psychiatric disorders.
- Psychosis does not equate with schizophrenia, though it may.

Notes

1. Hallucinations may be more prevalent in children than is commonly thought. As reported by Schreier (1999), Garralda (1984a, 1984b) distinguished nonpsychotic children who hallucinate from psychotic children: nonpsychotic children 1) are not delusional, 2) do not exhibit disturbance in language production, 3) do not exhibit decreased motor activity or incongruous mood, and 4) do not evidence bizarre behaviors or social withdrawal. Long-term follow-up of hallucinations has little prognostic

significance. In Schreier's (1999) view, "Hallucinations of critical voices or of those demanding that the patient do horrific acts to the self or to others do not predict severity or necessitate a poor prognosis" (p. 624). The presence of a single voice seems to indicate a good prognosis. The presence of internal versus external voices does not have any predictive value. Hallucinations may persist for several years without a major role in the child's functioning. Schreier (1999) has found an association between nonpsychotic hallucinations and migraine.

CHAPTER 9

Evaluation of Internalizing Symptoms

For didactic and organizational purposes, we distinguish in this book between internalizing and externalizing symptoms. The distinction often is not clear because of the intrinsic nature of a given disorder. Internalizing symptoms mostly affect the self and bring about subjective distress; externalizing symptoms mostly impact others and the environment due to acting-out behaviors. For example, in bipolar disorder, internalizing and externalizing symptoms are usually mixed. The distinction may also be blurred because of comorbid disorders (e.g., suicidal or depressive features in children who have conduct disorder). A mix of internalizing and externalizing symptoms is the rule rather than the exception in children and adolescents with psychiatric disorders.

Evaluation of Suicidal Behaviors

Suicide is the third leading cause of death in the United States for individuals ages 10–14 years, but the second leading cause of death for those ages 15–24 years (Centers for Disease Control and Prevention 2016). The most common methods of suicide are firearms, suffocation (including hanging), and poisoning (including overdosing). Whereas in the period from 1994 through 2012, the rates of suffocation increased for females (about 6.7% annually vs 2.2% for males), the rates of suicide by firearms decreased for both males and females from 10.9 to 5.9 per 100.000 and from 1.5 to 0.8 per 100.000, respectively (Wagner 2015, p. 50). Although it is good news that rates of suicide by firearm in their homes are decreasing, it is concerning that about one third of adolescents, at risk of suicide, have access to functioning firearms in their homes (Wagner 2015, p. 54) (see Note 1 at the end of this chapter). Following a decade of steady decline, the rate of suicide among U.S. youths who are younger than 20 years increased by 18% from 2003 to 2004. The rates of suicide for 2004 (4.74 per 100,000) and 2005 (4.49 per 100,000) were significantly greater than the expected rates based on 1996–2003 trends (Bridge et al. 2008).

Depression is a strong predictor of suicide attempts or completion; 79% of youths reported severe depression, and depression increased as youths, particularly males, progressed along the adolescent age along the continuum of suicide risk. Comorbidity was very important: 58% of youths had symptoms that fulfilled criteria for externalizing disorders, 53% had posttraumatic stress disorder, 30% displayed thought disorder problems, and 17% reported probable substance abuse problems (Asarnow et al. 2008) (see Note 2 at the end of this chapter). Consistent with a stress vulnerability model, increasing suicidal behavior risk was predicted by greater psychopathology, more life stresses, and particular stressors. Recent exposure to suicide, a breakup of a romantic relationship, a pregnancy event, and posttraumatic stress disorder increase an individual's suicide risk (Asarnow et al. 2008). Brent et al. (2015) demonstrated that children of parents with a history of suicidal behavior are about five times more likely than control children to display suicidal behavior; these children had an underlying impulsive aggression trait and developed a mood disorder during the study interval (5.6 years). Family and peer invalidation is another significant factor in adolescents' suicide. Surprisingly, a history of abuse (of any kind) did not reach a level of significance. Perceived family invalidation predicted suicidal events in males, and peer invalidation predicted self-mutilation in both males and females (Wagner 2015).

Suicidal crises are self-limiting and usually related to immediate stressors, such as a breakup with a boyfriend or girlfriend, conflicts with the family, school problems, or issues with drugs. As the acute phase of the crisis passes, so does the urge to attempt suicide: 90% of people who survive a suicide attempt, even a lethal attempt, do not go on to die by suicide (Miller and Hemenway 2008).

Pfeffer (1986) recommended that "all suicidal ideas and actions of children should be taken seriously and evaluated thoroughly and repeatedly" (p. 174). The evaluation of suicidal behavior entails the exploration of the what, how, when, where, how often, and why of suicidal behavior.

What refers to the nature of the suicidal behavior, including what the patient wishes to do and what he or she expects will happen if the action is accomplished. After the patient discloses that he or she wants to commit suicide in a particular way, the examiner needs to continue exploring alternative plans the patient may have (as in Matthew's case; see Chapter 2, "General Principles of Interviewing" [Case Example 3]). Consideration of multiple methods of suicide correlates with the child's determination to end his or her life; this indicates a great deal of hopelessness and despair and heightens the seriousness of the intent. An equally important exploration is whether the child expects to be rescued. High levels of aggression and impulsive traits increase the likelihood that suicidal ideation will progress to a suicide attempt. Furthermore, behavioral or conduct problems, substance abuse, and thought disorder are associated with lethal suicide attempts (Asarnow et al. 2008).

How refers to plans the child has conceived or steps the child may have already taken to kill himself or herself. The examiner assesses prior suicidal behaviors and the seriousness of current plans. Although death by firearm remains the most common mechanism for suicide among males ages 10–24, for females in the same age group, suffocation (including hanging) surpassed firearm as the most common mechanism for completed suicide (Sullivan et al. 2015). The examiner should carry out a detailed assessment of the means by which the child wants to actualize his or her intentions and pay particular attention to the child's access to weapons, medications, or toxic substances. The examiner determines how close the child is or has been to killing himself or herself so that necessary steps can be taken to ensure the child's safety.

When and *where* relate to the time and place planned for the suicide. Suicidal behavior may be connected temporally to significant events in the patient's life. As stated previously, common precipitating events include conflicts with the family or a recent breakup with a girlfriend or boyfriend. The recent death of someone close to the patient is a frequent precipitating event, particularly if the person died by suicide or died suddenly. If one of the patient's close friends has died by suicide, the examiner should ask the patient whether he or she had prior knowledge of the event or had ever made a suicide pact with the deceased. The examiner should explore the degree of guilt that the patient feels over the friend's death. Patients who have a depressive background are at greater risk of suicide following a close friend's suicide. Anniversaries are times of emotional reactivation of painful memories and unresolved guilt, and these occasions may activate suicidal behavior or fantasies of reunion with the deceased. When the patient is deeply emotionally connected to a dead person (e.g., grandparent, other relative, friend), the examiner should rule out the presence of psychotic features.

How much or *how often* relates to the frequency of the suicidal thoughts. The frequency correlates with the risk. The more the suicidal thinking erupts in the mind, the higher the suicide risk. Equally important is to know how long the suicidal thoughts "stick around"— "When the suicidal thoughts come to mind, what do you do with them? Do you let them be? Do you fight them?"— This exploration indicates how syntonic or dystonic these thoughts are.

In relation to *why*, the examiner should explore psychological factors that motivate the patient's suicidal ideation and behavior. Suicidal behaviors may be activated by many emotional states: helplessness; emotional pain; anger; worthlessness or devaluation; shame or humiliation; emptiness; nihilism; rejection or abandonment; loneliness or feelings of being unloved; disappointment or feelings of failure; hopelessness, despair, or futility; fears of a mental breakdown; feelings that a handicap or a medical illness is unacceptable; self-hatred; guilt; and many other negative, self-blaming, disorganizing, and pain-inducing subjective states. For a mnemonic tool regarding factors that need to be considered in the assessment of children and adolescents, refer to Table 9–1.

The systematic interviewing described above parallels Shea's (1998) Chronological Assessment of Suicidal Events (CASE) approach for the evaluation of suicidal behavior, which is described in Chapter 2, "General Principles of Interviewing." The questioning techniques of the CASE approach are used to explore the what, how, when, where, how often, and how "sticky" the suicide thoughts are. Table 9–1 addresses, as part of a mnemonic, areas of inquiry that are pertinent in the evaluation of suicide risk in children.

Individuals with a history of multiple suicide attempts are more likely to make subsequent attempts than are those with a history of a single attempt or no attempt. Some multiple suicide attempters wish to die, time their attempts so the interventions to help them are less likely, and regret recovery/survival from a suicide attempt. Multiple suicide attempters have more psychopathology at baseline (anxiety, mood, or substance abuse disorders); the presence of an anxiety disorder at the time of the attempt, along with a defined or uncertain wish to die, confers risks for future attempts. Single attempters and ideators do not differ regarding baseline diagnosis (Miranda et al. 2008). Single attempters and ideators deal with acute stressors that are likely to resolve more readily, whereas multiple suicide attempters deal with acute and chronic stressors and dispositional traits, such as impulsivity and aggression, as well as skills deficits such as limited problem-solving skills (Miranda et al. 2008).

In the evaluation of suicidal behavior in a child or adolescent, the examiner needs to consider the factor of intentionality. The intention to commit suicide is the source from which all suicidal behavior and a great deal of destructive behaviors derive. The following suicide letter, written by Myriam, expresses unambiguously what she had in mind when she attempted to end her life with a serious Tylenol overdose:

Table 9–1.   Mnemonic for suicidal assessment: THIS PATH IS DEATH

T houghts of suicide, suicide planning

H omicidal ideation, anger control difficulties

I nsomnia, feeling ineffective, feeling a burden

S substance abuse and alcohol problems

P rior suicidal attempts; psychosis

A buse history (physical, sexual, emotional abuse; neglect)

T erminations, losses, break ups, relocations, deaths

H opelessness, anticipating a bleak future

I mpulsivity, reckless behavior

S elf-esteem problems, narcissistic injuries, stressors: bullying, feeling unloved

D epression, irritability, hypomania

E lation, mania; eating disorders, low energy level

A anxiety, alienation, academic problems

T ired of life, feeling helpless, poor problem solving skills

H ome conflicts, family dysfunction; peer problems

Source.   Modified from Taliaferro et al. 2012.

To those it may concern,

If you are reading this I'm already dead. And IT WAS NOT AN ACCI-DENT! I didn't do this with selfish intent, I promise. Well, maybe a little.

I guess I'll go into my regrets and promises. My regrets are important but I have many confessions. Then I'll talk about my stuff. I want my stuff to go to some friends.

I regret not telling Mitchell how I felt about him. Just let him know how I reacted when he called, when he didn't, what I said about him, the effect he had on me, and how much he meant to me. Tell him…that he was the most important thing to me in the world. Tell him I love him more than life itself.

I also want to say I HATE MY SISTER! She's stupid, choking, competitive, snotty, bratty, bitchy, and kicks me whenever she can. I HATE HER!

Tell Mitchell I said thanks for always being there for me. Tell Theresa (my friend) thanks for always making me smile. Haley gets a thanks for letting me borrow her things and being my friend no matter what. Tell Emily . . . [unreadable]

I want to be buried six feet under with lilies and roses. I want all my friends there and teachers too. I want to be pretty, please, just to be nice. (Put on one of Mitchell's shirts.) Give Mitchell my penguins and let him go through my room to see what else he wants. Then show him this note and my poems in my purple and blue folders. Then let Emily look around please. Then Haley and everyone else.

I would like for you to call everyone in my address book and tell them I am gone. Please?

Just…I love you mom, but Dad…Heh.

Just tell Mitchell I love him and sort everything out! I love you.

Myriam

On another page, Myriam wrote the following list:

Reasons:
Guilt about Daniel
Ron's shit
Can't face school
No friends
Screwed-up family
So much stress
No comfort
Unloved
Too much pain
Too much hate
No point to keep going
I'm worthless
So much anger
My addictions
Ugly
Dad
Dad took Mitchell away

Confessions:
love Mitchell
hate my sister
words to friends

Wishes:
My funeral

Friends:
Eva
Mac
Emily
Haley
Mitchell
Jacob
Gregory
Jennifer
Robert

Myriam had been sexually assaulted 3 months before her suicide attempt, and her father was about to be deployed to the Middle East the following week. She took the overdose of acetaminophen after being punished by her dad for going to Mitchell's house and leaving her siblings unattended when she was supposed to babysit for them.

The examiner should explore whether the patient is experiencing auditory, commanding hallucinations, such as "voices" telling her to kill herself or

Table 9–2. Factors that affect bereavement risk after parental death

Poor outcome

    Loved one died suddenly

    Psychiatric history in the surviving parent

    Mother or caretaker is the parent who died

    Deceased parent had a high level of emotional involvement prior to death

    Child is from a higher socioeconomic bracket

No significant outcome

    Child's age or gender

Improved outcome

    Child has access to higher social supports, resilience in the surviving parent

Source.   Adapted from Schneiderman et al. 1996. Modified from Cepeda 2010, p. 203.

to commit other acts (e.g., to kill others). The voices may also tell the patient to join the deceased. The examiner should determine whether the patient is able to suppress these commands or is helpless against their overpowering influence. When suicidal behavior is unrelenting, the examiner should explore the possibility of psychotic guilt or other obsessive or delusional features (see Donna's case [Case Examples 4 and 11] in Chapter 2, "General Principles of Interviewing" and Chapter 8, "Documenting the Examination").

Another important line of questioning relates to recent deaths of loved ones. Schneiderman et al. (1996) reviewed a number of studies to determine factors that increase or lower the bereavement risk when a parent or child dies. These factors are listed in Table 9–2.

In assessing a child's current suicide risk, the examiner needs to evaluate the child's current psychological status and consider the ongoing family and environmental conditions. Pfeffer (1991) warned that "the status of these variables may change rapidly, so…a repeated, comprehensive discussion with a suicidal youngster is necessary" (p. 670). Pfeffer stressed the need to assess the family's level of functioning and the circumstances surrounding the child: "It is important to determine whether the family can provide a consistent, stable environment or whether there is a high intensity of stress, violence, and psychopathology and unavailability of relatives. Positive social supports are critical in diminishing suicide risk among children and adolescents with suicidal intentions" (p. 670).

Since the risk of suicidal ideation and aggression is doubled in children and adolescents taking antidepressant medications compared with those taking placebo, the psychiatric monitoring should be increased to identify these negative side effects (Sharma et al. 2016). An editorial by Moncrieff (2016) regarding the Sharma et al. (2016) article detailed glaring discrepancies between results reported in the clinical study reports and data from individual patients' listings and narratives. There was clear evidence of underreporting of suicidal ideation and behavior.

Because suicidal behavior and self-abusive behavior do not necessarily belong to the same psychopathological domains, they need to be examined separately. The management and prognosis of these behaviors are very different.

Explanations offered by the child or the family should not derail the examiner from exploring the motivations or reasons for the child's suicidal behaviors. Following a child's serious suicidal behavior, parents sometimes claim that the child was simply seeking attention. Children often offer the same excuse. Less commonly, children blame dissociative episodes in which they disconnect with or deny the seriousness of suicidal experiences. The examiner should not ask the child, "Did you really intend to kill yourself?" This judgment is the examiner's to make, not the child's. Revelations of abuse should not be disregarded after the patient recants them; the same holds true for statements that a suicidal behavior lacks intent. The factors considered in the evaluation of suicide attempts are also relevant to the overall assessment of suicidal behavior (Spirito et al. 1989). Table 9–3 summarizes the areas the examiner should consider in evaluating a child's suicide attempts.

Family conflicts, family disorganization, or major stressors within the family have direct influence in the child's suicidal actions. Berman and Carroll (1984) discussed family factors that contribute to suicidal behaviors: "The motives for suicide attempts of adolescents appear largely directed towards effecting change in or escape from an interpersonal system" (p. 60). On dealing with the close relatives of suicidal children, Berman and Carroll (1984) wrote,

> As essential as it is to view parents as "first finders," to identify and provide assistance to the precipitously or potentially suicidal child, these parents may be [the] least equipped to accomplish these tasks. Because of their own pathology; their intimate relationship with and, therefore, blind spots to their children; and/or the implicit and explicit blame levied by having a suicidal child, most parents deny, minimize, distort, etc. and only notice after (and, perhaps, only because of) a suicide attempt. (p. 60)

The psychiatrist has a duty and professional responsibility to take all the necessary steps to prevent a patient from killing himself or herself. This goal needs to be tempered, however, by the psychiatrist's limited capacity to pre-

Table 9–3. Pertinent areas of inquiry in examining children who have attempted suicide

Suicidal fantasies and actions

Anticipations and consequences of the suicidal act

Circumstances at the time of the suicidal behavior

Motivations for suicidal behavior

Experiences and concepts of death

History of suicide in the family or in close friends

Exploration of depression and other affective states

Exploration of family and environmental circumstances

History of a recent loss (e.g., break up with a loved one)

Use of alcohol or drugs

History of physical or sexual abuse

Family conflict, domestic violence

Exploration of recent and ongoing stressors

Source. Adapted from Pfeffer 1986. Modified from Cepeda 2010, p. 201.

dict suicidal behavior. Shaffer (1996) offered a thoughtful reminder: "In even the most troubled patient, suicide is a rare event whose eventuality and precise timing defy accurate prediction. Although a well-supervised environment may significantly reduce opportunities to commit suicide, a determined patient may circumvent supervision by feigning recovery and denying suicidal preoccupations" (p. 172). To this, he added a sobering comment: "For both the clinician and the public health official the message could be that we do not currently have a scale that will predict either a further suicide attempt or ultimate death by suicide with any useful accuracy" (Shaffer 1996, p. 173). This assertion is still true today (2016).

Goodyer (1992) also offered some caveats about the identification of suicidal behaviors:

> The presence of dysphoria may increase and maintain the risk for suicidal behavior in the population at large. Both clinical and community studies indicate, however, that in adolescents major depression is not a prerequisite for suicidal behavior. In addition, the association between thoughts and acts of suicide in this age group remains unclear....By contrast, complete suicide appears to be commonly associated with features of major depression....Such cases [completed suicide] appear likely to be comorbid for antisocial and interpersonal aggression [impulsive aggression]. (p. 589)

Therefore, family factors related to suicidal behaviors need to be examined carefully and exhaustively. The examination of suicide risk demands a thorough assessment of the family's functional level, family factors that contribute to precipitating events, the family's understanding of its role in the child's suicidal behavior, the family's commitment to ensuring the child's safety, and the family's determination to prioritize its emotional and financial resources for the treatment of the child and the improvement of the family's functioning.

When the child psychiatrist concludes that the child is actively suicidal and that the family cannot guarantee the child's safety (e.g., because of denial or minimization of the suicidal experience), measures should be taken to safeguard the child's life (e.g., hospitalization or involuntary commitment).

Evaluation of Depressive Symptoms

The identification of mood disorders (i.e., depression and mania) poses significant clinical challenges to the child psychiatrist. Mania poses more challenges than depression does. (Mania is discussed more fully in Chapter 10, "Evaluation of Externalizing Symptoms.")

Clinical depression varies in the nature and intensity of its presenting symptoms. The examiner should attempt to elicit as complete a picture of a child's depressive syndrome as possible by identifying a variety of symptoms associated with this disorder and by estimating their severity.

Cardinal Features

The examiner should explore the cardinal symptoms of depression. In exploring a patient's depressive mood, the examiner should inquire about the presence of sadness. Unlike depression, sadness is a word universally recognized by children. When the examiner is exploring sadness with the child, pertinent questions include the following: "Do you feel sad?" "How often do you feel sad?" "When do you feel sad?" "How bad does it get?" "What is the worst it has ever been?" "How long does it last?" "When you feel sad, what do you feel like doing?" "When you feel sad, is there anything that helps you to feel better?" Because crying is common in children who are depressed, the following questions should be asked: "How often do you cry?" "When you feel like crying, what comes to your mind?"

Also pertinent are questions aiming to ascertain how long the child has been sad. "How old were you when you started to feel sad? Since you started feeling sad, has there been any time when you have not been sad?" In the same vein of questioning, the examiner may ask, "How old were you when you thought about suicide for the first time?"

Feeling Unloved

In general, small children feel depressed when they feel or believe they are unloved, whatever the reasons may be. Serious family events—such as parental desertion, neglect, or discord; family violence; physical abuse; and other adversities—need to be identified. Deployment of a parent is a major event in the lives of military families. This event is fraught with a high level of anxiety and fear.

Many parents are late in recognizing depression in their children, in spite of obvious signs. These parents may not realize the magnitude of depression until their child's adaptive behavior at home and school seriously deteriorates, until the child has expressed his or her despair in the form of suicidal or other self-destructive behaviors, or until the child has fallen victim to a devastating drug abuse problem.

Constitutional Factors

Constitutional dysregulation of affect is an important factor in the origin of depressive affect. This problem starts very early in life and is manifested by irritability, temper tantrums, low tolerance for frustration, unhappiness, and limited response to soothing and loving care. The disturbance is enduring and creates a great deal of distress in caregivers because nothing seems to soothe these children. Children with a difficult temperament are usually a bad match for impatient parents, more so if the parents have mood dysregulations of their own. Akiskal (1995) described the concept of *temperament dysregulation*, also called *subaffective temperament.* He noted that these concepts refer to specific constitutionally based affective dispositions (e.g., melancholic-dysthymic, choleric–irritable, sanguine-hyperthymic, cyclothymic) that are manifested predominantly at the subclinical level. These dispositions "are distressing and disruptive and are in a continuum with major mood states" (p. 756). Thus, moody behavior, angry outbursts, and explosive episodes must be explored. Marked irritability is a behavioral change that many parents observe in their depressed children. For example, children may start displaying verbally, if not physically, abusive behavior toward their parents and siblings. (In the current diagnostic era [DSM-5; American Psychiatric Association 2013], the evaluator needs to consider Disruptive Mood Dysregulation Disorder, which is discussed below.) Other forms of aggressive acting-out behaviors, such as defiant and rebellious behaviors, are also common complaints.

Irritability

Irritability is a prevalent mood in depressed children and often generates a stable dysphoric affect. Many children identify this mood as soon as they wake up in the morning. The following question may be helpful: "When you first open your eyes in the morning, how do you feel?" These children are hyperreactive; anything can set them off. Any demand is upsetting, and any expectation is too much for them. These children are prone to exhibit explosive behavior or to lose control. Parents frequently complain that these children are moody, if not violent. Pertinent questions to ask include the following: "How often do you feel grouchy (irritable)?" "What does it take for you to feel grouchy?" "When you feel grouchy, how long do you feel like that?" "Is there anything that makes the grouchy feelings go away?" "Do you have a temper?" "What happens when you lose your temper?" These questions may be followed by exploration of potential aggression against the self (suicidal, self-abusive behavior), against others (violent and assaultive behaviors), or against the physical environment (e.g., destructiveness, vandalism).

Guilt

Guilt and its sources need to be identified. Children often feel responsible for things they have not caused. The following questions are helpful in identifying guilty feelings: "Is there anything for you to feel bad about?" "Is there anything you feel you need to be punished for?" In extreme cases, guilt takes a psychotic quality, as when the child feels responsible for the ills of the world and beyond. The following case example illustrates a form of psychotic guilt.

Case Example 1

Salim, the 8-year-old son of a Lebanese father and an American mother, was hospitalized for unrelenting suicidal ideation. He had overt psychotic features: he complained that aliens were after him. Salim's parents were divorced but maintained a bitter and hostile relationship. Salim's custody was still an issue, and he was caught in a loyalty conflict between his parents.

When watching television programs about the country's most wanted criminals, Salim would ask his mother to call the FBI to report that he was the person they were looking for. He also blamed himself for the war in the Middle East, for worldwide pollution problems, and so on. These delusional beliefs were impervious to reassurance or to reality testing.

At other times, guilt is latent but can be brought readily to the surface, as illustrated in the following case example.

Case Example 2

Fred, a 12-year-old Caucasian male, was admitted to an acute psychiatric setting because he set fire to the blankets and mattress where his younger brother was sleeping. His brother sustained second- and third-degree burns. During the interview, Fred appeared sad and downcast. The examiner told Fred that he didn't look happy and asked, "When was the last time you were happy?"

Fred became tearful but tried not to cry. Upon seeing this emotional struggle, the examiner said, "Can you share with me what is going on in your mind right now? You are trying very hard not to cry." Fred attempted to control his tears but finally broke down, and tears started pouring down his cheeks. Holding his head in his hands, he said, "I can't believe what I did to my brother." He continued sobbing and expressing sorrow, saying, "I burnt my brother."

Fred began displaying signs of genuine emotion; the emotional abreaction was clearly associated with guilt. Fred revealed that he had heard voices commanding him to kill his brother. This revelation clinched the diagnosis of a psychotic depression.

The concept of a bad parent is an alien concept for a child. A great deal of psychological growth and cognitive development are needed to appreciate that one's parents have flaws. Children who endure parental abuse usually blame themselves for the abuse. Similarly, if a parent abandons a child, the child usually feels that she did something that pushed the parent away.

Emotional Withdrawal

Emotional withdrawal occurs in many depressed children. Depressed children seek solitude and withdraw from family and peer interactions. Parents report that such children do not participate in family activities or that they withdraw to their rooms, refuse to be with friends, and so on. Helpful questions include the following: "Do you have any friends?" "How are you getting along with your friends?" "Do you have a best friend?" "How much time do you spend with your best friend?" "Do you enjoy your friends?" "What kind of groups or fun (social) activities do you participate in?"

Anhedonia

Anhedonia is evidenced when the child no longer feels happy, cannot have fun anymore, or cannot join in pleasurable activities. Pertinent questions include the following: "When was the last time you felt happy?" "In a given week, how many days do you feel happy?" "What kinds of things can you do to feel happy?" "Is it OK for you to be happy?" The child's history will indicate whether previous interests in sports or in other activities are no longer important to the child. Formerly athletic children no longer display interest in their favorite sports. When invited to participate in games, they refuse, or when they do agree to take part, their participation is perfunctory; they simply go through the motions.

Hopelessness

Hopelessness needs to be identified. Signs of hopelessness include behaviors that indicate the child feels there is nothing worthwhile to live for anymore;

these children may attempt to dispose of valuable belongings (e.g., giving away music compact discs, baseball cards, or other collectibles). Hopelessness is obvious in the presence of unremitting suicidal behavior or when the child considers multiple alternatives for committing suicide. Typically, when the child is experiencing such feelings—no matter how good the options presented to the child are and no matter how positive some alternatives may be—the child's characteristic and disheartened response is, "I don't care" or "It doesn't matter."

Feeling Tired

Depressed children complain of being tired; this complaint is present from the moment they wake up and usually remains throughout the day. The sense of tiredness contributes to the depressed child's lack of motivation, loss of interest in school, and problems with concentration. Tiredness is also secondary to sleep problems that are common in depressed children.

Sleep Problems

Depressed children frequently have marked difficulty with sleep. Falling asleep (initial insomnia) may be the most significant complaint. When they do fall asleep, they frequently wake up during the night and have trouble going back to sleep (middle insomnia). Problems with terminal insomnia occur when depressed children wake up very early in the morning (e.g., at 4:00 A.M.) and are unable to fall asleep again. For depressed children, sleep is seldom refreshing. When the time to wake up arrives, depressed children prefer to stay in bed, in part because getting up requires effort. Not surprisingly, many depressed children fall asleep during school or invert their biorhythm (i.e., by sleeping during the day and staying up at night). Many parents struggle every morning to get depressed children ready for school. Tardiness and absenteeism from school may be revealing. Frequently, parents are unaware of the presence or severity of their child's sleep difficulties. Tiredness in a child who has no known medical problem should raise suspicion of a depressive disorder. In atypical depressions, children display hypersomnia and sleep a great deal.

Weight Changes

Another contributor to tiredness is limited food intake due to a lack of appetite. Many depressed children lose weight even though they are not making any conscious effort to do so. Failure to gain weight in small children is an equivalent sign. Children with atypical depressions may show an appetite increase and may gain weight.

Academic Problems

Deterioration in academic performance or behavior at school is a common complication of depressed mood. The child's grades suffer for a number of reasons: poor motivation (lack of interest), tiredness, or impaired concentration. This last impairment is common in depressed children. Bad conduct in school is a consequence of dysphoria (e.g., due to irritability and low tolerance for frustration).

Psychomotor Activity

Hyperactivity, restlessness, and agitation sometimes occur in depressed children. These symptoms may be intrinsic to the disorder or may represent the expression of associated comorbid conditions, such as attention-deficit/hyperactivity disorder (ADHD) or anxiety disorders. More frequently, depressed children display slowness in psychomotor activity. Children with prominent melancholic features exhibit a marked decrease in the psychomotor sphere; in extreme cases, the examiner may observe signs of catatonia.

Negative Cognitions

Negative cognitions (e.g., feelings of worthlessness, personal devaluation, and poor self-concept), concentration or memory difficulties, and suicidal ideation are common in depressive disorders. Suicidal ideation and suicidal behavior must be explored systematically in all depressed patients.

Illegal Drug Use

In an attempt to deal with dysphoric affect, depressed children may start using alcohol or drugs. When they do not get the nurturing and understanding they need in their home environment, some children seek a sense of belonging in alternative family groups, such as gangs or cults.

Comorbidities

Because the length of depression and the number of depressive episodes have diagnostic, therapeutic, and prognostic implications, the examiner should strive to determine these factors. Depressive disorders are commonly associated with anxiety disorders, oppositional defiant disorder, conduct disorder, substance use disorders, obsessive-compulsive disorder (OCD), and ADHD.

Psychotic Features

When working with depressed children, the examiner needs to pay particular attention to psychotic features (i.e., auditory and visual hallucinations and paranoid features), which are common in severe depressions. Of particular importance is the identification of auditory hallucinations that command the patient to kill himself or herself. If these perceptual disturbances are identified, the examiner should ask whether the voices also command the patient to hurt or to kill anyone else. Suicidal and homicidal auditory commands frequently coexist.

Family Factors

A question that typically comes up concerns what role a parent's or grandparent's depression has on a child's mood disorder. Tully et al. (2008) found that having a depressed mother increased the risk of psychopathology during adolescence, but having a depressed father produced no such a risk. The noxious maternal effect was present even in families in which mother and child shared no biological relationship, indicating that a depressed mother posed a significant environmental risk for the offspring (Tully et al. 2008). A significant interaction also occurred between grandparents' and parents' major depressive disorder and young children's internalizing symptoms (Olino et al. 2008). Grandparents' major depressive disorder, even in the absence of major depressive disorder in the parents, was associated with an increase in internalizing symptoms in the grandchildren. Major depressive disorder can have effects that persist for multiple generations, and clinicians should obtain an extended family history to evaluate the effect on children (Olino et al. 2008).

Maternal Depression

The majority of investigations show that improvement in mothers' depression as a result of either medication or psychosocial therapy is positively correlated with improvements in their children (i.e., reduction of psychopathology and improvement in key areas of functioning) (see Note 3 at the end of this chapter). Consistent evidence indicates that the reduction or remission of parental depression is related to the reduction of children's symptoms and that these child effects are maintained (Gunlicks and Weissman 2008). According to Swartz et al. (2008), brief psychotherapy in mothers whose children were receiving psychiatric treatment lowered the levels of symptoms and increased the levels of functioning in their children. The positive impact of improvement of maternal depression on the child lagged by 6 months (Swartz et al. 2008). The inclusion of a history of parental mental health treatment (previous and ongoing) should also occur (see Note 4 at the end of this chapter).

Mood Disorders in Father

The role of fathers in childhood depression is rarely studied, although fathers may have a significant impact on depression in their offspring. A clear association between depression in fathers during the postnatal period and later psychiatric disorders in their children was demonstrated in a cohort population study (Ramchandani et al. 2008). This association was independent of maternal postnatal depression, psychosocial risk, and depression in the father after the postnatal period (when the child was age 21 months). Depression in men is relatively common; depression in fathers during the postnatal period was associated with oppositional defiant disorder and conduct disorder in children 7 years later (Ramchandani et al. 2008). Depression in fathers was associated with behavioral and peer relationship problems (antisocial behavior), whereas maternal depression appeared to be associated with a broad spectrum of child disturbances (Ramchandani et al. 2008). The findings of these various studies obligate the child psychiatrist to explore and to identify depression in the parents and grandparents and to recommend appropriate and prompt treatment when indicated.

Differential Diagnosis

In the differential diagnosis of depression, bipolar disorder poses the biggest challenge. Accurate identification of bipolar disorder is necessary because of the heightened suicide risk, the declared risks associated with antidepressant treatments, and the difficulties associated with achieving mood stabilization. The severe clinical course and complications associated with bipolar disorder increase the patient's risks of suicidality, psychosocial dysfunction, and comorbidity risks (e.g., conduct disorder, substance abuse, school and family dysfunction). About one-third or more of the children who are diagnosed with depression eventually develop bipolar disorder. Bowden and Rhodes (1996) highlighted the following features commonly associated with bipolar depression: positive family history of bipolar disorder, psychomotor retardation rather than agitation, psychotic or delusional features, hypersomnia, and a rapid onset rather than an insidious presentation.

DSM-5 (American Psychiatric Association 2013) now includes the diagnosis of disruptive mood dysregulation disorder (DMDD). The criteria for this disorder differ from those of other depressive disorders or intermittent explosive disorder in that hallmark features include frequent (at least three times a week), disproportionately intense outbursts of physical and verbal aggression that occur within the context of a persistently irritable, angry mood in between tantrums. These outbursts should be developmentally inappropriate; therefore, an age less than 6 is an exclusionary criterion for this diagnosis. The clinician should ascertain developmental level, mood between tantrum episodes, and dimensional aspects of the tantrums (frequency, intensity, and duration) to assist in distinguishing DMDD from a more discrete depressive episode.

An important clinical caveat in the evaluation of depression in children is that some children do not display depressive features during the psychiatric examination (are they cancelling them?), but this does not mean that they do not have a depressive disorder. Consider the following case example.

Case Example 3

Lillian, a 14-year-old Caucasian female, was evaluated for episodes of running away, aggression toward her mother, and rebelliousness and defiance directed at her parents. Lillian had threatened her mother a number of times and had become progressively more violent toward her. Lillian was markedly ambivalent toward her mother: when feeling close to her mother, she began to act out against her or ran away. Sometimes she ran away to avoid striking her mother.

Lillian's mother reported that her daughter had become increasingly dysphoric over the preceding 5 months, especially during the prior 2 months. Lillian had become irritable, explosive, and even physically abusive toward her younger half-siblings, too. Her academic performance had deteriorated: she was getting D's and F's, although previously she had gotten A's and B's. She had lost about 20 pounds in 4 months. Lillian had begun to defy her parents' rules and to confront her parents regarding curfew and other restrictions.

Lillian had befriended gang members and experimented with marijuana and drinking. She had no legal problems other than the charge of running away. Lillian was still a virgin; however, she confessed that her current boyfriend had been putting pressure on her to have sex. Lillian was about 7 years old when her stepgrandfather fondled her. He was prosecuted and sent to prison for fondling Lillian and other granddaughters.

Lillian reported that a number of her friends had died. Most recently, two teenage friends had been killed in a drive-by shooting. A rival gang member had killed her closest friend, a 16-year-old gang member whom she considered a brother. This had been a significant loss for her; she dreamed about her dead friend and mentioned him frequently in her writings, letters, and poetry.

Lillian had no psychiatric history despite two previous suicide attempts. In the latest attempt, she had overdosed on many over-the-counter pills while under the influence of alcohol and marijuana. The first attempt occurred a year earlier, when she had overdosed on over-the-counter medications. Lillian's 18-year-old sister had a stormy adolescence that included multiple hospitalizations and extensive psychiatric treatments. She had been given the diagnosis of bipolar disorder, which was being treated with lithium.

Lillian appeared somewhat older than her stated age. She was not very attractive; she had a prominent forehead and a conspicuous overbite. She was anxious and fidgeted throughout the examination. Her mood was considered anxious—there were no obvious depressive features, but her affect was constricted in range and intensity. She denied suicidal and homicidal ideation. She appeared to be intelligent. Her language was unremarkable for receptive and expressive functions. Her sensorium was clear. Her thought content related to her conflicts with and anger toward her mother, the loss of her close friends, and issues related to her discontent with her body (she had a well-endowed bosom and was self-conscious about it). She exhibited no evidence of hallucinations or delusional thinking. She had some degree of insight, but her judgment was impaired.

Even though Lillian appeared euthymic during the mental status examination, her history and overall clinical picture, plus the family history of affective disorders, were compatible with a depressive disorder. Lillian displayed a number of atypical depressive features and was given the diagnosis of mood disorder, unspecified. A number of factors may have influenced the patient's deceptive emotional display: drugs, a mixed mood state, an attachment disorder, and others.

The examiner needs to keep in mind some additional information about depression. Depressive disorders have a variety of negative prognostic features (Table 9–4). Even in manic patients, depression is a prevailing symptom; despair, hopelessness, and suicidal behavior are either overt or close to the surface in every patient with mania or hypomania. Also, up to 20% of schizophrenia cases have an onset after a depressive episode (Remschmidt 2008).

Evaluation of Anxious Symptoms

The following case example illustrates many issues common in anxious children. It also depicts the relationship between anxiety disorders and depressive disorders.

Case Example 4

Glenn, a 9-year-old Caucasian male, was referred for a psychiatric evaluation because of concerns about a progressive depression with ongoing suicidal verbalizations. Glenn, his mother, and her male friend sat down for the family evaluation, and Glenn began to present his concerns in a very coherent and articulate way. He became the main spokesperson for the group. As he was talking and responding to minor cues, Glenn's mother and her friend assented to most of what he said. Their nonverbal behavior indicated that they supported his disclosures and history presentation. At no point did Glenn's mother contradict him. He spoke with significant anxiety and with marked intensity. A child is rarely so active during a psychiatric examination.

Glenn reported that he began to feel depressed about 2 months prior to the psychiatric assessment. He had become very grouchy, and when upset, he would hit walls and stomp his feet. He was assaultive toward his younger brothers (ages 5 and 6). Glenn was moody and had problems falling asleep; he woke up in the middle of the night and complained of nightmares. Glenn also had difficulties with his appetite. He had been thinking about suicide with increasing intensity but had developed no plans. He cried on a regular basis.

A tense custody dispute occurred when Glenn's parents divorced 5 years earlier. Glenn's mother remarried but then divorced her second husband a year before this evaluation. Glenn stated that he would rather kill himself than go to live with his father. Glenn's father had been very abusive to his mother; Glenn had seen his mother being beaten many times. Glenn had also wit-

Table 9–4.   Negative prognostic features of depressive disorders

Affective disorders are frequently recurrent conditions.

Depressive disorders increase the risk of suicidal behaviors.

Depressive disorders are frequently associated with comorbid conditions such as oppositional defiant disorder, conduct disorder, substance use disorders, anxiety disorders, and even psychotic features.

Depressive disorders have a detrimental effect on psychological and interpersonal development.

Depressive disorders interfere with school academic progress and other adaptive functions.

Children with depressive disorder have a significant risk of developing bipolar disorders with added risks of suicide and other comorbidities.

Depressive disorders are associated with suicidal and homicidal behaviors.

Source.   Modified from Cepeda 2010, p. 205.

nessed his father attempting to kill his mother on more than one occasion (his father had shot, stabbed, and battered Glenn's mother in front of him). According to Glenn, his younger brothers were equally afraid of their father, and their father shot Glenn's dog in the head right in front of him. There were also reports that Glenn had got drunk once after his father gave him alcohol. There were no indications that Glenn had tried or used any other substances.

Glenn worried a lot about his mother. He was afraid something bad could happen to her and was protective of her. His mother said that she had post-traumatic stress disorder secondary to physical, sexual, and emotional abuse perpetrated by Glenn's father. She worked at a nightclub. Glenn didn't like her job and worried about it. The mother came to the evaluation inappropriately dressed in revealing shorts and blouse.

Glenn's mother broke down when her son revealed that his father had sexually abused him. She needed a great deal of reassurance and support, both from her male companion and from the examiner. The mother had initially misrepresented the companion as a brother; he was her current boyfriend. Glenn's mother appeared helpless and on the verge of tears throughout the interview. She changed the focus from Glenn's concerns to her own a number of times.

Glenn felt very close to his grandparents, but his mother had concerns about them because of their drinking. The most recent stressors for the family had been the family's recent relocation from Okinawa, Japan, and the mother's separation from her second husband.

Two years prior to the evaluation, Glenn saw a psychiatrist after one of his younger brothers had been sexually molested by his stepfather's brother. Glenn had been diagnosed with a gastric ulcer a year and a half earlier and was taking antacids on a regular basis. Glenn had been educated abroad because of his father's military career; he completed third grade in Okinawa and was currently attending advanced classes in fourth grade at the local school. Because of ongoing somatic complaints, Glenn was absent from school at least once a week. He enjoyed sports, including hockey and swimming.

The mental status examination revealed a handsome, well-dressed, and articulate 9-year-old boy who appeared to be his chronological age. He was cooperative and was an excellent historian. He gave a coherent account of his problems and fears, with minimal participation from his mother. He appeared depressed, tense, and anxious. His affect was increased in intensity but appropriate. He reported passive suicidal ideation with no plans. His thought processes were unremarkable; there was no evidence of delusional or hallucinatory experiences. His thought content centered on fears about his natural father, fears about his mother, worries that something bad would happen to him, and bad feelings in his stomach. Glenn's level of intelligence appeared above average. He appeared to have excellent verbal skills and good receptive language. His sensorium was intact, and his judgment and insight were good. Glenn had indicated to his mother that he needed psychological help.

In Glenn's case, a depressive disorder could be considered the predominant condition, and an anxiety disorder could be considered its major comorbid condition; however, the clinical picture could have been interpreted the other way around. Anxiety features had been the most prominent psychopathology throughout Glenn's life. Somatization had been a major problem, and a physician had diagnosed Glenn's anxious epigastric distress as a manifestation of a gastric ulcer. Obviously, Glenn qualified for a PTSD diagnosis.

Not all anxious children are as forthcoming as Glenn. The examiner more frequently encounters patients who become electively mute during the psychiatric examination. Verbally engaging these children can be a challenge. The examiner needs time and patience and may also need to engage the nonverbal child with use of nonverbal techniques (see Chapter 3, "Special Interviewing Techniques").

Anxiety symptoms that are commonly endorsed by preadolescents are excessive concerns about competence, excessive need for reassurance, fear of harm to an attachment figure, fear of the dark, and somatic complaints (Bernstein et al. 1996). The most frequently endorsed anxiety symptoms by adolescents are fear of heights, fear of public speaking, blushing, excessive worrying about past behavior, and self-consciousness (Bernstein et al. 1996).

Children who develop anxiety disorders have antecedents of *behavioral inhibition*. This condition should be considered an enduring temperamental trait. Behavioral inhibition is indicated by a tendency to withdraw, to be unusually shy, and to show fear in the presence of novelty. Demonstrable physiological markers include higher stable heart rates during tasks that require cognitive effort; tension of the larynx and vocal cords; elevated salivary cortisol levels; elevated catecholamine levels; and pupillary dilation during cognitive tasks (Bernstein et al. 1996). Attachment difficulties in infancy probably predispose children to the development of anxiety disorders later in childhood (Bernstein et al. 1996). The following areas of symptomatology need to be explored on a regular basis in anxious children.

Separation Anxiety

Anxious children display separation difficulties. Frequently, school refusal problems bring these children to the child psychiatrist for the first time. These children are afraid of being alone and are clingy and dependent on their caregivers. Anxious children are unable to enjoy the thrills of a slumber party because they are uncomfortable venturing beyond their own homes. They have great difficulty sleeping in their own beds and often go to the parents' room to sleep with them. Separation anxiety is a nonspecific precursor for a number of adult psychiatric conditions, including depression and a variety of anxiety disorders (Bernstein et al. 1996). Separation anxiety in adolescence is a very serious and incapacitating condition.

Worrying

Worrying is a common symptom. Anxious children worry that something bad may happen to their parents or complain of vague or ill-defined apprehensions. For example, they fear that "something bad" may happen to them or their primary caretakers or their family as a whole.

Fears

Fears of the dark or of storms and other specific phobias are common. Fear usually intensifies at night; a child may want to sleep with parents because of fear that something bad might happen to him or her or to the parents. Schildkrout (2015, p. 5) states that clinicians need to differentiate anxiety from fear; fear may be associated with seizures. If the patient experiences fear or a sense of dread or impending doom, sensations in the chest or abdomen, frequent déjà vu experiences, and/or alterations in one's sense of reality (including dissociative experiences, olfactory, gustatory or sound hallucinations, and kinesthetic or visual illusions or hallucinations), he or she needs a neurological workup.

Social Phobia

Social phobia is a common impediment for anxious children. They are very self-conscious and prone to feelings of embarrassment and shame. These children suffer a lot when asked to go in front of the class or to speak in front of a group. Anxious children are doubtful, are insecure, and have poor self-esteem; they need frequent reassurance and support; and they commonly have problems initiating and maintaining friendships. Social phobias that begin in early and middle adolescence are particularly problematic. Anxious adolescents display excessive anxiety about social situations or performing in front of others because they fear scrutiny by and exposure to unfamiliar persons. For this diagnosis to apply, the anxiety should occur in peer situations, and the ability for age-appropriate relationships with familiar people must be evident (Bernstein et al. 1996).

Somatization

Somatization is a common phenomenon in anxious children. Nausea, vomiting, and epigastric pain or distress frequently accompany anxiety disorders. As Glenn's case illustrated (see Case Example 4), these children are often incorrectly diagnosed with medical illnesses, such as peptic ulcers or irritable bowel syndrome. Anxious children also complain of chest pain, dizziness, headaches, and other somatic symptoms. Many anxious children with epigastric distress undergo unnecessary X rays, endoscopic procedures, or cardiovascular evaluations. Other anxious children make multiple visits to the pediatrician or family physician for somatic complaints. Panic symptoms are increasingly being recognized in pediatric populations.

Elective Mutism

The evolving consensus is that elective mutism represents an anxiety disorder. Black and Uhde (1995) reported that "in 97% [of cases], there was clear evidence of significant social, academic, or family impairment due to social anxiety, other than that attributable to the failure to speak, sufficient for a diagnosis of SP [social phobia] or avoidant disorder" (p. 854).

Physical and Sexual Abuse

Many anxious children have a history of physical and sexual abuse and have been raised in environments in which marital discord and overt family dysfunction are commonplace. Evaluation of symptoms of abuse is discussed in Chapter 11, "Evaluation of Abuse and Other Symptoms."

Anxiety Features Within the Family

Children who have severe anxiety disorders often have other family members who exhibit incapacitating anxiety symptoms. The examiner should inquire if the parents are anxious or depressed. The family exploration regarding the presence of mood and anxiety disorders should be extended to the two prior generations. The following case exemplifies this situation.

Case Example 5

Aurora, a 9-year-old Hispanic female, was evaluated for school refusal. She had prominent somatic complaints and, because of persistent epigastric discomfort, had been diagnosed with a peptic ulcer. She had undergone endoscopy and an upper gastrointestinal series. Aurora's mother had a crippling anxiety disorder with prominent agoraphobic features. Her maternal grandfather had quit grammar school and never returned because of severe anxiety features; he had remained agoraphobic most of his life.

Mood Disorders

Anxiety disorders are commonly comorbid with mood disorders, and vice versa. Judd and Burrows (1992) proposed three models to explain the relationship between depression and anxiety: 1) the unitary model proposes that anxiety and depression are variants of the same disorder; 2) the dualist model advocates that depression and anxiety are different entities; and 3) the anxious-depressive position proposes a mixture of the two models in which the anxiety and depression are phenomenologically different from primary anxiety or primary depression.

Evaluation of Obsessive-Compulsive Behaviors

With the publication of DSM-5, obsessive-compulsive disorder was removed from the category of anxiety disorders and grouped with a set of related disorders (obsessive-compulsive and related disorders) in which certain features predominate: "preoccupations and…repetitive behaviors or mental acts in response to the preoccupations" (p. 235). The preoccupations and behaviors are developmentally inappropriate and result in significant emotional distress and dysfunction (see Note 5 at the end of this chapter). According to a new analysis, one or more obsessive-compulsive symptoms may increase the risk of suicide among U.S. college students. Obsessive-compulsive symptoms were more common in subjects with depression; obsessions about speaking and acting violently were independently significant associated factors with suicidal ideation (Huz et al. 2016).

In adults, OCD is two to three times more common than schizophrenia and takes, on average, two decades from the onset of the disorder until it is appropriately diagnosed and treated. The delay in diagnosing OCD is similar when it starts in adolescence; however, children with severe obsessive-compulsive features in latency age and preadolescence are referred more quickly for a psychological or psychiatric evaluation because of their broad dysfunction and broad adaptational handicaps. Making the diagnosis in these cases is a major challenge. The delay in diagnosis may be shortened by a systematic exploration of obsessive-compulsive symptoms in children and adolescents. OCD in preadolescence probably is about 10 times more frequent than schizophrenia.

A four-factor (ordering, checking, symmetry, and aggression) category-based OCD symptom dimension model provides an adequate but limited quantitative representation of symptomatology in children, adolescents, and adults (Stewart et al. 2008). Significant prevalence differences were found across age groups in the categories of obsession/aggression (adults > children > adolescents), compulsion/ordering (children > adults), and compulsion/checking (adults > children) (Stewart et al. 2008).

In a study of OCD symptom dimensions, hoarding tended to be associated with longer illness and higher levels of depression, and both parents and children endorsed greater emotional problems and emotional difficulties (Mataix-Cols et al. 2008). The symmetry/ordering dimension was more likely to be associated with Tourette's disorder or a tic disorder, whereas the contamination/cleaning dimension was more often associated with higher avoidance scores (Mataix-Cols et al. 2008). Hoarding symptoms are more common in children than in adults, and these symptoms are associated with greater comorbidity, disability, and poor compliance with and response to conventional drug and cognitive-behavioral treatments. In the Mataix-Cols et al. (2008) study, checking symptoms loaded on the same factor as hoarding; this was unexpected.

When evaluating a patient for obsessive symptoms, the examiner should ask about unwelcome and recurring thoughts: "Do any thoughts keep coming to your mind in spite of your efforts to get rid of them? What are they?" Because of the irrational nature of the intrusive thoughts, many obsessional adolescents fear they are becoming insane or "going mad." Some may respond affirmatively when the examiner asks, "Do you fear you are going crazy?" The examiner should determine the context in which the symptoms worsen or reappear.

As reported by Mataix-Cols et al. (2008), boys were found to have more sexual obsessions than girls (34% vs. 18%), but girls had more sexual rituals than boys (53% vs. 36%). The most common obsessional symptoms are concerns about dirt and germs, fears of an ill fate befalling loved ones, preoccupations with exactness or symmetry, and religious scrupulousness (Swedo et al. 1989). Concerns over bodily functions, preoccupations with lucky numbers, sexual or aggressive preoccupations, and fear of harm to oneself are less common (Towbin and Riddle 1996). Obsessional thinking related to forbidden, aggressive, and sexual content (e.g., perverse sexual thoughts) is infrequent in adolescents but occurs more commonly in adults.

Prominent obsessive-compulsive symptomatology occurs in a variety of psychiatric and neurological disorders. Depressed children frequently struggle with obsessional ideas about committing suicide and ruminate a great deal about their self-worth and lovability. Some aggressive children have recurrent homicidal ideations. Obsessional features are also common in adolescents who have addictive tendencies or perverse proclivities. Obsessive-compulsive features are also prevalent in children with eating disorders. Obsessional concerns with weight and body image, often of a quasi-delusional proportion, are prominent symptoms in children with severe cases of dysmorphic disorders and eating disorders. These symptoms need to be explored exhaustively. In children with OCD, the examiner needs to explore the possibility of Tourette's disorder.

Hollander and Benzaquen (1996) proposed organizing OCD spectrum disorders in three overlapping clusters. Table 9–5 illustrates this concept.

Compulsive features are more common than obsessional thinking during childhood, and compulsive features are more common in children than in adults. The examiner needs to ask children about ritualistic behaviors such as hand washing, taking a number of showers a day, changing clothes many times during the day, doing and undoing behaviors (e.g., tying and untying shoes, checking and rechecking doors and windows), fussiness with food while eating, collecting and hoarding, orderliness, and so forth.

When careful investigation does not reveal the presence of overt repetitious activities, the examiner should proceed with sensitive probing to rule out the presence of less obvious compulsive activities. The exploration of compulsive symptoms can be initiated by asking the following questions: "Are there any silly habits that you cannot stop?" "Are there any habits you do in secret that you do not want people to know about?" Children commonly respond by mentioning nail biting or hair pulling (trichotillomania). Skin picking (excoriation disorder) is another compulsive symptom (see Britt's case [Case Example 3] in Chapter 16, "Countertransference"). Table 9–6 summarizes the compulsive features that Swedo et al. (1989) identified as the most common in children with OCD. In children and adolescents, rituals are more common than are obsessions, and pure obsessional presentations are rare.

Some children spend a great deal of time readying themselves for school in the mornings, and their grades may suffer when their compulsive repetitive behaviors interfere with their academic work. The following case illustrates many of the features commonly described in adolescents with OCD.

Case Example 6

Ann, a Caucasian female, was 16 years old when her parents requested a psychiatric consultation. Ann's grades were deteriorating, her fears and inhibition were increasing, she was becoming socially withdrawn, and she was demonstrating an increased need for her mother's assistance in both personal care and homework assignments. Ann had been shy all her life, but her social isolation had become progressively more noticeable. She had begun to refuse to leave home during the weekends and was feeling progressively un-

Table 9–5.   Obsessive-compulsive disorder spectrum

Cluster	Characteristics	Examples
1	Marked preoccupation with body and sensations with associated behaviors performed with the goal of decreasing anxiety brought on by these preoccupations	Body dysmorphic disorder
		Depersonalization disorder
		Somatic symptom disorder (hypochondriasis), illness anxiety disorder
		Anxiety disorder
		Anorexia nervosa
		Binge-eating disorder[a]
2	Impulse-style disorders	Intermittent explosive disorder[b]
		Pathological gambling[b]
		Compulsive buying[a]
		Sexual compulsions[b]
		Kleptomania[a]
		Pyromania[b]
		Trichotillomania (hair-pulling disorder)[a]
		Excoriation (skin-picking) disorder[a]
		Self-abusive behaviors[a]
		Substance-induced OCD
		Psychotic disorders

Table 9–5.   Obsessive-compulsive disorder spectrum (*continued*)

Cluster	Characteristics	Examples
3	Neurological disorders with compulsive features	Autism spectrum disorder
		Tourette's disorder
		Sydenham's chorea
		Huntington's disease
		Torticollis
		PANDAS
		Seizures

Note.   An overlap is suggested between OCD and somatic symptom, dissociative, eating, tic, neurological, autism spectrum, and impulse-control disorders. OCD=obsessive-compulsive disorder; PANDAS=pediatric autoimmune neuropsychiatric disorders associated with streptococcal infections).
[a]Disorder is more common in females.
[b]Disorder is more common in males.
Source.   Adapted from American Psychiatric Association 2013; Hollander and Benzaquen 1996; and Phillips and Stein 2015. Modified from Cepeda 2010, p. 223.

Table 9–6. Common compulsive disorder symptoms in children and adolescents

Behavior	Percentage of cases involving this behavior, %
Excessive and ritualized hand washing, showering, bathing, tooth brushing, and grooming	85
Repeating rituals (e.g., going in and out of the door, up and down from a chair)	51
Checking rituals (e.g., checking doors, windows, locks, appliances, emergency breaks, paper route, homework)	45
Miscellaneous rituals (e.g., writing, moving, speaking, moving body parts)	26
Rituals to avoid contact/contamination	23
Touching	20
Counting	18
Hoarding and collecting	11

Source. Adapted from Swedo et al. 1989. Modified from Cepeda 2010, p. 224.

easy in social situations. She was intelligent and had striking artistic talents. Her parents had noticed that her need for perfection had intensified during the preceding 3 months, coinciding with the observation that she got "stuck" more frequently in the mornings when she had to get ready for school. She often missed the school bus because it took her a long time to get ready in the morning.

Ann's problems in the morning started with difficulty finishing her shower. She would spend a great deal of time soaping herself over and over; she couldn't stop doing this. While dressing, she would get stuck buttoning her shirt and could not finish tying her shoes because she needed to tie them over and over again. Sometimes she got stuck putting her shoes on because of her compulsion to align the creases of her socks with certain features of her shoes. To cope with Ann's worsening behavioral paralysis, her mother had begun to wake Ann very early and had taken a progressively more active role in helping Ann to keep moving and to not get stuck. Her mother's assistance included bathing her, dressing her, and so on. Ann's mother also participated actively in her homework, because Ann had similar difficulties finishing this task. The intensification of Ann's regressive and dependent behaviors was wearing her mother's patience very thin. Ann was unable to explain her peculiar behaviors and denied any significant ongoing concerns. Ann's progressive incapacitation affected her whole family, and her mother in particular.

When children and adolescents have impulse-control features, the examiner should ask whether they have any urges they cannot control. The urges could be of a diverse nature: urges to perform inappropriate sexual acts, to hurt others, to purge, to eat, to steal, to use drugs, to commit self-injurious acts, and so forth.

Transitory but pronounced obsessional and compulsive features are common in patients undergoing profound psychotic regressions (e.g., in those with schizophrenia or bipolar disorder). Frequently, these transitory clinical pictures are misdiagnosed because of the prominent nature of the obsessive-compulsive features. Consider the following case example.

Case Example 7

Ramona, a 13-year-old Hispanic female, presented for treatment in a florid manic state. She displayed conspicuous compulsive traits, and her mother reported that Ramona was preoccupied with dirt and that she went around the house cleaning and vacuuming. She also spent an inordinate amount of time picking up things from the floor and tidying up the place.

An alternative interpretation to Ramona's clinical picture is that she had bipolar disorder and OCD; such comorbidity is common in patients with bipolar disorders. Anxiety disorders may be forerunners of mood disorders, particularly bipolar disorder.

The examiner should inquire about the presence of comorbid conditions because the majority of children with OCD have associated comorbidity. Frequently associated conditions are depressive and anxiety disorders (e.g., elective mutism, separation anxiety, social phobias), disruptive behavior disorders, and developmental language or learning disorders. A compulsive personality disorder is uncommon. Soft neurological and neurocognitive deficits are observed in some children with OCD. The examiner should also determine whether OCD features are present in other family members, because such features are common in close relatives of children with OCD.

Evaluation of Eating Disorders

Eating disorders are relatively common and serious psychiatric disorders that often have an onset during adolescence and young adulthood. These disorders can be life threatening. Anorexia nervosa and bulimia nervosa are the two specific DSM-5 eating disorders, but the broader category of unspecified eating disorder is the most frequent eating disorder presentation in children and adolescents. Binge-eating disorder will be discussed below. Regardless of the diagnosis, patients with eating disorders have severe difficulties maintaining both normal patterns of eating and a normal weight range.

Patients with eating disorders often try to control or lose weight by exercising excessively; using laxatives, diuretics, or other medications; or practicing other types of behavior (e.g., purging). Many of these patients have a persistent distortion of body image. Individuals with anorexia nervosa tend to be obsessive and perfectionistic; they have low self-esteem and display difficulty in recognizing their feelings (alexithymia). Subjects with bulimia nervosa tend to be impulsive and self-critical. These issues need to be explored. The predisposing role of childhood experiences, including sexual abuse, is uncertain. Weight gain and changes in body shape due to puberty may contribute to the onset of the eating disorder (Fleitlich-Bilyk and Lock 2008).

Anorexia nervosa is characterized by four major symptoms: 1) weighing less than 85% of expected weight; 2) fear of gaining weight or becoming fat, even though underweight; 3) disturbance in perception of one's body or body shape; and 4) amenorrhea in postmenarche females (Fleitlich-Bilyk and Lock 2008). Many adolescents while still menstruating have symptoms that fit the diagnosis of anorexia. An accurate parameter to measure weight loss in children and adolescents is a decline in weight percentile. A decrease in body mass index is not suitable for premenarche individuals (Fleitlich-Bilyk and Lock 2008).

Bulimia nervosa is characterized by 1) recurrent episodes of binge eating and 2) recurrent compensatory behavior to avoid gaining weight (e.g., purging, use of laxatives or diuretics, fasting, excessive exercise). In binge-eating episodes, during discrete amounts of time, an individual consumes a larger amount of food than most people. The person has a sense of lack of control over eating during these episodes. The examiner needs to explore and identify these features. Commonly, the individual has an increased focus on weight and body shape, followed by an increase in dieting and exercise. Concerns about weight or shape may be so extreme that the patient develops unhealthy strategies for weight loss, such as severe restriction, excessive exercise, and purging. A vicious cycle of dieting, binge eating, purging, and anxiety about weight and shape is perpetuated (Fleitlich-Bilyk and Lock 2008).

DSM-5 now recognizes binge-eating disorder as a new diagnostic entity (American Psychiatric Association 2013, pp. 350–353). *Binge eating* is defined as the episodic intake of large amounts of food in association with a sense of loss of control over eating during the episode. The binge-eater consumes a larger amount of food than other individuals would eat in similar circumstances, and they have a sense of loss of control over eating during the episode. Lack of control is the hallmark of the disorder because neither size or amount of food nor the frequency of the intake has been documented with regularity. Prospective longitudinal studies of subjective binge eating (loss of control) and objective binge eating have documented that loss of control in children predicts adiposity and psychiatric symptomatology. Objective binge eating in adolescents and young adults predicts incidence of depressive feelings and obesity (Marcus and Wildes 2014, p. 444).

Common comorbid conditions with eating disorders are depression, anxiety disorders, and personality disorders. Affective disorders co-occur with or appear after the eating disorder in 52%–98% of the patients, and approximately 65% of individuals with anorexia nervosa have some form of anxiety disorder. OCD is commonly associated with anorexia nervosa, and social phobia often co-occurs with bulimia nervosa. Comorbid disorders persist after recovery from eating disorders and are appropriate targets of treatment (Fleitlich-Bilyk and Lock 2008).

Evaluation of Psychotic Symptoms

Psychotic symptoms are rather common in the overall psychopathology of childhood and adolescence. Affective psychoses (i.e., psychoses associated with mood disorders) and dissociative psychoses (i.e., psychoses associated with posttraumatic stress disorder or dissociative identity) are rather common in clinical practice. Psychoses associated with complex partial seizures are probably seen more frequently than schizophrenia. Very-early-onset schizophrenia (VEOS) disorder, formerly called *childhood schizophrenia*, is a rare psychiatric disorder. Not all psychotic symptoms have a progressive or negative prognosis.

VEOS has an onset before age 13 years. Early-onset schizophrenia (EOS) has an onset between 13 and 17 years of age. The prevalence of VEOS is 1/ 10,000 (far higher than Remschmidt [2008] mentioned; see below). The prevalence of EOS is estimated to be 1–2/1,000. VEOS and EOS are considered more disabling disorders than adult-onset schizophrenia (Armando et al. 2015, p. 312).

van Os (2016) proposes that the label of schizophrenia be abandoned in favor of *psychotic spectrum syndrome*. He reasons that schizophrenia is not a diagnosis of a disease but a grouping of symptoms. He further notes that 70% of psychoses are not schizophrenia-related; van Os asserts that people with psychosis spectrum disorder display extreme heterogeneity, both between and within people, in psychopathology, treatment response, and outcome. He advises that the mental health community should forget about the devastating category of schizophrenia as the only condition that matters, and start attending to a variety of diverse conditions that really exist.

Clinicians seldom encounter preadolescents with schizophrenia, except in inpatient settings. Even among the most seriously disturbed children, schizophrenia is an uncommon illness in preadolescence. Remschmidt (2008) asserted that VEOS is rare, occurring in 2 per 1 million children. We agree that

VEOS is rare, but not as rare as Remschmidt stated. Remschmidt quoted Gillberg (2001), who speculated that schizophrenia before age 15 is about 50 times more rare than after that age, and that in child and adolescent inpatient psychiatric settings, up to 5% of patients ages 13–19 years are typically diagnosed with schizophrenia (Remschmidt 2008).

VEOS and some forms of EOS are now considered to be neurodevelopmental and neurodegenerative disorders. In Harris's (1995a) opinion, "although childhood onset schizophrenia seems to be on a continuum with adult schizophrenia, it represents the more severe neurobiologic presentation" (p. 411). This disorder is commonly described as causing multidimensional impairments (i.e., children with schizophrenia demonstrate functional disturbance in many developmental domains). The schizophrenic process is insidious, and more often than not, the affected child comes to the child psychiatrist only after many years of developmental disturbance. Table 9–7 outlines a number of developmental events and precursors for VEOS and EOS.

In a study of patients with pediatric bipolar disorder, Pavuluri et al. (2004) found that the early onset of psychotic features puts those patients at risk for a poor long-term outcome. Adolescent mania requiring hospitalization appears to have a poorer short-term prognosis than adult-onset mania. Psychotic disorders in patients with bipolar disorder are considered an indicator of poor interepisodic functioning. Also, psychosis associated with pediatric mania is unrecognized or overlooked (Pavuluri et al. 2004). Compared with patients with adolescent-onset bipolar disorder, patients with prepubertal and early-onset bipolar disorder had higher incidence of irritability, mixed features of depression, poor interepisodic recovery, and rapid cycling. Higher rates of grandiose and paranoid delusions also occurred in patients with prepubertal and early-onset bipolar disorder. The prevalence rate of psychosis in patients with prepubertal and early-onset bipolar disorder ranged between 61% and 87.5%, depending on the assessment instrument used (Pavuluri et al. 2004).

For some patients, the examiner may need to differentiate between VEOS and pediatric mania. Table 9–8 is useful in this differential diagnosis.

Examiners should ask the following questions if a child is suspected of having schizophrenia: Does the family have a history of schizophrenia? Have any family members had difficulties relating to others? The following questions are pertinent regarding the child's developmental history: How was the pregnancy? Were there any problems during labor and delivery? Were there any neonatal complications? Was the baby responsive to the mother (or primary caregiver)? Did the child cuddle? Did he or she mold into the mother's arms? When did the major developmental milestones occur? In particular, when did social smiling and stranger anxiety first occur? When did the child begin to talk? What was the child's socialization progress? What progress has the child made in the process of separation-individuation? What autonomous

Table 9–7.   Developmental events and precursors of very-early-onset and early-onset schizophrenia

Developmental

    Pandysmaturation (neurodevelopmental delay)

Neurodevelopmental

    Soft neurological signs: gross motor and fine motor coordination difficulties

    Deviant patterns of brain maturation

Autonomic reactivity changes

Premorbid conditions

    Premorbid anxiety and social withdrawal

    Hyperactivity in boys

    Withdrawal in girls

    Depression

    Transient symptoms of pervasive developmental disorder (now autism spectrum disorder)

School difficulties

Social difficulties

Psychotic features

    Global negative and positive thought disorder

    Negative symptoms years before onset of schizophrenia

Cognitive deficits

Source.   Adapted from Remschmidt 2008. Modified from Cepeda 2010, p. 229.

behavior is the child able to demonstrate? What self-care behaviors is the child capable of? Is the child able to sleep alone in his or her own bed? Does the child demonstrate consistent behavioral organization (see section "Using AMSIT" in Chapter 8, "Documenting the Examination")? Is there any harmony in the progress of the developmental lines (see Chapter 13, "Comprehensive Psychiatric Formulation")? If the child demonstrates affect disturbance or mood dysregulation, the history and evolution of these disturbances must be explored.

Relevant questions regarding psychosocial development include the following: Does the child play with other children, or does the child prefer to be alone? Is the child able to share? How easy is it for the child to make friends? Is the child able to keep the friends that he or she makes? Is the child invited

Table 9–8. Differential diagnosis between pediatric mania and very-early-onset schizophrenia

	Pediatric mania	Very-early-onset schizophrenia
Prevalence	Uncommon	Rare
Mood-incongruent delusions	Uncommon	More common
Mood-congruent delusions	Common	Uncommon
Grandiose delusions	Common (50%)	Uncommon (11%)
Hallucinations	Hallucinations and delusions are common during mood episodes*	Common (80%)
Thought disorder	Pressured speech	Loose associations
Nonpsychotic	25%	7%
Mood	Irritability, elation, depression, and mixed	Depression in prodromal/residual phase
Family history	Commonly homotypic	Less commonly homotypic
Chronic impairment	25%–40%	90%
Episodicity	20%–50% AO-BD 0%–16% PEA-BD	Non-episodic
Promptness of diagnosis and treatment	May be short	Usually long

Note. AO-BD=adolescent-onset bipolar disorder; PEA-BD=prepubertal and early-adolescent bipolar disorder.

Source. Adapted from Pavuluri et al. 2004 and *Youngstrom et al. 2009. Modified from Cepeda 2010, p. 230.

to birthday or slumber parties? Does the child behave or play in a gender-appropriate manner? Does the child demonstrate empathy or a concern for others? Does the child demonstrate any realistic self-esteem or self-worth? These questions are equally relevant in the evaluation of profound developmental disturbances such as autism and pervasive developmental disorders.

Fundamental observations during the psychiatric examination focus on the child's overall demeanor, the degree and appropriateness of the child's relations to the family and to the examiner, the propriety of the child's social behavior, the range and appropriateness of the child's affective display, and the nature of the child's thought processes. The following case example illustrates the clinical presentation of VEOS in a child of middle latency age.

Case Example 8

Rick, a 9-year-old Caucasian male, would wake up around 6:30 A.M. every morning, but he was very slow in getting ready for school. His mother provided a great deal of assistance with his hygiene and dressing, even though Rick could do those tasks by himself (cognitive dyspraxia). Rick was a fussy eater and was very thin. There were always questions about his health. In the past, Rick's food intake had been supplemented with Ensure. His mother also complained that her son got easily upset and that he would become enraged at minor provocations. Anger dyscontrol was a significant problem. He regularly focused his anger on his younger brother. Rick had become progressively more aggressive with his brother and had attempted to choke him. The day of the examination, Rick had attacked his mother as well.

Six months before the evaluation, Rick had disclosed that he began hearing voices when he was 8 years old. He claimed he heard a mean voice telling him to do bad things like hitting and kicking his brother hard. This voice also told him to hurt his 17-year-old sister and asked him to be mean to the family dog. He said that sometimes he could make the voices go away, but sometimes he couldn't.

Rick was born prematurely and experienced respiratory distress. He spent 11 days on a respirator and stayed in the neonatal unit until he was 4 weeks old. His language development was precocious: Rick began to talk by age 8 months and spoke in full sentences by age 18 months. He did not start walking until after he was 12 months old. Rick's father had always felt very proud of his son's intelligence. When his mother expressed concerns about Rick to her husband, he disregarded her anxieties.

Rick's mother first became concerned about her son when he was 4 years old. At that time, she heard from other mothers and friends that there was something unusual about Rick. She heard similar concerns from the day care center staff; in particular, she was told that Rick had problems socializing with other children. At times, Rick complained that other kids made fun of him, in part because he frequently told stories about aliens. His mother described Rick as introverted; he didn't initiate play with his peers and tended to play by himself.

Rick had been on the honor roll in first and second grades, but his academic performance had deteriorated. At school, Rick was described as oppositional and had problems doing schoolwork, but there had been no reports of physical aggression or explosive outbursts. Rick had required one-to-one teaching during kindergarten.

Rick's parents had been married for 12 years. Rick's mother had two children from her first marriage: a 21-year-old son and a 17-year-old daughter. The son had stayed with the father, and the daughter had lived with her mother until she was 15 years old, at which time she decided to live with her father. She had moved back to her mother's home 4 months before Rick's psychiatric evaluation. Apparently, Rick had taken it very hard when his sister left 2 years earlier; he had become depressed, stopped eating, and cried a great deal. His mother reported that Rick had returned to "normal" after his sister came back. Rick's parents reported no history of physical or sexual abuse. Their marriage was described as stable. His mother reported being markedly stressed about Rick's problems to the point that she had feared hurting him.

The mental status examination revealed a thin, almost emaciated, and peculiar looking boy who looked and acted younger than his age. Rick clutched his teddy bear, called Hypo, all the time. Rick smelled Hypo frequently and kept it close to his chest. Rick had big, unexpressive eyes and big ears. His eye contact was erratic. At times, he stared blankly at the ceiling or the wall. Occasionally, he would display unusual eye movements and would converge his eyes in a peculiar fashion. His posture was unusual. He slouched in the chair despite his parents' prompting him to sit upright. Rick would often bend over and seemed able to rest his chest on his lap. He also displayed unusual finger movements, mostly stereotypic, in both hands. He sucked his thumb sporadically. Rick would stay in abnormal positions for extended periods of time. He was also very fidgety.

Rick didn't display any spontaneous speech. When he was asked a question, there were prolonged latencies. Both the parents and the examiner often needed to repeat a question before he would start talking. His responses were simple and unelaborated, and he spoke in a halting and hesitating manner. Rick remained indifferent, if not detached, in his manner of relating to the examiner. He sometimes appeared vacant and distant. Rick's mood appeared euthymic, but his affect was markedly constricted and remained so throughout the psychiatric examination. The range and intensity of his affect were markedly decreased. No evidence of inappropriate affect was observed. It was questionable if the examiner ever achieved engagement.

When asked about the incident with his brother, Rick said that a voice commanded him to push his brother down the stairs. Rick said that he had been hearing four kinds of voices for a long time. A mean voice asked him to do mean things and got him in trouble all the time. Rick added that he wanted to block this voice, but often he couldn't. He described the second voice as the "wacky one": that voice asked him to do funny and silly things (e.g., make noises). He said he could block this voice but did not want to. The third voice was a kind one. A fourth voice, a "weird one," sounded like a vampire that could predict the future. This voice told him to go to the bathroom to do either "number one" or "number two" and talked to him about eating. Rick reported visual hallucinations; he saw animals from time to time. Rick also believed that he had a person in his stomach that pushed his stomach to one side.

Rick also said that his teddy bear talked to him. Rick's responses to the examiner's questions were disjointed and rambling, and often it was hard to follow what he was saying. He displayed a thought disorder. His sensorium was clear; there were no signs of any overt expressive or receptive language difficulties. [See Note 6 at the end of this chapter.]

On the basis of Rick's developmental history, his difficulties with interpersonal relatedness, the presence of stable regressive behavior, and his long history of psychosis, a diagnosis of VEOS was made. Rick displayed pandevelopmental disturbances. His clinical presentation met DSM-5 criteria for the diagnosis of schizophrenia: Criterion A (psychotic symptom lasting more than 1 month), Criterion B (social and occupational dysfunction), and Criterion C (the disturbance having persisted for more than 6 months). This child's diagnosis was based on a comprehensive assessment. The diagnosis of schizophrenia in childhood and adolescence is based on clinical observations, predominantly.

The child in the preceding case example has features similar to those described in EOS:

With the early onset of schizophrenia, there is a higher frequency of premorbid developmental disorders; rates of 54% to 90% have been reported, depending on the study; the earlier the onset, the more likely the developmental disorder. Premorbid schizoid and schizotypal personality features are commonly reported; the child is seen by others as odd, anxious and socially isolated. (Harris 1995a, p. 411)

Rick's case is an interesting example of disharmony in the unfolding of the developmental lines (see Chapter 13, "Comprehensive Psychiatric Formulation"). He exhibited precocious cognitive and linguistic development, while other lines lagged behind or did not develop at all.

The diagnosis of VEOS should not be made without a comprehensive assessment, including a detailed developmental history, a detailed psychosocial assessment, a methodical psychiatric examination, a physical and neurological examination, and related tests and procedures. Complete psychological testing (psychoeducational and projective) is mandatory. In any given case, other testing and examinations may be deemed necessary (e.g., speech and language assessment, OT assessment, neuropsychological testing, further neurological evaluations such as an electroencephalogram or neuroimaging studies). (For a list of instruments used in the diagnosis of schizophrenic disorders in childhood and adolescence, see Table 9–9.)

Although the presence of thought disorder is necessary for the diagnosis of schizophrenia, this criterion is not sufficient to make such a diagnosis. In the absence of any significant medical or neurological disorder, the child must show persistent developmental deviation or developmental arrest (or marked

Table 9–9.   Instruments used in the diagnosis of schizophrenic disorders in childhood and adolescence

Assessments	Age range (years)
Clinical Interviews	
Child and Adolescent Psychiatric Assessment	8–18
Diagnostic Interview for Children and Adolescents–IV	6–17
Interview for Childhood Disorders and Schizophrenia	6–18
NIMH Diagnostic Interview Schedule for Children–IV	9–17
Schedule for Affective Disorders and Schizophrenia for School Aged Children	6–17
Scales	
Children's Psychiatric Rating Scale—Child	5–13
Children's Psychiatric Rating Scale—Interviewer	Up to 15
KIDDIE–Positive and Negative Syndrome Scale (PANSS) Interviewer Parent/Child	6–16

Source.   Adapted from Remschmidt 2008. Modified from Cepeda 2010, p. 235.

loss of the adaptive capacity), profound problems in interpersonal relationships, disturbance in affect and emotional development, and clear evidence of thought disorder. (For the differential diagnosis of psychotic symptoms in children and adolescents, see Cepeda 2007, Chapters 6 and 7.)

Schizophrenia in childhood is associated with unspecific neurological findings, language disorders, cognitive impairments, ADHD, and other disorders. The psychiatrist should exhaustively rule out medical and neurological conditions. Finally, the examiner needs to heed Volkmar's (1996) advice: "If psychosis is suspected, consideration of the patient's safety—and, as appropriate [imperative], that of others—should be the initial consideration" (p. 848).

The following case example illustrates the development of schizophrenia in middle to late adolescence (i.e., EOS).

Case Example 9

Troy, a 17-year-old Hispanic male, had been referred by the local school district because of concerns over bizarre behaviors that included inappropriate sexual verbalizations and open masturbation. He had been verbalizing homosexual intentions and had spoke about having sex with a dog. It had been reported that Troy kept checking his "belly," even in front of people. Before the evaluation, Troy had inappropriately grabbed a teacher's hand. Teachers and classmates felt uneasy about him.

Troy's mother complained that her son had problems with hygiene and personal care. She also reported that Troy frequently got angry and that he was self-abusive. According to his mother, Troy had demonstrated disturbed behavior for the past few years. Troy had undergone his first psychiatric evaluation the previous Christmas (1 year before the current evaluation). Three months before the first psychiatric examination, he had spent 3 weeks in a program for adolescents at the local state hospital after he stopped eating.

Troy was conceived out of wedlock, and the pregnancy was uneventful. Troy's father was described as alcoholic. His mother reported no significant problems with her son during childhood. Apparently, Troy had been sexually abused (anal penetration) by one of his maternal uncles when he was 10 years old. The family also reported a history of physical abuse. Troy's mother reported that one of her brothers and an uncle were mentally ill. The precise nature of those illnesses could not be ascertained. Troy had tried a number of drugs in the past, including LSD, marijuana, alcohol, and tobacco products.

Troy's mother reported changes in his behavior after she had a stroke, 2 years before the evaluation. After the stroke, the mother was paralyzed on her right side for months. During that time, she had severe expressive language difficulties. She still had problems with word finding (the examiner also felt that she had difficulties understanding the seriousness of her son's psychiatric problems).

Troy was born abroad but had been brought to the United States when he was about 5 years old. At the time of the psychiatric evaluation, Troy was living with his mother and his stepfather. The relationship between stepfather and stepson was not positive because the stepfather was in charge of limit setting, and he had to discipline Troy for his inappropriate behaviors, which included open disrespect and overt indiscretions toward his mother. Although Troy had opportunities to see his natural father, he had shown no interest in doing so.

During the previous year, the parents had noticed a progressive deterioration in Troy's behavior. Troy's mother had observed him masturbating openly and without any discretion or sense of propriety. Troy often made inappropriate sexual comments to his mother. When his attention was called to these improprieties, he blandly responded by saying, "There was nothing wrong with that." During the previous year, Troy had developed an infatuation with Salvador Dali's art; he spent a lot of time drawing surrealistic drawings of body parts with explicit sexual content. Troy took offense when his family called his attention to the impropriety of his art. His dream was to become an artist like Dali, and he daydreamed of exhibiting his artwork.

The mental status examination showed a tall, Hispanic male who looked younger than the stated age. Troy displayed an inappropriate smile throughout the examination. Troy's grooming and hygiene were poor. He wore baggy pants and a T-shirt with M.C. Escher drawings on the front and back. His medium-length black hair was tucked behind his ears, and his fingernails were painted black. Troy walked slowly, and his posture was stooped.

As soon as Troy and his mother entered the interviewing room, he sat down and began to touch and inspect his abdomen. His mother asked the examiner why Troy kept looking at and touching his belly. The examiner told the mother in a playful and humorous manner that maybe Troy thought he was pregnant. Upon hearing this, Troy smiled and, expressing a sigh of relief, he said, "You see, mom, this doctor makes a lot of sense."

Troy remained aloof and distant throughout the interview, and the examiner could not develop rapport with him. Troy was unfriendly and had very poor eye contact. He was also evasive and secretive. He looked mildly depressed, and his affect was grossly inappropriate: he displayed a silly, sardonic smile throughout the interview. The range and intensity of his affect were decreased. Troy was oriented to time and place. His memories were intact, and his intellectual functions appeared average.

In the area of thought processes, Troy was not logical and at times was incoherent. Troy exhibited very loose associations. He claimed that he heard and saw his own thoughts. He was markedly delusional; his delusions related to the end of the world and were blasphemous in nature. He made innumerable references to feces, body orifices, and primitive sexual misconceptions. For instance, he thought that Jesus was made of the "crap that comes from the butt." There was also repeated telescoping (e.g., merging, confusion) of psychosexual issues. He talked about a girl who was born from the butt of the cross. A repeated theme was that of a child who is being delivered vaginally to become the leg of his mother. He wondered if he was pregnant. He advanced that he would like to be a girl when he dies and wished he had his whole body full of penises and wished that girls had multiple vaginas. He wished he could die and have sex.

He declared that Satan had sex with Jesus. In reference to the latter, he brought to the examination a picture he was very proud of: a large poster, of fair artistic quality, in which Satan was sodomizing Jesus. Troy seemed pleased to be showing his artwork and was completely unaware of the offensive nature of its content. He seemed very surprised when the examiner asked him to think about the implications of such a picture in a very religious Catholic and Christian community. Troy didn't see anything wrong with it. Troy stated that when he masturbated, he became God; he also saw God. When he was questioned about suicidal ideation, he responded that he thought about it. When asked if he had any plans to kill himself, he was secretive and evasive. He denied any homicidal ideation. His judgment and insight were nil. (See Note 7 at the end of this chapter.)

Troy's symptoms fulfilled the diagnostic criteria for schizophrenia. He had a history of active symptoms (hallucinations and delusions) for more than 1 year (Criterion A). Residual symptoms (i.e., affective flattening) and marginal educational and interpersonal functioning (i.e., significant compromise of the level of adaptive functioning, including a decline in self-care and minimal social adjustment) were also present (Criterion B). Troy demonstrated serious impairment of reality testing, and he lacked insight and a sense of social propriety (judgment impairment). He also displayed a conspicuous thought disorder. Finally, the global disturbance had lasted for over 1 year (Criterion C).

The caution expressed regarding the diagnosis of VEOS applies equally to the diagnosis of EOS. A complete medical and neurological examination is mandatory before EOS can be diagnosed, because medical and neurological conditions can mimic schizophrenic disorders. Consider the following case example.

Case Example 10

Myra, a 16-year-old Caucasian female, was brought for a psychiatric examination by her natural mother, who had been followed by the examiner for paranoid and dysphoric features. Myra's mother complained that Myra did not show any initiative in taking care of herself and that she needed to be "on her" about basic personal care, including hygiene. At school, Myra refused to participate or to do any schoolwork; at home, she wanted to stay in bed or in her room most of the time. She had been evaluated by a psychiatrist a number of months before the current evaluation and had received the diagnosis of chronic schizophrenia. Olanzapine had been prescribed for her, but her mother had interrupted the neuroleptic treatment because Myra became sedated. Myra did not have a history of seizures or head trauma or a history of fainting or blacking out. She had no significant medical history.

According to Myra, she regularly saw Jesus and her dead baby brother. She had been experiencing those perceptions for 5 years. Both Jesus and her baby brother said to her, "You will be dying soon…you will be reuniting with your brother." Myra enjoyed hearing these voices, claiming that they were soothing. She wanted to join her brother in heaven and anticipated she would die in a few years.

The mental status examination revealed a quiet, withdrawn, nonspontaneous adolescent who appeared somewhat older than the stated age. Her psychomotor activity was decreased, and her speech was dysprosodic. She spoke in a monotone with no emotion. Her mood appeared depressed, and her affect was markedly blunted. Myra denied homicidal or suicidal ideation. She was illogical but goal directed. She endorsed auditory, visual, gustatory, and olfactory hallucinations. Besides hearing and seeing her dead brother and Jesus, she reported a periodic experience of "an awful smell, like a skunk," and "a taste, like throwing up." During those experiences, Myra felt confused. She also endorsed strong and prominent paranoid delusions. She believed that many people wanted to kill her and that people had guns and knives for that purpose. Myra believed she had been in danger since she was 3 or 4 years old. Her sensorium was clear.

Because of the diagnostic consideration of a complex partial seizure, Myra was referred to a neurologist. Her mother refused to comply with the consultation and also refused to consider neuroleptic medications, claiming that previous experiences with those medications had been negative. Because the examiner thought that the probability of a complex seizure was strong, he prescribed valproic acid. When the examiner saw Myra 2 weeks later, the sense of confusion and the olfactory and gustatory hallucinations had improved. Although Myra was still seeing her brother and Jesus, these experiences and the voices associated with them were less frequent than before. The changes in Myra's mood and in her emotional display were most striking. She was more expressive and displayed a broader range and richer intensity of affect. Her paranoid feelings had decreased, and she felt less suspicious and more at ease. The dosage of valproic acid was adjusted, and Myra's psychotic and paranoid symptomatology further improved.

Although Myra's symptoms fulfilled the criteria for a diagnosis of paranoid schizophrenia, she probably had a neurological disorder—a complex partial seizure disorder. An alternative explanation is the presence of a mood disorder with psychotic features, with a very good response to valproic acid.

What are the psychotic clinical symptoms that have the most predictive power for the diagnosis of schizophrenia? Two recent articles address this question. Perkins et al. (2015) assert that illogical thoughts and suspiciousness are symptoms most predictive of schizophrenia in patients at high risk to develop the disorder. Furthermore, concentration difficulties and reduced ideational richness are further predictive of schizophrenia. Perceptual disturbance, such as hallucinations, did not have a predictive power in a 2-year follow-up study. In a second study, Bedi et al. (2015) noted that subtle changes in semantics and syntax can differentiate which individuals are at the greatest risk of developing schizophrenia. This study was based on automated speech analysis: when plotting three semantic variables—frequency of determiner words ("that," "which"), coherence between phrases, and phrase length—the algorithm discriminated subjects at risk of developing schizophrenia from other subjects.

Evaluation of Schizoid Symptoms

In the differential diagnosis of depression, questions regarding how to separate affective disorders from schizoid disorders are frequently raised. Close attention to the patient's history and affective display and close monitoring of the examiner's own emotional reactions during the interview (see Chapter 16, "Countertransference") are helpful in differentiating this diagnostic complexity.

The patient's social developmental history is of great assistance in the differential diagnosis (see previous section, "Evaluation of Psychotic Symptoms"). Has the child been a loner? Does the child prefer to play by himself or herself? Attachment difficulties need to be considered in the differential diagnosis of schizoid disorders (Volkmar 1995). The following case example is typical of children with schizoid disorders.

Case Example 11

Kurt, a 14-year-old Caucasian male, was admitted to a local psychiatric hospital after making a suicidal gesture. He had a history of extensive conduct disorder, including regular use of his mother's car without permission. He would sneak out at night on a regular basis. During the interview, Kurt appeared meek and behaved oddly. He constantly attempted to hide his hands in the long sleeves of his sweater. His eye contact was erratic, and his speech was monotonous and dysprosodic. His mood was very constricted, and he did not seem to be in touch with his feelings. When asked to describe his mood, Kurt said he was happy. He immediately corrected himself and said he was sad. He showed no modulation of affect throughout the interview except, for a short moment, when he declared that he missed home. At that moment, he became tearful, helpless, and childish. He did not endorse any psychotic features. At no point during the interview did the examiner feel that he had made emotional contact with Kurt, and there was no countertransference response concordant with the diagnosis of depression.

Children with language disorders and other neuropsychological deficits—particularly nonverbal learning disabilities due to problems in decoding and expressing affective communication—display difficulties in interpersonal communication; these situations create diagnostic confusion. Such difficulties complicate the identification and assessment of depressive affect. This observation is in agreement with Cummings's (1995b) assertion that "right-hemispheric damage sustained in childhood may result in a schizoid type of behavioral pattern, perhaps because the inability to perceive or to execute emotional cues limits the child's ability to engage in interpersonal relationships" (p. 185).

When working with children with schizoid disorders, the examiner may encounter difficulties in establishing rapport because of the children's inability to perceive and to express affect, peculiarities in these children's affective display, or the degree of inappropriate affect. Some children with neuropsychological difficulties want to connect with others and are interested in people; however, they either do not know how to go about doing so or use means that put other children off.

When examining children with schizoid features, the evaluator senses their inability to link emotionally to others, their sense of isolation, and their difficulty warming up to social interactions. The examiner's subjective response is of immense diagnostic value. In general, when the patient is depressed, the patient stimulates depressive feelings in the examiner. As expressed by Akiskal and Akiskal (1994), "The depressed person's dejection and pain tend to be communicated to the clinician and elicit emotional as well as intellectual empathy. Admittedly, this criterion is subjective, but is invaluable in the hands of experienced clinicians" (p. 43).

Children with schizoid disorders have long-standing difficulties with interpersonal relationships. These children typically are unable to initiate friendships. Commonly they are loners, and more often than not they are ostracized and ridiculed by peers. Children with schizoid disorders are frequently odd looking, and their affective communication is atypical. Often their affect is constricted, and at times their emotional display is inappropriate. Comorbid cognitive, language, and psychotic disorders are common. Soft neurological deficits (e.g., in gross and fine motor coordination) and other deficits may be present.

Key Points

- Internalizing symptoms are very common in clinical practice.
- Internalizing symptoms relate to psychiatric conditions that cause subjective distress or psychological pain; the most common conditions that bring about these symptoms include depressive, anxiety, obsessive-compulsive, and psychotic disorders.
- Evaluating internalizing symptoms requires a broad knowledge base about the configuration and components of internalizing disorders as well as a strong familiarity with DSM-5.
- A comprehensive assessment that includes a detailed developmental and psychosocial history as well as a complete medical and psychological evaluation is key in delineating the relationship between symptomatology and specific disorders. Such comprehensive assessment is especially critical prior to the diagnosis of schizophrenia in children and adolescents.

Notes

1. According to data compiled by the Centers for Disease Control and Prevention, suicide is the 10th leading cause of death among all Americans (Centers for Disease Control and Prevention 2016). For Americans of all ages, 51% of completed suicides involved a gun. Suicides are impulsive: of individuals who attempted suicide, 24% took less than 5 minutes between the decision to kill themselves and the actual attempt. The recent U.S. Supreme Court decision supporting gun ownership may lead to higher rates of gun-related suicide (70% took less than 1 hour; Miller and Hemenway 2008). More than one-third of U.S. households own a firearm. Compelling evidence links firearms to suicide. The presence of a firearm in a house increases the odds of suicide from two- to tenfold. The higher incidence of suicide is not restricted solely to the gun owner but also applies to the spouse and children. The risk is higher if the gun is kept loaded and unsecured (Miller and Hemenway 2008). International experts have concluded that the restriction of access to lethal means is one of the few suicide prevention policies with proven effectiveness.
2. The diagnoses of disruptive disorders and substance dependence (other than alcohol or marijuana) were predictive of increased noncompliance with individual psychotherapy, and affective/anxiety disorders were predictive of increased noncompliance with medications at 6 months (Burns et al. 2008).

3. The contrary is also true: the treatment of pediatric depression decreases the level of maternal depression, even when the mothers are not treated. Kennard et al. (2008) reported that 30% of mothers reported moderate to severe depression at the beginning of their child's treatment, but only 17% reported it at the end of treatment. The level of depression severity in a child correlated with the mother's depression severity; by the end of the study, children of mothers with more severe depression had higher levels of depression than children with less depressed mothers (Kennard et al. 2008).

4. In another study, mothers with major depressive disorder were treated, and their offspring (ages 7–17 years) were followed for up to 1 year after the initiation of maternal treatment. At baseline, about one-third of the children had a current psychiatric disorder. At 3-month follow-up, maternal remission from depression was associated with a significant decrease in children's diagnoses. One year after the initiation of treatment for maternal depression, the mothers' depression severity and the children's psychiatric symptoms continued to show decreases; most of the functional improvement occurred within the first 3–6 months of the 1-year follow-up interval. Decreases in the child's psychiatric symptoms were significantly associated with decreases in maternal depression severity, as reflected in scores on the Hamilton Rating Scale for Depression, and these decreases tended to precede symptom and functional improvements in children (Pilowsky et al. 2008). No change in symptoms was observed in children of nonremitting mothers, and no change in the degree of disruptive behaviors was seen in the children of either remitting or nonremitting mothers. Plausible explanations regarding why maternal depression improvement has an impact on children's psychopathology include the following: diminished marital discord, improved parenting, and a less critical attitude by the mother toward the offspring (Pilowsky et al. 2008). Developmental factors and gender were also found to be important in regard to the impact of maternal depression on offspring: maternal depression during children's late childhood was associated with an increase in girls' internalizing symptoms over time and a decrease in boys' symptoms. During early to middle adolescence, girls showed greater vulnerability to the adverse effects of maternal depression when compared with boys, but these interactions explained only a small amount of the variance (Jenkins and Curwen 2008).

5. Other diagnoses in this category include body dysmorphic disorder (preoccupation with perceptions of physical defects or flaws); hoarding disorder (preoccupation with accumulating items resulting from an inability to discard them); trichotillomania (hair-pulling disorder) (recurrent hair pulling despite multiple attempts to decrease or discontinue the behavior);

and excoriation (skin-picking) disorder (recurrent picking of skin despite multiple attempts to decrease or discontinue the behavior). Obsessive-compulsive and related disorder (OCRD) induced by medications or substances, OCRD due to another medical condition, other specified OCRD and unspecified OCRD are also included (American Psychiatric Association 2013).

6. Further diagnostic assessment on Rick:

- **Physical examination.** *Positive findings:* a very thin child with elongated fingers and inwardly curved fifth fingers on both hands.
- **Neurological screening.** *Positive findings:* dysgraphia, balance difficulties, apraxia (had difficulties putting on his shoes).
- **Psychological testing.** *Positive findings:* deficits in written expression. He obtained a superior score on Letter-Word Identification and an average score on Passage Comprehension.
- **Projective testing.** *Positive findings:* deficits in perceptual accuracy consistent with impaired reality testing. Rick misinterpreted and/or distorted perceptual stimuli. Serious problems in thought processes, mainly discontinuity, were observed; at times his thinking was incoherent and overtly concrete. Rick evidenced significant social and emotional immaturity; this was reflected in his social ineptness and the problems in establishing and maintaining rapport with others. He showed very little interest in approaching and being close to others and had a very unrealistic view of self and others. Rick's Rorschach responses had very little human content but prominent ambiguous and solitary "alien" beings. Also, Rick had a very inaccurate perception of how others perceive and relate to him and a poor awareness of the extent and significance of his problems. His aggression was poorly neutralized, and he was delayed in the process of separation and individuation from the parents.
- **Occupational therapy assessment.** *Positive findings:* poor to fair kinesthetic abilities; significant difficulties with visual-motor control and fine-motor manipulation of objects; problems in sensory-motor processing. Sensory-motor testing revealed visual crossing midline problems (e.g., he ignored the right side of the page while copying geometric shapes until he shifted the paper to his left side). Did Rick have symptoms of hemispatial neglect?

7. Further diagnostic assessment on Troy:

- **Physical examination.** *Positive findings:* Troy had multiple self-inflicted injuries on the anterior aspect of both forearms.
- **Neurological screening.** *Positive findings:* Troy was left-handed. Evidence of difficulties with praxis and some degree of dysprosody were present.

- **Psychological testing.** *Positive findings:* Troy used a neologism during the examination: he used the word "insormal" to indicate parent-approved incestuous relations between siblings. He told the tester his idea for an art piece: to cut off one of his fingers and mount it on cardboard. Troy's thought processes were tangential and rambling. The thought content was consistently dominated by bizarre, morbid, and often perverse themes. His ideas frequently involved the condensation or fusion of opposite qualities, activities, ideas, and feelings (e.g., good/evil, procreation/killing, pleasure/pain). He often condensed sexuality with religious symbolism and a personal sense of alienation. He often seemed fascinated and perplexed by his bizarre musings, which took on a stereotyped and perseverative quality over the course of the evaluation. He said his main interests were in being "bizarre" and "weird."
- **Projective testing.** Troy's self-image was distorted and conflictive. He appeared to reject all conventional aspects of his identity and life, including identifications with the family, in favor of an intense identification with countercultural ideas and values (i.e., the "bizarre"). He entertained grandiose fantasies (e.g., "being famous someday and producing great works of art") while simultaneously being preoccupied with masochistic themes of humiliation and self-abuse. Troy was very conflicted about gender identification. He was comfortable with social isolation and alienation and appeared indifferent to others, except as they provided stimulation for his fantasy life and nourishment of his fascination with the bizarre. Troy's inner life was characterized by pervasive boundary confusion in which conflicted ideas, tendencies, and feelings were resolved or negated in fantasy through the fusion or merger of conflicted opposites. His internal representations were poorly differentiated and lacked substance and diversity. Troy's intense fantasy preoccupation with sexual and religious conflicts may represent primitive denial and distortion defenses, which provided a means of dealing with early trauma. For example, he wondered aloud if death might consist of continuously repeated sexual activity with transvestites that creates "straight good feelings, no bad feelings or thoughts, just good." Troy's thinking disturbance significantly impaired his capacity for adaptive social and educational functioning and self-care and adversely impacted his motivation for conventional pursuits. On the positive side, Troy's artistic abilities were well developed and represented a potential strength for him that should be further developed.
- **Cognitive testing.** Troy's level of intelligence was in the low average range. Troy demonstrated a learning disability in written expression.

CHAPTER 10

Evaluation of Externalizing Symptoms

Evaluation of Hyperactive and Impulsive Behaviors

Although distractibility was traditionally considered the core feature of attention-deficit/hyperactivity disorder (ADHD), researchers, more recently, have proposed that the central deficit in ADHD is a problem of behavioral inhibition that involves a delay in the development of self-control and self-regulation. The behavior of children with ADHD is regulated more by immediate circumstances (i.e., external sources) and less by executive functions and considerations of time and the future. As Barkley (1997, p. 313) stated, "ADHD is far more a deficit of behavioral inhibition than of attention."

DSM-5 (American Psychiatric Association 2013) distinguishes three types of ADHD: inattentive, hyperactive-impulsive, and combined. The inattentive type predominates in pediatric populations, whereas the hyperactive-impulsive and combined types are more prevalent in child psychiatric populations. The ADHD types are associated with different clinical, comorbid, and prognostic courses. According to Faraone et al. (1998), children with the combined type have the highest rates of comorbid disruptive, anxiety, and depressive disorders. In comparison with children who have the combined type, children with the inattentive type have similar rates of comorbid anxiety and depressive disorders but lower rates of disruptive disorders. Children with the hyperactive-impulsive type, compared with children with the other subtypes, have the highest rates of externalizing disorders but lower rates of associated anxiety and depression. Children with the combined or inattentive types have higher rates of academic problems than do children with the hyperactive-impulsive type. Compared with children with the other two types, children with the combined type have higher lifetime rates of conduct, oppositional, bipolar, language, and tic disorders; they also have the highest rate of counseling and multimodal treatments. Few differences were found between the hyperactive-impulsive and the inattentive types, although children with the inattentive type had a higher lifetime prevalence of major depressive disorder (Faraone et al. 1998). In the case of moderate to severe symptoms noted in preschoolers, the ADHD diagnosis appears stable into later childhood. In children diagnosed with ADHD as preschoolers, the Preschool Attention-Deficit/ Hyperactivity Disorder Treatment Study (PATS) found that at 6-year follow-up, 89% of the children who were not lost to follow up and had been diagnosed with moderate to severe ADHD as preschoolers continued to have symptoms that met ADHD diagnostic criteria (Riddle et al. 2013).

In a 5-year prospective study by Hinshaw (2008), nearly two-thirds of females with ADHD showed depression at some point during the study; this rate was several times higher than that in the non-ADHD comparison group. Depressive symptomatology in females with ADHD was more severe (i.e., earlier onset and longer duration, higher levels of irritability and suicidal ideation, and greater need of multiple types of treatment) than in the comparison group. Major depression also predicted continuity of depression, onset of anxiety, and substance use disorders (Hinshaw 2008).

Longitudinal studies of boys with or without ADHD revealed that major depression at baseline predicted syndrome-congruent outcomes 4 years later. Boys with major depression and comorbid ADHD were at significant risk for bipolar disorder, psychosocial dysfunction, and psychiatric hospitalizations. Boys with a clinical presentation meeting the criteria for major depression had prototypical symptoms of the disorder, a chronic course, and severe psychosocial dysfunction (Biederman et al. 2008). In contrast, females with ADHD were 5.1 times more likely to develop major depression than were control females. Biederman et al. (2008) reported that major depression in females with ADHD, compared with major depression in control females, was associated with an earlier onset and greater duration of the major depression, as well as more severe associated major depression impairment, including psychiatric hospitalization and increased suicidal ideation. ADHD in females significantly increased the risk for mania, conduct disorder, and oppositional defiant disorder (ODD) independent of the major depression status. Parental history of major depression and the subject's history of mania were predictors of major depression among females with ADHD. Having ADHD at baseline is a significant predictor for major depression in females.

A robust bidirectional overlap occurs between ADHD and major depression, and mania in childhood is a significant predictor for major depression at follow-up for females. An emerging literature also documents a bidirectional association between ADHD and bipolar disorder in pediatric subjects and adults with ADHD, as well as in pediatric and adult patients with bipolar disorder (Biederman et al. 2008). Major depression is also associated with an increased risk for anxiety disorders. The comorbidity of ADHD and major depression thus indicates high morbidity and disability, as well as a poor prognosis (Biederman et al. 2008).

In evaluating children who have the hyperactive-impulsive type of ADHD, the examiner should inquire about the onset of the hyperactivity and impulsivity. Commonly, the origin of these symptoms can be traced to early preschool age. Some mothers report hyperactivity during the child's gestational or early neonatal life. Parents may complain that these children were hyperactive, willful, obstinate, or disobedient from an early age, or that they got into everything without any forethought (e.g., they were frequently moving, never finishing anything they started). Many of these children have no sense of danger and require close and ongoing supervision. A low tolerance for frustration and dysregulation of emotional states are common. Some of these children have difficult temperaments and demand inordinate amounts of attention; they lack self-soothing regulatory mechanisms and are prone to intense and prolonged temper tantrums. These tantrums easily escalate into dyscontrol, and when this happens, it takes the child a long time to regain self-control. In severe cases, biorhythm dysregulation may be present, as evidenced by sleep difficulties.

Symptoms of ADHD are conspicuous in the classroom. Children with ADHD are distractible and disruptive. They demonstrate off-task behaviors and are unable to remain seated. They commonly have difficulty completing assignments, and they have problems taking turns and sharing with peers. Some of these children are intrusive and have limited social skills, whereas others have poor problem-solving abilities. Some children with ADHD develop early comorbidity. Children with the hyperactive-impulsive or combined types have problems with anger control and with affective modulation; these deficits contribute further to their limited social success.

Cantwell (1996, p. 982) recommended a comprehensive assessment for children and adolescents suspected of having ADHD. This assessment includes the following components:

1. A comprehensive interview with all parental figures. This interview should be complemented by a developmental, medical, and school history of the child and a social, medical, and mental health history of family members.

2. A developmentally appropriate interview with the child to assess his or her view of the signs and symptoms and to screen for comorbidity.
3. An appropriate medical evaluation to screen for health status and neurological problems.
4. An appropriate cognitive assessment of ability and achievement.
5. The use of both broad-spectrum and more narrowly focused (i.e., ADHD-specific) parent and teacher rating scales.
6. Appropriate adjunct assessments, such as speech and language assessment and evaluation of fine and gross motor function.

Because children with the combined type of ADHD require frequent corrective feedback (as a result of their impulsivity), they evolve a negative self-view that contributes to the early development of dysphoric affect. Frequently, children with ADHD develop a defective self-concept and a poor sense of competence. According to O'Brien (1992), self-esteem difficulties are the core psychological problems for these children. The examiner needs to explore these complications to determine the extent of additional psychopathology to formulate a comprehensive treatment program. The examiner should ask the child to explain the reasons for the psychiatric examination and should help the child to explain, in his or her own words, the nature and extent of the problems.

The examiner should consider the following questions: Does the child display problems with hyperactivity-impulsivity only in certain circumstances or at certain times? Are the problems evident in most of the child's daily activities? Is the child able to concentrate in the classroom? Is the child able to stay on task? Does the child finish assignments? Does the child show behavioral disorganization? Do any activities grip the child's attention (e.g., playing certain games, watching television)? What television programs does the child watch? How are the child's social and problem-solving skills? This information has significant clinical relevance.

As soon as the interviewer detects that the child is too hyperactive or impulsive and lacks means of self-regulation, self-structure, or self-control, he or she should structure both the physical space and the activities in which the child is permitted to engage. Restricting spatial boundaries and controlling the quality, quantity, and modality of stimulation are mandatory to maintaining a safe and productive interview. Such control will help the child to focus and concentrate on structured tasks (e.g., those involving building blocks, puzzles, or table games).

If the child is easily distracted, the examiner should reduce the amount of stimulation by limiting the number of items available at any given time. Limiting and structuring the elements for specific tasks is important: a box full of crayons and an unlimited amount of paper are too distracting for an inattentive and disorganized child. Such a child should receive one crayon or one pencil and one piece of paper at a time. Similarly, the examiner should limit the number of blocks or other items that the child can use at any given time.

If the child is too fidgety or has difficulty remaining seated, the examiner should pull the child's chair close to the interviewing table so that the chair and table form a physical boundary. The examiner should instruct (and encourage) the child to concentrate on only one task at a time. The examiner should encourage and help the child to complete the assigned task before moving on to a new one. Throughout the interview, the examiner should note the child's response to structure and limit setting; these observations have important diagnostic and therapeutic implications. Ongoing support should be given when the child meets the examiner's expectations and abides by the provided structure. The examiner should help the child concentrate on the project at hand and should give support and reinforcement each time the child finishes a task. Transitions from one activity to the next should be handled with care, because the child may have problems with moving on to new tasks.

The length of the interview is an important factor; brevity is the goal. After 15–20 minutes of active interviewing, the child needs a break (e.g., a trip to the bathroom). In an intensely structured setting, the patient and the clinician tire easily. The amount of structure needed in subsequent sessions will indicate how well the child is responding to ongoing behavioral and psychopharmacological interventions. Observations made during structured interviewing, as well as changes observed in ratings on specific checklists completed by the examiner, teachers, or parents, are helpful in ascertaining whether changes at school, at home, or in other settings have been made in response to treatment.

Additional deficits may also emerge in the course of the initial evaluation and subsequent visits. Social skill difficulties are significant problems for some children with ADHD. Cantwell (1996) described this comorbidity as an inability to pick up social cues, which leads to interpersonal difficulties. In a child who has responded well to treatment and has demonstrated behavioral improvements (decreases in hyperactivity and impulsivity but not attention or academic improvements), the examiner also needs to rule out nonverbal learning disabilities. Finally, rating scales should be used to support the diagnosis.

Galanter and Leibenluft (2008) provided a number of considerations for the examiner faced with differentiating ADHD from bipolar disorder. First, ADHD is far more common than bipolar disorder. Second, the venue of the assessment is important: bipolar disorder is more likely in an inpatient psychiatric unit than in a pediatric clinic. Third, the examiner should explore for an episode of mania or hypomania. If such an episode is not uncovered, the examiner should search for an episode of irritability that is greater than the child's baseline. ODD, conduct disorder, anxiety disorder, and major depressive disorder also produce irritability and are more common than bipolar disorder. Fourth, the examiner should consider the DSM-5 Criterion B symptoms for mania (symptoms that are not present in ADHD), such as grandiosity, flight of ideas or racing thoughts, decreased need for sleep, and hypersexuality.

Evaluation of Aggressive and Homicidal Behaviors

According to Ash (2008), violence is surprisingly common among children and adolescents. Longitudinal studies using youth self-reports indicate that by age 17 years, 30%–40% of boys and 16%–32% of girls have participated in a serious violent offense (i.e., aggravated assault, robbery, gang fight, or rape). Homicide is the second cause of death for youths ages 15–19 years, second to accidents and ahead of suicide; it accounts for about 2,000 deaths a year. The homicide rate stands at 9.3 deaths per 100,000 youths. Adolescent dating violence is also frequent: up to 9% of boys and girls reported being physically hit by a boyfriend or girlfriend during the previous year (Ash 2008). Ash (2008) asserted that children first learn to manage their aggression from their parents during toddlerhood and that poor parenting (abusive parenting, neglect, coercive parenting, rearing by antisocial parents, poor limit setting, or general family dysfunction) during toddlerhood sets the stage for the children's later problems with aggression or violence. ODD is a frequent precursor of more serious aggression; about 30% of individuals with early ODD progress to conduct disorder, and 40% of those with conduct disorder progress to antisocial personality disorder. The most potent risk factors for preadolescent violence are general nonviolent criminal offenses and preadolescent substance abuse, whereas peer effects are the most influential factors for adolescent-onset violence. For both preadolescent-onset and adolescent-onset violence types, a developmental progression of offenses is common, beginning with minor crimes such as vandalism and shoplifting, then progressing to aggravated assault, followed by robbery, and then rape. That robbery precedes rape in 70% of cases is the strongest evidence that rape is a criminal violent offense and not a crime of sex (Ash 2008).

Dating violence should be explored. According to Wolitzky-Taylor et al. (2008), older age, female sex, and exposure to previous and recent stressors were associated with greater risk for experiencing dating violence. Experience of severe dating violence (i.e., physical assault causing harm, threat with a weapon, rape or forced sexual activity) was estimated, conservatively, to be 2.6% for girls and 0.6% for boys, representing 335,000 girls and 78,000 boys in the United States. (Verbal threats, hitting or slapping without injury, and verbal aggressiveness were not considered in the study.) Sexual assault was the highest act of violence, followed by physical assault and drug- or alcohol-facilitated rape. Dating violence is associated fourfold with posttraumatic stress disorder and major depressive episodes. Also, an association exists between dating violence and having experienced a prior traumatic event (Wolitzky-Taylor et al. 2008).

The examiner should explore aggressive behavior at school. Results from a 1995 survey of students ages 12–18 years indicated that 2.5 million students were victims of some crime at school. Serious crimes (i.e., rape, aggravated assault, sexual assault, and robbery) accounted for 186,000 victims in schools; 47 of the crimes resulted in 47 school-associated deaths, including 38 homicides (Malmquist 2008).

As Tardiff (2008, p. 4) noted, "The evaluation of violence potential is analogous to that of suicidal potential. Even if the patient does not express thoughts of violence, the clinician should routinely ask the subtle question, 'Have you ever lost your temper?' in much the same way as one would check for suicide potential with the question, 'Have you ever felt that life was not worth living?' If the answer is yes in either case, the evaluator should proceed with the evaluation in terms of how, when, and so on with reference to violence as well as suicidal potential." Tardiff added, "When making decisions about violence potential, the clinician also should interview family members, police, and other persons with information about the patient and about violence incidents to ensure that the patient is not minimizing his or her dangerousness" (p. 4). Ash (2008) advised, "Whenever risk of predatory violence by an adolescent is a serious consideration, if at all possible some friend should be talked to…[because] the evaluee's friends are most likely—more so than parents—to have heard the youth express threats, even if the friends did not take the threats seriously" (p. 371).

The examiner should keep in mind, when evaluating violence, that the standard unstructured assessment interviews have limited diagnostic validity and no predictive validity: "Research has not been kind to unstructured violence risk assessment" (Monahan 2008, p. 19). For predictions of violence, "actuarial" methods are recommended (see Note 1 at the end of this chapter).

An important consideration in assessing an adolescent's risk for violence is where he or she is on the violence pathway or trajectory: fantasies about killing, initiation of planning, increased interest in weapons and how to use them, interest in how others have committed mass murders, use of the Internet for this purpose, and detailed preparation (obtaining weapons, scouting out sites, and stalking potential victims). The farther along this path the adolescent is, the higher the risk he or she poses. A person does not have to make a threat to be a threat. The examiner should also explore the motivation, including why people are included on the "hit list" (Ash 2008). Ash (2008) stated the importance of reducing the availability of weapons, but many parents do not comply with the recommendation to dispose of weapons.

For the evaluation of short-term violence risk in adults, Tardiff (2008) recommended the importance of the following factors: 1) appearance, 2) presence of violent ideation and degree of formulation and/or planning, 3) intent to be violent, 4) available means to harm and access to the potential victims, 5) past history of violence and other impulsive behaviors, 6) history of alcohol or drug abuse, 7) presence of psychosis, 8) presence of personality disorder, 9) history of noncompliance with treatments, and 10) demographic and socioeconomic characteristics. These factors have a parallel importance in the assessment of violence in children and adolescents.

In an article on assessing violence risk in children and adolescents, Weisbrot (2008) discussed infamous school shootings. Warning signs are evident, and the interviewer needs to confront the child's denial or minimization of these issues. "Leakage" relates to clues signaling a potential violent act, including feelings, thoughts, fantasies, attitudes, and intentions expressed via direct threats, boasts, doodles, Internet sites, songs, tattoos, stories, and yearbook comments with themes of death, dismembering, blood, or end-of-the-world philosophies. School shooters indicated their plans before the shootings occurred via direct threats or by implication in drawings, diaries, or school essays. Prior to school shootings, other students usually know about the impending attacks (in 75% of cases, at least one person knew; in about 66% of cases, more than one person knew), but this information was not communicated to adults.

Weisbrot (2008) advised that threat assessment requires a thorough psychiatric diagnostic evaluation, including fundamental assessments of suicidality, homicidality, thought processes, reality testing, mood, and behavior. A detailed developmental history should be gathered, with a specific focus on abuse, past trauma, school suspensions and expulsions, school performance, and peer leadership. A red flag for potential violence is the history of trauma or violence, either as a victim or as a perpetrator. Attackers feel teased, persecuted, bullied, threatened, or injured by others before the attacks. Important issues to cover in the assessment include verification of the threat, as well as exploration of the ongoing intent, the focus on the threat, the intensity of the threat preoccupation, the access to weapons, and the concern expressed in the child's environment. Parents may demonstrate pathological levels of denial, indicating a chaotic home environment, a highly conflicted parent-child relationship, and inadequate limit setting.

Contemporary models of antisocial behavior recognize both social and biological factors, reflecting the assumption that both types of factors interplay in a complex fashion to influence the development and persistence of antisocial behaviors. Genetic influences are suggested for lifelong, persistent antisocial behaviors rather than for adolescence-limited behaviors (Popma and Vermeiren 2008) (see Note 2 at the end of this chapter). Research increasingly shows that multiple genes are simultaneously involved to create the susceptibility for antisocial behavior.

Otnow Lewis's (1991) advice to clinicians working with children with conduct disorder is particularly applicable to those dealing with aggressive and violent behaviors: "Clinicians are obliged to attempt to overcome the negative feelings toward the child that may be aroused by the child's frightening and obnoxious behaviors. One must embark on the evaluation of a behaviorally disturbed child with curiosity and an open mind" (p. 571). Negative responses toward the patient (i.e., countertransference) may interfere with the clinician's ability to thoroughly and systematically assess these children.

If the clinician knows in advance that the child is likely to be aggressive or self-abusive, he or she should make preparations beforehand to meet the child's special needs. No matter how syntonic a child's aggression seems to be, the clinician should assume that the child is anxious about, if not afraid of, the possibility of losing control. If the child appears to have this anxiety, the examiner should reassure the child that every effort will be made to help him to stay under control or to regain control, if needed. The examiner may need to consider psychopharmacological interventions, hospitalization, or other options. The diagnostic interview should be stopped if the examiner becomes concerned with his or her personal safety. If this happens, the examiner should take the steps needed to prevent the patient from injuring anyone.

During the evaluation of a volatile, labile, or aggressive adolescent, the examiner should avoid provoking the patient any further. The examiner should also be attentive to signs that the patient is about to lose control. Regardless of the etiology of the aggressive behavior, all communications and interventions need to take into account that the patient is struggling to maintain self-control and is experiencing an ongoing disturbance with his or her sense of self—a narcissistic disturbance that needs to be identified, abreacted, understood, and if possible repaired. Something has injured the patient's self-esteem and the patient's narcissism to the point that he needs to resort to aggressive behavior to restore his self-worth (i.e., to repair the perceived injury). If the examiner knows the nature of the injury, he should offer empathic comments regarding the perceived injury, evaluate the patient's response to such comments, and explore alternatives to deal with the identified injury. The examiner will be more successful if he assesses aggression in this broader context and prudently assumes that the patient may lose control at perceived provocations.

Depending on the individual case, the patient may appear defensive, suspicious, fearful, or ashamed. If the patient feels humiliated or has been humiliated, he or she may anticipate further humiliation or even retaliation for aggressive, hateful, and vengeful feelings. Some adolescents who are struggling with aggressive feelings may experience shame or guilt secondary to intense anger and the fear of losing control. The examiner should explore paranoia and other psychotic features exhaustively.

The examiner's emphasis in dealing with aggressive adolescents is to determine their propensity for violence and to establish whether such adolescents are at imminent risk of losing control. If the examiner determines that the patient is on the verge of losing control, the examiner needs to be extra cautious in his or her approach and demeanor and should be particularly judicious with his or her words.

Regardless of the nature of the aggression, the examiner's priority is to help the patient regain a sense of self-control. Lion (1987) expressed this principle in the following manner: "The evaluator's goal [when meeting belligerent and violent patients], whenever possible, is to convert physical agitation and belligerence into verbal catharsis. This principle holds true irrespective of the etiology of the patient's violence" (p. 3).

Because a history of violence is the best predictor of future violence, the examiner should make a comprehensive inquiry into this area. The following questions may be pertinent: Has the child ever lost control? What has been the nature of the child's dyscontrol? Has the child ever hurt someone? Does the child intend to harm someone? Has the child developed a plan to kill someone? The examiner should remember his duty to protect potential victims.

Many adolescents exhibit a facade of bravado or a bullish attitude. The examiner should take these surface behaviors seriously. An attempt to challenge these defenses carries a serious risk and is not recommended; the child might act out to prove to the examiner that she can do what she says. By stressing the dangerousness of threatened behaviors and highlighting the potential risks of what the adolescent is contemplating or the repercussions of the intended behaviors, the examiner may help the adolescent to take another look at his intentions and may also help the adolescent to better understand his potential for acting out.

Being honest, direct, and compassionate are indispensable qualities in building trust with aggressive children. When adolescents have grown up in deceptive and manipulative environments, they expect that everyone else (the examiner included) will try to put something over on them or to "con" them. If being honest and direct are indispensable qualities, they are of particular importance when dealing with hostile and assaultive adolescents. Issues need to be discussed plainly and directly.

When the examiner meets the adolescent, the examiner should make explicit what she already knows about the adolescent and should encourage the adolescent to present his side of the problem. The following case example demonstrates this practice.

Case Example 1

Todd, a 13-year-old Caucasian male, came reluctantly for a psychiatric evaluation. He said to the examiner, "I don't have to see you. I don't need any help." He was evaluated because of physically abusive behavior toward his mother. He had also threatened to kill her. Recently, Todd had brought a loaded gun into his house and had threatened to use it against his mother. Todd had beaten his mother many times before. He was unruly and at home did pretty much what he wanted. He was the only male in the household.

The interviewer focused on Todd's homicidal intentions toward his mother:

INTERVIEWER: I understand you want to kill your mother.
TODD: I don't like that bitch.
INTERVIEWER: You have threatened to kill her.
TODD: She gets on my nerves. I hate her.
INTERVIEWER: You took a loaded gun and threatened to kill her.
TODD: I was joking.
INTERVIEWER: You seem to be capable of killing her.
TODD: I just wanted to see what she was going to do.
INTERVIEWER: Sounds like you are looking for reasons to kill her.
TODD: She makes me so mad!
INTERVIEWER: You are looking for excuses to do it.

Todd started feeling anxious and smiled nervously. He said that he didn't want to live at home anymore. The examiner said, "There is a part of you that does not want to lose control."

At this point, Todd let his guard down, and his bullish facade faded. He acknowledged that he had problems controlling himself and was receptive to the examiner's recommendations. The interview proceeded in a more comfortable tone, and Todd's interest and participation in the diagnostic assessment improved.

Although psychiatric examiners pay attention to issues of aggressive behavior (e.g., physical and sexual abuse) perpetrated against children, they are less attentive to the aggressive and other abusive behaviors that children perpetrate against their parents and siblings. Also of concern are children's behaviors against themselves. These aggressive behaviors need to be explored on a regular basis.

The following case example illustrates an interview with a primitive, aggressive, and self-abusive female adolescent.

Case Example 2

Sally, a 17-year-old Caucasian female, had been admitted to the state hospital many times for severe episodes of explosive and assaultive outbursts accompanied by self-abusive behaviors. She had severe impairments in interpersonal relationships: she was markedly withdrawn and stayed away from people most of the time. Although endowed with normal intelligence, she had major problems in school because of her pervasive dysphoria and temper outbursts. As she grew older, her attendance at school became a regular problem because she had difficulties waking up in the mornings. She had an "awful" mood in the mornings, but her mood and attitude would improve somewhat by noon each day. Her school schedule had been adjusted accordingly.

Sally's self-abusive behavior consisted of savage self-biting and self-cutting of the forearms and self-inflicted injuries to the hands and knuckles that resulted from hitting walls. She had been assaultive to many members of the hospital staff and to peers. She had been put in restraints and had received additional medications as needed on numerous occasions. Many psychopharmacological treatments had been tried unsuccessfully.

The psychiatric consultant was asked to ascertain whether Sally exhibited evidence of an affective disorder. About a dozen clinical staff members attended this consultation. Upon arriving to the consultation area, Sally refused to sit in the designated chair. She was a heavyset adolescent with ambiguous secondary sexual characteristics: her haircut, facial appearance, and demeanor lacked femininity. Shortly after sitting down, she stood up and said, "Fuck you," to the group; began to suck her right thumb; and exited promptly from the room, grumbling on her way out. The consultant felt that the large audience had overwhelmed her and that a more private evaluation was needed.

The consultant found Sally sitting with a nurse in the hospital lobby area. She was sucking her thumb again and was also rubbing her eyebrows, rituals she performed regularly when she felt anxious or overwhelmed. The consultant attempted to engage her in a verbal exchange while allowing her to keep her distance (the consultant sat at least 15 feet away from her). Sally acknowledged that too many people made her nervous. The interaction continued at a distance, with Sally and the consultant speaking loudly to each other.

The consultant, sensing that Sally was not amenable to a variety of topics, chose to test the waters by bringing up the topic of discharge. Initially, Sally said that she was never going to leave, but when the nurse said that she thought Sally had been working on this goal, Sally agreed to discuss what she needed to do to leave the hospital.

The consultant asked Sally if he could sit closer to her. She said it was fine with her. He sat one chair away from her and continued the psychiatric interview. She said she wanted to go home but her family was not looking forward to her return. The consultant asked Sally what was expected of her before she could go home. She spoke about the need to control her anger and to be less self-abusive. The consultant then asked what kind of progress she had made in those areas. She lifted the left sleeve of her shirt, showing him thick resolving scabs from recently inflicted self-injuries. Sally indicated that she was now less self-abusive than before. She also said that she was trying to control herself better and was doing so by staying away from people.

The consultant asked Sally if she could talk about her mood in the mornings. She nodded and said that she had a very bad mood in the mornings; she felt very angry and feared losing control and hurting someone at those times. To control these feelings, she would try to sleep until noon because by midday she felt in better control of herself. She denied feeling suicidal and said that she did not want to hurt anyone but acknowledged that she felt very nervous around people.

The consultant had observed by this time that any topic that raised Sally's level of anxiety would simultaneously elicit the self-regulatory behaviors of thumb sucking and eyebrow rubbing. The consultant asked Sally who her best friend was, and she said it was her 4-year-old cousin, who liked her and played with her. Her second best friend was her father. The consultant had learned that Sally's mother, who had abused drugs, abandoned Sally in early infancy. He did not ask Sally to discuss anything related to her mother.

Sally refused to say whether there were any other important persons in her life. When the consultant approached the issue of medications, she said that they did not help. She reluctantly acknowledged that one antipsychotic medication had helped. She denied experiencing any hallucinations. She even denied feeling paranoid. When asked what activities she enjoyed, she said that she liked to take care of plants.

By this time, she was smiling occasionally and even became playful by making fun of the consultant. After the consultant asked Sally about the presence of paranoid feelings, he asked her if she had any unusual experiences. She said she had "EPS" [extrapyramidal symptoms]. The consultant thought she had said "ESP" [extrasensory perception] and continued without catching his mistake. When the consultant realized that Sally had said EPS, Sally began to laugh. She said that she had fooled the consultant. Both Sally and the consultant laughed. Sally then said that sometimes she knows what the other person is going to say. The consultant replied that ESP is important in dealing with people. As the interview proceeded, Sally agreed that she had a big problem with her mood and agreed to try some medications that might help her with this problem.

The consultant closed his contact with Sally on positive terms. When he was leaving the hospital building, he could see Sally at a distance. She waved at him, and he waved and smiled back at her.

This interview had been carried out in unusual circumstances; Sally was a very uncooperative and volatile patient. Because of her unpredictability, the consultant made a special effort not to aggravate her more and took great care in forming and maintaining an alliance with her. The consultant was deliberate in the selection of areas or issues that he felt were appropriate and safe to discuss. Despite these difficulties, a genuine engagement occurred, and the evaluation was helpful and productive. The information and observations gathered during the interview helped the consultant to conclude that Sally exhibited evidence of mood and anxiety disorders.

The examiner should strive to determine the history and epigenesis of aggressive behaviors. Aggressive children frequently have a history of problematic temperament, persistent oppositional behaviors, impulsiveness or conduct problems, poor social cognitions, coercive discipline (i.e., involving physical punishment), and peer relationship problems. Self-abusive behavior is a common symptom in impulsive-aggressive children.

Loeber and Hay (1994) proposed an epigenesis of aggressive behavior that starts with the infant's difficult temperament and an unsuitable caregiver (poor infant-caregiver matching). This poor match is followed by the persistence of oppositional behaviors, which produces a developmental arrest in the socialization process in a variety of ways. The parental figure then gives up out of frustration. The parent begins to pay attention exclusively to the child's negative behavior and becomes unresponsive or stops giving positive feedback. This parental behavior alters the child's social cognitions. The child begins to perceive bad intentions from others and to display aggression as a means to solve problems because he or she lacks adaptive problem-solving skills. This pattern of response creates rejection from the peer group. At this point, association with deviant peer groups is an expected step.

In evaluating a patient who exhibits aggressive or assaultive behaviors, the examiner should obtain the patient's passive and active histories of violence. The passive history relates to victimization (e.g., the patient's history of physical or sexual abuse); the active history refers to violence perpetrated against others, including physical or sexual violence (e.g., physical assault, rape).

The examiner should strive to link a patient's aggressive behavior to specific psychiatric syndromes and other comorbid conditions (e.g., ADHD, conduct disorder, bipolar disorder, psychotic disorders, substance use disorders) that may contribute to aggressive dyscontrol. Aggressive children demonstrate serious deficits in problem-solving skills and peer relationships. These deficits should be addressed in a comprehensive treatment plan that focuses on aggressive behaviors and related problems.

Otnow Lewis (1996) described evidence in violent youths of psychosis (e.g., paranoid delusions), affective disorders, neuropsychological dysfunction (e.g., language and cognitive deficits), brain injury (e.g., psychomotor seizures associated with epilepsy), hyperactivity, impulsivity, and other signs of brain dysfunction (so-called organicity). The dyscontrol of these individuals is an end-pathway deficit resulting from brain injury related to a variety of causes. These violent persons have a history of head trauma as a consequence of physical abuse. Evaluation of the presence of brain injury and dysfunction in violent adolescents must be pursued systematically. Otnow Lewis (1996) added dissociative disorders to a number of comorbid conditions the examiner should scrutinize methodically in children with behavioral dyscontrol.

Biederman et al. (1996) addressed the role of bipolar disorder as a cause of aggression and behavioral dyscontrol: "Since juvenile mania has high levels of irritability that can be associated with violence and antisocial behavior...

this overlap between BPD [bipolar disorder] and conduct disorder is not surprising....If this overlap continues to be confirmed, these findings may provide some new leads as to the possibility of subtypes of mood-based antisocial disorders not previously recognized" (p. 1006).

Children with so-called borderline disorder psychopathology display a broad spectrum of functional impairments. These include overwhelming rage and violent fantasies (with extreme anxiety and loss of control); rapid regression in thinking and reality testing; affective control difficulties; extreme vulnerability to stress with psychotic decompensation; chronic regressive states; severe separation anxiety; generalized restricted development (in relationships, affect, cognition, and language); and schizoid retreat into preoccupations with fantasy life and withdrawal from relationships (Lewis 1994).

The new DSM-5 diagnosis of disruptive mood dysregulation disorder (DMDD; American Psychiatric Association 2013) should be considered in the differential diagnosis of violence in childhood (see next section).

Evaluation of Bipolar Symptoms

The diagnosis of bipolar disorder in children is a major clinical challenge for psychiatrists because children do not display classically described symptoms of adults and the classical picture of this disorder may not easily be recognized in young patients. Controversy exists about the legitimacy or validity of the diagnosis in preadolescents (see Note 3 at the end of this chapter).

Clinical features of bipolar disorder in childhood and adolescence may often overlap with those of other disorders (such as ADHD) or be interpreted as extremes of "normal" childhood behaviors. Despite the heterogeneity in presentation of symptoms, the manic symptoms, as described in the DSM-5 diagnostic criteria for mania, remain consistent with those identified in adults (Van Meter et al. 2016). Bipolar disorder in its classical manifestations becomes even more common as the child advances throughout adolescence. During late adolescence, the clinical picture becomes progressively similar to that described in adults.

The diagnosis of bipolar disorder has become more common in recent years. In outpatient visits by patients age 19 and younger, bipolar disorder was diagnosed in 25 per 100,000 visits in 1994 and in more than 1,000 of 100,000 visits in 2003, representing a 40-fold increase. In inpatient populations, the diagnosis increased sixfold between 1996 and 2004 (Singh 2008). No doubt, there was an overextension of this diagnostic category, bringing unnecessary polypharmacy to a great number of children and adolescents so misdiagnosed. In an attempt to address the overuse of in the bipolar disorder diagnosis, DSM-5 introduced the diagnosis of disruptive mood dysregulation disorder to include clinical presentations of children and adolescents with history of chronic irritability and frequent aggressive outbursts in whom the more classic manic symptoms are not evident (Van Meter et al. 2016). These children have a different clinical presentation, clinical course and evolution, family aggregation, and genetic background than prima facie bipolar cases. The irritable or angry mood must be characteristic of the child, being present, most of the day, nearly every day, and noticeable by others in the child environment (Criterion D in DSM-5; American Psychiatric Association 2013, p. 156). In DSM-5, the term *bipolar disorder* is explicitly reserved for episodic presentations of bipolar symptoms (p. 157). Characteristically, DMDD is more prevalent in males, whereas in bipolar disorder, the prevalence is even for males and females (p. 158). Although DMDD is included in the depressive disorders, emerging data suggests that DMDD appears to have greater overlap with ODD symptoms (Freeman et al. 2016; Mayes et al. 2016) and that treatment of ADHD symptoms with stimulants significantly improves symptoms of aggression and mood (Blader et al. 2016).

Skeptical clinicians believe that early bipolar disorder in children is nothing more than a severe form of ADHD (so-called bad ADHD). About this controversy, Goodwin and Jamison (2007) wrote, "Overall, studies of manic symptoms in children and adolescents may indicate true bipolar disorders in some cases, but in other cases, these symptoms may be mainly markers of severe emotionality and disruptive behaviors" (p. 194). Post et al. (2002) described a series of developmental factors in the evolution of bipolar disorder (Table 10–1). The critical factor in the differential diagnosis of early-onset bipolar disorder is not the ADHD symptomatology, because manic children and children with ADHD have symptoms that overlap significantly in this area. The difference is in the mood presentation—mania and hypomania, explicitly—and, more importantly, in the history of mood dysregulation with episodicity.

Geller and Luby (1998; cited in Goodwin and Jamison 2007) described five symptoms that differentiate children with bipolar disorder from those with ADHD: elation, grandiosity, racing thought or flight of ideas, lack of need for sleep, and hypersexuality. In Geller and Luby's sample, 60% of children with bipolar disorder displayed psychosis, including 50% of children who showed grandiose delusions. Psychosis was a negative predictor of morbidity and incapacitation. The high frequency of psychoses in children with bipolar disorder is in accord with Pavuluri, who described a range of psychosis from 16% to 88% with a prominent prevalence of grandiose delusions (Pavuluri et al. 2004, p. 188).

When assessing children for bipolar disorder, examiners often ask parents and/or teachers about children's demonstration of symptoms. Requiring endorsement of manic symptoms from both parents and teachers leads to the diagnosis of children who have greater severity of impairment (Carl-

Table 10–1. Developmental factors in the evolution of bipolar disorder

Factor	Age at emergence, years
Irritability-dyscontrol (impulsivity, tantrums, aggression, hyperactivity)	1–3
History of violence	—
Depression	By 8–12
Mania (racing thoughts, grandiosity, mood elevation, bizarre behavior)	7–12
Psychosis–suicidal behavior	9–12

Source. Adapted from Post et al. 2002. Modified from Cepeda 2010, p. 269.

son and Youngstrom 2003). Considering the discrepancy of symptom endorsement by different observers, as Carlson and Youngstrom (2003) note, "two conclusions are warranted":

> First is that the stability, validity, and age-related aspects of these cardinal symptoms of mania are in need of greater attention, and, as with other childhood conditions, more than one source of information may be necessary for a better understanding of the phenomenology in question and the validity of the diagnosis. Second, hyperactive, irritable children who appear to be pervasively 'euphoric/elated/grandiose' constitute a more severe seriously disturbed population than children without those symptoms, regardless of whether they have episodes that meet stringently defined mania criteria. (p. 1055)

The following case example involves a preadolescent child whose manic condition had not been identified.

Case Example 3

Tony, a 5-year-old Caucasian male, had been admitted to an acute inpatient setting for evaluation of severe aggressive behaviors at home and at school. Tony displayed overt and inappropriate sexual behavior, including attempts to have sex with a dog. Tony had a history of mood fluctuations, unpredictable temper, clear depressive trends, and even suicidal behaviors. He had been neglected and had been sexually abused by his 16-year-old brother. At the time of admission to the acute inpatient psychiatric program, Tony was living with his maternal great-grandmother, who allegedly infantilized him. Tony's natural parents were psychiatrically ill: his mother had a diagnosis of bipolar disorder, and his father had alcoholism. There was a family feud regarding Tony's most suitable rearing environment because other relatives felt that the child's great-grandmother was senile and mentally unstable.

The therapist who sought the psychiatric evaluation had told the psychiatrist with amusement that Tony had the whole unit in stitches: he went around the unit cracking jokes and making everybody laugh. Tony's undeniable manic episode had not been recognized. He displayed euphoric mood and pressured speech and was driven and overly friendly; his history of hypersexuality and family background of bipolar illness had been overlooked.[1]

Early-onset bipolar disorder differs from the adult version of the disorder. According to Wozniak et al. (1995), "We found [children with bipolar disorder] to have a developmentally different presentation from adults with BPD [bipolar disorder] such that the majority of these children presented with irritable rather than euphoric mood disturbance, a chronic rather than an episodic course, and a mixed presentation with simultaneous symptoms of depression and mania" (p. 1577). Currently, Wozniak's patients would be diagnosed as having DMDD and not bipolars disorder. DSM-5 (American Psychiatric Association 2013) no longer supports statements like "It is developmentally possible for childhood-onset manic-depressive illness to be more severe; to have a chronic non-episodic course; and to have mixed, rapid-cycling features similar to the clinical picture reported for severely ill, treatment-resistant adults" (Geller and Luby 1997, pp. 1168–1169). It is most likely that these patients have DMDD.

Hypomanic features are sometimes disregarded because they can be mistaken for normative childhood behaviors. For example, silliness and clownlike behavior are often mistakenly considered normal behaviors of childhood. Parents of hypomanic children often report that their children are unusually happy or overly silly, laugh for no apparent reason, or show an unusual degree of expansiveness, often out of character with their more subdued, if not depressed, demeanor. More often, however, a protracted course of irritable mood and prolonged dysphoria is the rule. Some children with hypomanic features share symptoms with DMDD. The moods of these children shift unpredictably, and the children's negative moods are prolonged and intense, despite efforts by sensitive caregivers to soothe the children. Prolonged temper tantrums and bouts of violent, destructive, and uncontrollable behaviors are the norm rather than the exception in early-onset bipolar disorder. Parents report mood fluctuations, even during the same day, and these mood changes

---

[1]At the time of this writing, Tony is a 30-year-old young adult. He has displayed intermittent manic and psychotic behaviors over the years. From time to time, he becomes paranoid and aggressive in response to delusional perceptions. Tony's comorbid anxiety and somatoform symptoms continue to be incapacitating. He lives in a group home and has limited functional capacity. Tony has continued to receive psychiatric treatment since the initial contact.

often seem unmotivated. The clinician should suspect early-onset bipolar disorder when the following complaints are present: recurrent dejected states, prominent irritability, and proneness to angry outbursts in response to even minor provocations. Since clinicians need to consider DMDD in the differential diagnosis, longitudinal observations and an open mind will offer the best approach to insure a valid diagnosis.

The examiner should assess bipolar symptoms in terms of the child's developmental state. For example, a preadolescent with bipolar disorder explained his high energy level by saying that he felt like "I have 100 jet engines in my body." In Joe's case (see Case Example 5 later in this section), the adolescent exercised excessively for long periods of time without experiencing exhaustion.

Grandiosity may have age-related manifestations. Children with bipolar disorder frequently believe they are superheroes (e.g., Superman, Batman, Spiderman, Iceman, Wonder Woman). These children believe they can perform incredible feats, such as "defending the world from alien invaders," because they believe they have special strength or special abilities. Some children with bipolar disorder believe they can fly, have attempted to do so, and have been injured when they jumped from high places.

Most frequently, children with bipolar disorder display or verbalize aggressive themes (e.g., "I can beat anybody"). One 7-year-old child felt so strong and invincible that he said, "I can beat even God." Another 7-year-old girl expressed her grandiosity by boasting, "I have two thousand boyfriends." Yet another 7-year-old child claimed that he was a millionaire and kept making plans for all the money he expected to receive from his disability. Adolescents may be involved in schemes to get rich fast that are similar to the economic misjudgments made by manic and hypomanic adults. For example, a 16-year-old adolescent stole a number of checks from his grandfather and forged his signature with the idea of buying some stereo equipment at a cheap price. He was convinced that he could resell the equipment at a big profit.

Patients sometimes exhibit entrenched traits of arrogance and condescension (see Habib's case [Case Example 6], later in this section). These individuals believe they know more than their parents, teachers, or psychiatrists do. Because of their boastfulness and their persistent devaluation of others, they frequently clash with peers and with authority figures. Typically, these children lack friends and get into frequent conflicts with authority figures, including the law. Parents and other significant figures in these children's lives are often impressed by the children's display of knowledge or by their use of sophisticated language. Parents may believe that these children have superior intellectual abilities and become incredulous when faced with the reality of their children's abilities.

The expression of hypersexuality also needs to be assessed in reference to developmental norms. Several of the case examples in this chapter illustrate inappropriate sexual behavior or hypersexuality (see Tony's case [Case Example 3] earlier in this section, and Kathy's and Joe's cases [Case Examples 4 and 5, respectively], which follow). Compulsive masturbation, promiscuity, and other forms of sexual preoccupation must be explored. The examiner should pursue the possibility of sexual abuse as the cause of these abnormal behaviors. Because a mixed clinical picture seems to be the norm, the examiner must always inquire about depressive feelings when the child exhibits hypomanic traits, and vice versa.

The following cases are clear examples of bipolar disorder in children.

Case Example 4

Kathy, an 11-year-old Caucasian female, was being followed up for a mood disorder that had started about 1 year earlier. She appeared floridly manic. She was markedly euphoric (e.g., she laughed boisterously on an ongoing basis), was driven and restless (e.g., she was unable to sit still for a prolonged period of time), and was in need of continual redirection. She also had trouble sleeping at night. Kathy was sexually preoccupied, and the obsessional quality of her sexual thoughts was quite disturbing. At school, she had boasted in front of the class that she was Lorena Bobbitt [who was infamous for emasculating her husband]. One day, Kathy took a razor blade to school and announced, "I am going to cut the penises from all the boys." This created a great consternation among her classmates, and as a result, she experienced further rejection by her peers. Kathy also displayed conspicuous regressive behavior. Kathy would touch her mother repeatedly and would often tell her, in an endearing but childish manner, "You are so pretty!" or "You are so beautiful!" Occasionally, she would put her head on her mother's lap. When Kathy interacted with her mother, she would talk in a childish and regressive manner.

Kathy also exhibited significant depressive symptoms: she complained that she felt depressed; cried frequently; and was unhappy about her looks (she was overweight), her lack of friends, and her feeling that her peers rejected her. Frequently, she became withdrawn and said that she wanted to die.

Kathy's clinical presentation was not very different from Joe's.

Case Example 5

Joe was a 14-year-old Hispanic male who had been diagnosed at age 12 with bipolar disorder with mixed features. He had been hospitalized multiple times in acute psychiatric units for suicidal, homicidal, and psychotic behaviors. At the time of the last hospitalization, Joe complained of being very depressed. He said that he wanted to kill himself and had heard command hallucinations ordering him to do so. He had problems concentrating and had no motivation to do any homework. He felt very guilty, ashamed, and remorseful about the sexual feelings he had experienced toward his 37-year-old aunt. These feelings had a compulsive quality. In the past, Joe had complained about feeling like having sex with his dog, and he was also disturbed by these feelings. Joe reported feeling like Superman. He experienced a great deal of energy: on one occasion, he lifted weights for an entire day because he didn't experience any feeling of tiredness. At times, he felt that he was God and felt that his school classmates were his subjects who needed to pay homage to him because he was their master.

The following case example provides a dramatic illustration of mixed manic and depressive features.

Case Example 6

Habib, a 12-year-old male whose mother was Caucasian and whose father was Arabic, was admitted to an acute care psychiatric unit after he attempted to hang himself. He had tied his belt to a high bar in the bathroom of a psychiatric residential treatment facility, had put the belt around his neck, and was about to jump when he was found.

Habib had been admitted to the residential program 2 months earlier, because his mother believed she could no longer handle his aggressive, explosive, oppositional, and defiant behaviors. Nine months before that placement, Habib had been hospitalized for suicidal and homicidal behaviors. Before the residential placement, Habib had felt progressively depressed and hopeless, and he had had trouble sleeping. He had dreamed that his father was dying. In reality, his stepfather, who had been like a real father to him, was dying of terminal lung cancer. Since his first admission, Habib had been followed in outpatient therapy, and a number of psychotropic medications had been tried without significant benefits.

Habib was a very bright child and was an excellent student. He had very few friends because of his domineering, condescending demeanor and his low tolerance for frustration. He had particular problems with his 11-year-old sister, who apparently was afraid of him.

Habib's stepfather died 5 weeks before the most recent suicidal crisis. This was a major loss for Habib and his family. His mother was overwhelmed with her husband's death. Habib had been progressing satisfactorily in the residential program, and a discharge date had been set for him to return home, but his mother dreaded his return. Habib's mother, feeling incapable of handling him, told Habib over the phone that she was planning to put him in a shelter while he waited for a group home placement. It was at this point that Habib planned to commit suicide. He wrote the following suicide note:

> To whom it may concern, I have been torn to shreds emotionally, mentally, and spiritually. All the strings in my life have been cut. My mother, my own flesh and blood, has cut the last one today. Now I have no reason to live. There were many things I wanted to do that I will be able to do in heaven. I wanted to write the best book of all time. I wanted to play in the NFL and NBA. I wanted to be a star in the movies and a singer. I wanted to go to Harvard and Harvard Law to become a litigator. I wanted to be rich and not have to worry about money. I wanted to

skydive and bungee jump and go river rafting. I wanted to improve the world with my inventions. I wanted to fly a fighter jet in combat for the marines. I wanted to travel the world and beyond. But more than anything else I wanted a family, parents, children, and grandchildren. I wanted love. I refuse to live in this chaotic world. FUCK YOU, MAMA!

I love you Casey, Ebony, Meggy, Sleepy, Spike, Sugar, Fay, Thena, Precious, La'Britt, Goodwin, Matthew F., Troy, Ricky P., Brandon L., Scooter, Troy, and everyone from the Center [Habib listed all of the residential placement staff members].

Sincerely,
Habib

P.S. I also wanted to be a big-time artist, design shoes, and create games.

The reader of this letter will recognize Habib's pressured speech, marked verbosity, depression, sense of hopelessness, and boundless grandiosity. When Habib mentioned his inventions at the residential program and the therapist expressed curiosity about them, Habib asked the therapist to sign a letter in which the therapist would promise not to infringe on his patent inventions!

Constitutional and developmental affective dysregulation are implicated in early-onset bipolar disorder. Akiskal (1995), developmental considerations about the emergence of bipolar disorder are relevant:

From a very young age, children of bipolar parents evidence difficulty modulating hostile impulses, extreme emotional responses to relatively minor provocations such that the responses greatly outlast the provocation, and heightened awareness of and distress for the suffering of parents and others. ...By late childhood, they have significantly higher rates of comorbid depressive, anxious, and disruptive behavioral problems....Such comorbidity might be interpreted as an indication of emerging dysregulation along irritable-cyclothymic temperamental lines....These findings testify to the affective and behavioral liabilities, as well as the personal qualities of an emerging bipolar temperament. (p. 758)

To this, not surprisingly, the author added that for children with a bipolar profile, "Encounters with peers and adults, especially parents sharing the same temperamental dispositions, are bound to be intense, tempestuous and sometimes destructive" (p. 758). Akiskal concluded, "The profile of the child at risk for bipolar illness...suggests that whatever emotion—negative or positive—these children experience, they seem to experience it intensely and passionately. Their behavior is likewise dysregulated and disinhibited, which leads to an excessive degree of people-seeking behavior with potential disruptive consequences" (p. 758).

The difficulties in ascertaining the diagnosis of bipolar disorder, as expressed by Carlson in 1990, are still valid today:

> While the distinctions between normality, hypomania and mania reflect differences of degree of disorder, differences between mania, psychotic mania, schizoaffective mania and schizophrenia raise questions of different disorders. Moreover, there is still no unequivocal way to make distinctions. Such time-honored criteria as degree of thought disorder, or presence of Schneiderian first rank symptoms and mood incongruent with psychotic symptoms, at least during the manic episode, have not been reliable in distinguishing a manic course from a schizophrenic course. (Carlson 1990, p. 332)

Many times, longitudinal developmental follow-up will assist in deciphering the enigma.

Examiners should exercise caution when diagnosing first psychotic breaks during adolescence because many presentations appear to be schizophreniform in nature. The clinical picture changes into a bipolar presentation as the clinical course unfolds (see Note 4 at the end of this chapter).

The diagnosis of bipolar disorder is also missed in children who abuse alcohol and other substances. Alcohol abuse in preadolescents is closely associated with affective disorders. Famularo et al. (1985; quoted in Goodwin and Jamison 1990, p. 190) asserted that "seven of their ten cases of preadolescent alcohol abuse or dependence were bipolar or cyclothymic, and the remaining three had closely related disorders (major depression with conduct disorder, atypical psychosis, and atypical affective disorder)."

Table 10–2 lists the constellation of history, signs, and symptoms that raises the index of suspicion of a bipolar diagnosis in children.

Evaluation of Oppositional Behaviors

Children with ODD pose the greatest challenge for the examining psychiatrist. The challenge is not so much in formulating a diagnosis but in establishing a treatment alliance. These children most often arrive at the psychiatric evaluation already disgruntled, refusing to speak, and with a defiant and uncooperative attitude. The examiner quickly realizes that the interview will be a trying affair because the child avoids eye contact and exhibits a downcast and defiant demeanor and a tense, if not an angry countenance.

Because children with ODD are hypersensitive to authority figures and are prone to oppositional or defiant behaviors at the slightest perception of provocation, the examiner needs to avoid stimulating the child's oppositional and provocative defenses. Simply, the examiner needs to avoid falling into the provocative trap enacted by the patient. The child's refusal to talk or defiant mutism could stimulate angry counter-responses in the examiner; this

Table 10–2. History, signs, and symptoms associated with bipolar disorder

Evidence of elation during the mental status examination: Euphoria is usually infectious. Mixed mood, including depressive and hypomanic or manic mood may be present.

Evidence of grandiosity: Some children feel that they have special powers; they want to perform the feats of superheroes (e.g., Superman, Batman). Some have made attempts to fly. Other children are hard to teach because they "know it all." Frequently, these children have no friends because they have alienated peers with their devaluating and condescending attitude. Thus, delusions of grandeur, primary identification with superheroes, and paranoid symptomatology may be prominent.

Hypersexuality: Perverse sexual activity may be present.

Episodicity: In bipolar disorder; the mood disorder in major depressive disorder is chronic.

Positive family history: A family history of mood disorders—in particular, bipolar disorder (more so when a three-generation history of the disorder is present)—makes the diagnosis probable.

Judgment impairment: Hypomanic and manic states always involve impairment of judgment. Some patients develop ill-conceived financial schemes; frequent "joyriding" and other impulsive actions are commonly reported.

Mood dysregulation: Commonly, these children have a background of chronic mood disorder with mostly depressive symptomatology. Moodiness and irritability are commonly present. These children have histories of intense and prolonged temper tantrums and difficulties with anger control. Some symptoms overlap with those of disruptive mood dysregulation disorder.

— Depressive delusional manifestations have been considered to be predictive of a bipolar diathesis. Psychotic depressions are common: the earlier the presentation of depression, the greater the likelihood of psychotic symptomatology.

— Severe preadolescent depression with psychomotor retardation may be a forerunner of bipolar disorder.

— There is history of depression with marked psychomotor retardation or a history of atypical depression or of hypomania/mania in response to antidepressant treatment.

— Homicidal or suicidal behavior: frequently, these children have been violent, assaultive, suicidal, or self-abusive.

— Pressured speech and rushing thoughts may be present.

Table 10-2. History, signs, and symptoms associated with bipolar disorder *(continued)*

Psychomotor activation: These children are hyperactive if not driven and are restless and very impulsive. They may be distractible (many patients have been diagnosed with ADHD or may have comorbid ADHD). Other related symptoms are the lack of a need for sleep (i.e., insomnia) and a high level of energy.

Common comorbidities: ADHD, conduct disorder, substance abuse disorder, anxiety disorders, and borderline personality disorder.

Psychotic symptomatology: Psychotic features are common. Auditory hallucinations, often of a commanding nature, are present.

Note. ADHD = attention-deficit/hyperactivity disorder.
Source. Modified from Cepeda 2010, pp. 276–277.

behavior is due to the child's satisfaction in enacting a power struggle and his or her striving to be the victor. A common assumption of children with ODD is that nobody understands them or will be able to understand them. The examiner should be aware that the oppositional behavior may be related to a dysphoric state, an affective disorder, or another psychiatric or neuropsychiatric condition.

The examiner should attempt to moderate the child's provocative facade by relating to the child in a straightforward but caring and concerned manner. The child becomes a victor if the examiner falls into the child's trap or if the examiner gives up the interviewing effort out of frustration over the child's lack of cooperation. Facing an overtly uncooperative and defiant child, the examiner may feel great temptation to plead for cooperation, to give advice, or to become patronizing. These strategies must be avoided. Table 10–3 offers some suggestions on how to deal with and respond to a child with ODD.

The following case example illustrates some of these issues.

Case Example 7

Raul, a 12-year-old Hispanic male, was being evaluated for progressive aggressive behavior at home and at school. He had been involved in fights at school and had been suspended a number of times. He was suspended recently for physically assaulting a third grader. After assaulting the boy, he threatened to kill anyone who reported the incident. At home, Raul got into frequent fights with his younger brother and argued with, talked back to, disobeyed, and provoked his mother on a regular basis. The night before the evaluation, Raul threatened to run away and also threatened to kill himself. A short time before the evaluation, Raul's 8-year-old sister had been removed from the home because their 14-year-old brother had sexually abused her.

During the preceding 6 months, Raul's mother had noticed that he was becoming progressively irritable. She also reported that he had daily angry

Table 10-3. Productive and counterproductive approaches in dealing with children with oppositional behaviors

Productive approaches

Be conscious of your behavior with child.

    Approach the child in a matter-of-fact manner.

    Display warmth and benevolence.

    Give the child the benefit of the doubt.

    Exercise self-control: be aware of your tone of voice.

    Use a positive and assertive tone of voice.

    Be concise and to the point when you address the child.

    Do not give up; do not give in (giving up is akin to abandonment).

Model problem solving

Focus on the problem at hand, not on the child.

Foster the child's cooperation.

Engage the child in the solution of the problem.

Praise the child's steps toward resolving the problem.

Try playfulness and humor.

Do not miss any opportunity to praise or reward the child's prosocial behavior.

Be empathic toward the child's plight.

    Pinpoint your awareness that the child is hurting.

    Attempt to identify with the child's problems.

    Help the child to verbalize sources of distress.

    Assist the child in regaining control.

    Give the child opportunities to save face.

Use sensitive redirection.

    Keep behavioral expectations.

    Emphasize the child's strengths and positive expectations.

    Make child aware of behavioral consequences.

    Exercise consistent limit setting.

    Focus on the here and now.

    Reverse roles (help the child to verbalize the experience).

Table 10-3. Productive and counterproductive approaches in dealing with children with oppositional behaviors *(continued)*

Counterproductive approaches

Negative emotional tone

Critical attitude

Insensitive confrontation

Engaging in power struggles

Taking a threatening or intimidating stance

Ignoring the child

Dramatizing or patronizing

Personalizing the problem

Reminding the child of previous mistakes

Making the child feel bad

Source. Modified from Cepeda 2010, pp. 278–279.

outbursts toward her and his siblings. Raul had been in a psychiatric hospital for treatment of a major depressive episode with psychotic features 4 years earlier. He had been followed up in outpatient therapy on a weekly basis. At the time of the current evaluation, Raul was taking antidepressants.

Since Raul was 8 years old, his father had been in prison for dealing drugs. Raul was in the sixth grade in a special education program, but because of the recent episode of dyscontrol, he was referred to an alternative school. He had no significant medical or surgical history. According to Raul's mother, he had reached his developmental milestones in a timely manner. Raul's mother was afraid that her son had used drugs, and she suspected him of associating with gangs.

Raul was in a dysphoric mood when he entered the interview room. He wore casual clothes, and his hair was shaved on both sides of his head. He gave the examiner a defiant look. The interview proceeded as follows:

> INTERVIEWER: Why were you brought for this evaluation?
> RAUL (*responding in an irritated manner*): Go and ask my mother.
> INTERVIEWER: Do you know why you were brought to see a psychiatrist?
> (*Raul shrugged his shoulders and didn't say anything.*)
> INTERVIEWER: What problems do you have at home?
> (*Raul shook his head, made a gesture of displeasure, and shrugged his shoulders again.*)
> INTERVIEWER: What problems do you have at school?
> RAUL: Fighting.
> INTERVIEWER: Have you ever been suspended?

RAUL: Two times.

INTERVIEWER: I wonder if you have been expelled.

RAUL: No.

INTERVIEWER: What kind of fights were those?

RAUL (*shouting defiantly*): That is something private. That stupid teacher!

INTERVIEWER: Have you ever been in a gang?

RAUL: That's personal.

(*Because Raul had begun to answer some questions, the examiner repeated some of the earlier questions.*)

INTERVIEWER: What problems do you have at home?

RAUL: Fighting with my brother and arguing with my mother.

INTERVIEWER: Who lives at home?

RAUL: My mother and two brothers.

INTERVIEWER: Do you have a father?

RAUL: He is in prison. (*Raul looked down at his lap.*)

INTERVIEWER: Why is he in prison?

RAUL: That's personal. (*Raul gave the examiner a defiant look.*)

INTERVIEWER: Have you ever gone to see him?

RAUL: No. (*Raul became less confrontational.*)

INTERVIEWER: Does he ever write to you? Do you ever write back?

RAUL (*with sadness*): I can't read. (*Raul's face appeared downcast, and he rested his head on the table.*)

INTERVIEWER: You are sad.

(*Raul nodded but didn't say anything. His head was resting on the table at this time.*)

INTERVIEWER: Do you ever cry?

(*Raul nodded again.*)

By this time, Raul's demeanor had softened, and he was more amenable to an extended interview. By the end of the psychiatric examination, Raul was more animated and appeared less defiant. The interview was difficult and filled with tension, but as the engagement increased, the tension and pressure decreased. By the end of the interview, the examiner had empathic and positive feelings toward Raul. The examiner persisted in the goal of completing the psychiatric examination in spite of Raul's persistent defiance and obstructionism. The examiner was firm but related to Raul in a caring manner and avoided responding to his provocations.

ODD coexists with a variety of comorbid conditions, such as depressive disorders, ADHD, DMDD, and psychotic disorders. Oppositional behavior is not uncommon in children with anxiety and conduct disorders. Severe oppositional behavior is common in children with language disorders (particularly receptive disorders), cognitive deficits, limited problem-solving skills, and other neuropsychological deficits, and in children with narcissistic features. Many children with oppositional behaviors have a history of abuse, significant parental inconsistency, and exposure to parental discord or family violence.

Evaluation of Substance Abuse

Substance use disorders (SUDs) often co-occur with risk-taking, impulsivity, inattention, and conduct problems and a broad trait of personality and temperament termed *behavioral disinhibition.* This is a highly heritable general propensity to not restrain behavior in socially acceptable ways, to break social norms and rules, to take dangerous risks, and to pursue rewards excessively despite dangers or adverse consequences (Crowley and Sakai 2015, p. 931). SUDs have a strong association with conduct disorder and antisocial behavior. Youths with behavioral disinhibition do very dangerous things, such as driving under the influence, using multiple substances, carrying weapons, or fighting frequently, creating a serious risk for both homicide or accidental injury and premature death (Crowley and Sakai 2015). In the background of serious SUDs there are multiple drug use and conduct problems, other psychiatric disorders, a prolong relapse course, family substance and antisocial problems, and pursuit of exciting pleasures (novelty seeking), while danger or even mortal risk is ignored. The treatment goal is often to minimize psychological and physical morbidity and mortality (Crowley and Sakai 2015, p. 932).

Crowley and Sakai (2015) recommend the following mnemonic series of questions, CRAFFT, to screen for SUDs:

- **Car.** Have you ridden in a car driven by someone, including yourself, who was high on alcohol or drugs?
- **Relax.** Do you use alcohol or drugs to relax, change your mood, feel better about yourself or fit in?
- **Alone.** Do you use alcohol or drugs when you are by yourself, alone?
- **Friend.** Has a friend, family member, or any other person ever thought you have problems with alcohol or drugs?
- **Forget.** Have you ever forget or regret things you did while using?
- **Trouble.** Have you ever got in trouble while using alcohol or drugs, or done something you would normally not do like breaking the law, rules or curfew, or engage in behavior that put others or yourself at risk?

The authors state that there are 10 fundamental questions to ask to a youth being evaluated for SUD:

1. Are there serious life problems (e. g., frequent intoxications, intravenous drug use, fighting, carrying weapons, extensive truancy, runaway behaviors, criminality, unprotected sex, unplanned pregnancies, experiences of abuse or neglect, depressions, or suicidal behaviors)?
2. Has there been any emergency response needed?
3. Does alcohol or drugs contribute to your behavioral disinhibition?

4. What is the amount of the substance you use, and what is the route of administration?
5. Is there any history or alcohol or substance abuse in your family? Any history of behavioral disinhibition?
6. Has parental care, supervision, and monitoring been adequate?
7. Are the problems exacerbated or lessened by any ongoing environmental factors, such as, other family members, friends (including girlfriends or boyfriends), school, work, church, juvenile officers, therapists, or other agencies?
8. What may block or facilitate treatment with the patient and family?
9. If treatment were to work, what would be your reasonable goals, a year from now?
10. What modality of treatment including medications do you think will be needed to achieve the goal in a year and to maintain success there after?

The authors note that answers to these questions will provide information to recommend a treatment venue, and treatment selection and execution (Crowley and Sakai 2015, p. 939).

Usually, a person's first drug contact starts in adolescence; commonly, adolescents begin to experiment with so-called licit psychoactive substances such as alcohol and nicotine. Some youths go on to experiment with illicit drugs (Szobot and Bukstein 2008). The earlier the onset, the more serious the SUD; earlier onset is associated with sexual risk behaviors and teen pregnancy (Crowley and Sakai 2015, p. 934). The rate of SUDs is higher in children and adolescents with affective disorders, anxiety disorders, and bipolar disorder. Although the role of ADHD in substance use disorder is controversial, when compared with children without these disorders, persons who have experienced trauma in childhood are at a higher risk of SUD (Szobot and Bukstein 2008). Youths with SUDs may have a dysfunction in the brain reward system involved in motivation, salience, and capacity to delay gratification (Szobot and Bukstein 2008) (see Note 5 at the end of this chapter).

When assessing drug abuse in adolescents, the examiner should 1) assess the severity of the drug abuse problem (preferred drugs, past and present use, age at onset of abuse, frequency, quantity, consequences from use, treatment experience and response); 2) determine risk factors and protective factors; and 3) assess mediating factors (i.e., reasons for the substance use, drug preference, expectations, readiness to change behavior, self-efficacy) (Kaminer 2008). Self-reporting of drug use by adolescents is generally valid and detects more drug use than laboratory tests or collateral reports (Kaminer 2008) (see Note 6 at the end of this chapter).

Key Points

- Externalizing symptoms include hyperactive and impulsive behaviors, aggressive and violent behaviors, features of mania and hypomania, oppositional behaviors, and substance abuse.
- Externalizing disorders may exist as primary or comorbid disorders (see discussion in Chapter 9, "Evaluation of Internalizing Symptoms").
- The examiner is successful in interviewing children with externalizing symptoms by engaging them or by interacting with them with a helpful, hopeful, and noncritical attitude.

Notes

1. The most frequently used structured instruments for the "actuarial" assessment of violence are the HCR-20, the Classification of Violence Risk, and the Violence Risk Appraisal Guide. Although the HCR-20 was created for adults, this protocol has significant implications for assessment of violence in youths. The HCR-20 (Webster et al. 1997) includes 20 ratings addressing historical, clinical, and risk management. The 10 historical items are 1) previous violence, 2) age at onset of first violent episode, 3) unstable relationships, 4) employment (school) problems, 5) substance use problems, 6) major mental illness, 7) psychopathy (enduring conduct disorder behaviors), 8) early maladjustment, 9) personality disorder, and 10) supervision failure. The five clinical factors are 11) lack of insight, 12) negative attitudes, 13) active symptoms of mental illness, 14) impulsivity, and 15) no response to treatment. The five risk management factors are 16) feasibility of the plan, 17) exposure to destabilizers, 18) lack of personal support, 19) noncompliance with remediation attempts (medications, therapies), and 20) stress.

    The Classification of Violence Risk (Monahan et al. 2005) is an interactive software program designed to estimate the risk that an acute psychiatric patient will be violent toward others in the coming months. The program measures 40 risk factors. Three categories of risk factors are generated: 1%, 26%, and 76% likelihood of violence.

    The Violence Risk Appraisal Guide (Quinsey et al. 1996), which measures 12 risk factors designed to predict violence in offenders with mental illness, has impressive predictive validity. The authors of the assessment do not allow for any clinical review of the structured risk estimate generated by the instrument (Monahan 2008).

Two scales have the greatest psychometric support for adolescents. The Hare PCL: Youth Version (Forth et al. 2003) requires a 60- to 90-minute expert interview and provides a score but has no cutoff values for categorical diagnosis or risk of violence. The Structured Assessment of Violence Risk for Youth (Borum et al. 2005) guides trained evaluators in a systematic assessment of risk factors associated with violence. A final determination of risk as minimal, moderate, or high is reached. Prospective validity of these scales has not been demonstrated (Ash 2008).

2. An interplay exists between genetics and environment: a genetic susceptibility for antisocial behavior may remain latent in the absence of negative environmental factors, such as harsh parenting or living in a criminal neighborhood. Certain genotypes may be protective against or increase vulnerability for antisocial behavior; thus, maltreated children with a genotype conferring high levels of monoamine oxidase A (MAOA) expression were found to be less likely to develop antisocial problems than were maltreated children with a genotype conferring low levels of MAOA expression (Popma and Vermeiren 2008).

3. The controversy surrounding the diagnosis of mania in preadolescence is similar to the controversy surrounding the diagnosis of depression in preadolescence before it was recognized officially in the mid-1970s. Many clinicians do not accept that children of early latency or preschool age might exhibit such a severe symptom complex. Mania is both an internalizing and an externalizing disorder (Carlson and Youngstrom 2003). Hechtman (1999) explained that the bipolar disorder diagnosis is overused in children due to 1) modifications to DSM-IV (American Psychiatric Association 1994) diagnostic criteria (irritability for mania, chronic instead of episodic course); and 2) the overlap of diagnostic criteria between ADHD and bipolar disorder. Five of seven symptoms for the diagnosis of mania are shared with ADHD. Hechtman asserted that the diagnosis of bipolar disorder should not be made lightly and that it should require strong, sound evidence. She commented that no large epidemiological studies had been done supporting the over-inclusiveness of the bipolar disorder diagnosis. Pliszka (1999) supported the need for longitudinal studies and favored strict criteria for bipolar diagnosis. He pointed out diagnostic ambiguities between intermittent explosive disorder and bipolar disorder. Hechtman (1999) and Pliszka (1999) both warned that psychopharmacological response should not be considered confirmatory of bipolar disorder. The ongoing controversy notwithstanding, Kraepelin found that 0.4% of his patients (i.e., 1 in 200 cases) had displayed manic features before age 10 years

(Goodwin and Jamison 1990). The new DSM-5 DMDD will allow clinicians to find diagnostic alternatives for children and adolescent who were previously and easily diagnosed as bipolar.

4. When parents of high-risk offspring were queried about how early they would approve intervention in their children, 60% thought that acute medication interventions were warranted at the onset of moderate symptoms; in very high risk, 70%; the approval rate increased to 80% at the onset of severe symptoms and to 99% when a definite diagnosis was made. For long-term treatment, the rates are lower: 45% of parents would approve medication use for the onset of moderate symptoms, 65% for onset of severe symptoms, and 93% for a definite diagnosis. Only 7.1 of the parents would wait for the occurrence of multiple episodes or a definite diagnosis (Post et al. 2002).

5. Why are some adolescents and not others at higher risk for drug use? The ventral striatum (nucleus accumbens) activates vigorously when rewards are expected. For adolescents not exposed to drugs, the risk taking is negatively correlated with the strength of the anticipated excitement. That is not the case in adolescents exposed to drugs. So differences in striatal structure and function are neural markers for individual differences in risk taking, including drug risk taking. In addition, when attempting to inhibit a behavior, these youngsters have diminished neural activation in numerous brain regions, and such hypoactivation predicts drug and conduct problems several years later (Crowley and Sakai 2015, p. 936).

6. Administration of screening instruments is the first step in assessing drug abuse. Reliable and valid screening tools include the Personal Screening Experience Questionnaire, Substance Abuse Subtle Screening Inventory, Drug Use Screening Inventory—Revised, and Problem Oriented Screening Instrument for Teenagers. Measures for the assessment of drug abuse severity include the Teen Addiction Severity Index, Adolescent Drug Abuse Diagnosis, and Personal Experience Inventory (Kaminer 2008).

CHAPTER 11

Evaluation of Abuse and Other Symptoms

We discuss in this chapter issues related to the exploration of abuse and a number of other symptoms that do not fit well into the categories of either internalizing or externalizing symptoms. The assessment of these symptoms may involve agencies such as the legal system.

Evaluation of Bullying

The assessment of bullying should be a regular component of a comprehensive psychiatric evaluation of preadolescents and adolescents. The experience of bullying is implicated in a multiplicity of mental health issues in the victims, including an increased incidence of suicides and homicides (see Note 1 at the end of this chapter). Longitudinal studies have demonstrated the long-term effects of bullying beyond childhood and adolescence on physical and mental health and even on socioeconomic status, social relationships and overall quality of life (Takizawa et al. 2014). Indicators that should raise the index of suspicion that bullying might be taking place are listed in Table 11–1.

Malmquist (2008) discussed bullying as a major school problem. Bullying includes 1) being called names, being made fun of, or being insulted; 2) being subjected to rumors; 3) being threatened with harm; 4) being pushed, shoved, tripped, or spit on; 5) being made to do things one does not want to; and 6) purposefully being excluded from groups or activities or purposeful destruction of personal property. A student survey indicated that 16% of chil-

Table 11–1.   Behaviors that indicate that a child may be experiencing bullying

Abrupt decline in school function

Development of suicidal thoughts or self-harm behaviors

Withdrawal from family and friends

New-onset anger outbursts or depressive symptoms

School avoidance or refusal

Sudden dissatisfaction with or desire to change appearance

Refusal or avoidance of previously enjoyed social activities

New concerns with looks or body appearance

dren endorsed being bullied during the current school term and that up to 30% of students in grades 6–10 reported they had been involved in a bullying incident as a bully or as a target.

According to Barker et al. (2008), most adolescents follow a low or declining trajectory of bullying and victimization from early to mid-adolescence, indicating a decrease in the prevalence of victimization and bullying with age. The inclusion of a category of "high/increasing bullying and high/decreasing victimization" suggests that some students transition from victim to bully status during adolescence—a rather common trajectory for bullying victims to turn passive into active and become bullies themselves. Although not all bullies are victimized, victims have a high probability of engaging in bullying behaviors. Those transitioning from victimization to bullying learn to modulate anger in favor of more planned, instrumental aggression. In Barker et al.'s study, those boys and girls who engaged in greater bullying behavior were higher in overall delinquency and self-harm.

Bullying is a form of interpersonal aggression focused on peer victimization (see Note 2 at the end of this chapter). The three characteristics differentiating bullying from other types of interpersonal aggression are intentionality, repetition, and an imbalance of power (Hymel and Swearer 2015). As a result, when assessing bullying, the interviewer should explore the frequency of episodes (repetition), whether the bullying statements or behaviors are directed toward a single individual or group in general (intentionality), and the perceptions of status (power imbalance). The assessment of power imbalance should include exploration of topics such as physical size and strength and social and economic status, as well as use of and access to weapons. In boys, bullying frequently takes the form of physical aggression (assaultive behaviors or threats of violence), whereas girls are more prone to relational aggression (exclusion or emotional/verbal abuse). Although bullying has traditionally been considered a hallmark of "life on the playground," the advent of mobile technology, the Internet, and social media has extended the reach of bullying and has brought about the concept of *cyberbullying*.

Cyberbullying is also named *electronic aggression, cyber aggression*, and *online harassment*. Common electronic aggressive behaviors include hostility (e.g., insults, threats), humiliation (e.g., posting an embarrassing picture), obsessive monitoring or control (e.g., intrusive texts), deception (e.g., using a fake social media profile to interact with another), and exclusion (e.g., unfriending). The estimates of the prevalence of cyberbullying among children and adolescents in middle and high school fall between 10% and 40% (Ramos and Bennett 2016). It appears that electronic aggression during adolescence continues into college (Ramos and Bennett 2016, p. 24). The most common platforms for bullying include message boards, social networking sites, blogs, Twitter, and Web pages. Adolescents who have been cyberbullied report becoming more withdrawn, losing self-esteem, and feeling uneasy. There are adverse effects in relationships with friends and family. Therefore, mobile phone, social media, and Internet usage should also be assessed during a psychiatric evaluation.

In light of the intensified focus on bullying as a risk factor for completed suicides in children and adolescents, the emerging research assists in elucidating the factors that increase the risk for victimization. In the TRAILS (TRacking Adolescents' Individual Lives Survey) study, researchers assessed the impact of preschool behaviors, family characteristics, and parental mental health on bullying. They determined that early risk factors for victimization included poor motor function and low socioeconomic status; these were statistically significant risk factors at age 11; preschool aggressiveness was a statistically significant risk factor at age 13 (Jansen et al. 2011). Poor motor function may increase the risk for victimization because of the social and self-esteem implications. That is, children with poor motor performance may not perform well in sports or other games that require motor competence and may suffer exclusion or poor acceptance by peers.

Children who experience frequent bullying and are targeted by more than one peer experience greater levels of social anxiety, depressive symptoms, and poor well-being at school (van der Ploeg et al. 2015). Bullying victims also express higher levels of anger and internalizing behaviors (Lovegrove et al. 2012).

The following is an example of a male adolescent who announced his death to a number of friends. The mother of one of one these friends, upon reading the letter, ran over to this adolescent's home to alert the child's parents about the imminent risk. The child was saved. The message reveals many issues related to bullying and adolescents' struggles; the letter is unedited, except for the adolescent's name.

Im writing this letter so you don't end up asking any questions when I'm gone. If you're reading this that means you care enough to know that I'm quitting. If you're mentioned in this letter that means I care about you and I don't want you to cry or be sad because I can rest in peace finally. I just want everyone to know that if I'm going to hell then so be it. That is my just punishment, but both ends of the knife were in favor of this act, suicide is a shot with a very high price. It is not murder, it is not self respect. I just wanted to live a normal life. A normal brother, normal parents, normal school, just to be average, standard. I used to hate that but its better than being a fat emo freak who cuts himself for the stupidest reasons. So let my death not be a sad one. But a reminder that you can push someone off a ledge without laying a hand on them. I'm going to start this letter by talking to my friends giving them clarity.

Dear Mary, I wrote you first because I know this is hitting you the hardest. Please don't cut or cry or even die over me. I know I have fallen but you have to keep moving. You will be a beautiful smart girl in Juilliard whose dream is to bring a smile to others and yourself through music. Keep moving Soaps, I know this might psychologically damage you permanently but I'm so, so sorry. I broke the promise I made to you that I said I would keep living. I will always be with you to protect you when you are threatened, comfort you when you are sad, and make you smile with thoughts of happiness. Stay alive. I love you like a sister.

Dear Judy, please don't think that I will ever leave you. You are a sweet, funny, and loving girl and your scars will kin you with rejoice in the future. Don't cut no more. Don't get worse, it would hurt me even if I was dead. I feel so sorry if I ever hurt you or made you feel excluded to the point of you mentally and physically hurting yourself. Stay strong, I can tell if you ever have kids they will love you so much.

Dear Bob, I've been through two-thirds of my middle school experience with you. We've switched through different squads, hung out a lot, hated some people, but I never left your side. You would remind me constantly to put my dark thoughts where they can't hurt me or anyone else but I just couldn't win the battle this time. I have tried to pull through but so many people want to hurt me and I feel so much pain every day I can't handle this shit anymore.

Dear Hank, I've never hated you or been mad at you even for the slightest second. Even though every time I hear your name I think of that stupid letter. Ugh goddamn it I hate that letter. Maybe we would have gotten along sooner if that letter burned in hell before it even reached your hands. I have to admit I did cut myself when you found out I wrote that piece of shit, but I want you to know none of it was your fault. I was not sad because you said you were straight. I saw that coming. I was sad because it created eternal awkwardness between us. You have forgiven me for the letter already but I still feel like you would be a little more comfortable around me without it. I don't usually call it a letter I call it Lucifer's diaper. I hate myself for this. Anyway, you are funny, smart, artistic, thoughtful, and really fun to be around. Take care of my friend Mary, she might be taking this really hard. Reliving that horrendous mistake gets me thinking how you don't hate me after that extremely disturbing letter.

Dear Tom, can I just say that sometimes I took offense to some of your jokes, that never ended well. I remember in 2nd grade when I got you in trouble for no reason at all and to this day you still hold a grudge. I know I suck for quitting at life, but if you were in my position no thought would be different. I know I shouldn't starve myself, I shouldn't cut, I shouldn't be sad all the time but fuck it. I still think we got along better before I told you I was pansexual. Yes.. I seriously think you're homophobic. Even if it's just a phase, or a mental defect, even if I was just born with it I'm dead right now and I still don't give a fuck. Everyone hated me just because of a sexual orientation and that hurts. Its not a choice, being homosexual is the same reason for being straight. Love is love. Don't worry, one day not being gay will be as normal as being black.

Dear Shawn. You are funny, sensitive, smart, and different. Your silly bickering with Tom and Bob at the lunch table keeps me entertained. Although a lot of times I felt forced to choose side between my own friends when you really got mad at them. I honestly don't know who starts the arguments but I could care less because getting along is so much easier. I could never forgive myself for emotionally scaring you with my absence from life. I just struggled too much with everything. They can call it a phase, they can say I was just looking for attention, but that won't bring me back from the dead. Sorry triggering use of words. Anyway don't stop moving, you will be a wonderful person one day buddy.

Dear Sarah, you are hilarious, sweet, thoughtful, and some of the things you would tell me made my day. Through all the people that would spread crap about me I feel like I could tell you anything because you kept my secrets to the fullest. Im sorry I suck at comforting you when you were sad but I often felt I needed to cheer myself up before I could make others happy. I know you'd get mad at me when I would do suicidal things but I want to apologize for everything. We were very close and that will never change. Stay up and don't fall like I did.

Dear Louise, I wish you didn't have to hear this because I know this would hurt you a hella lot. But I am no longer physically here. At my point of view in writing this I don't know if I'm going to hell or heaven but I just feel so sorry for leaving you like this. I remember one day you were crying and I felt so bad because I was just sitting there because I suck ass at comforting people. I know that you have struggled with this stuff in the past. Please Louise, let it stay in the past. I want you to move on so that if you're ever sad again my ghost ass can climb out of my grave and give you a hug whenever and wherever you are. You are funny, supportive, sweet, pretty, and honestly (George didn't deserve you). We are really close and dead or alive it's gonna fucking stay that way so get comfortable. I love you like a sister and I would appreciate it if you kept on moving. I was so stupid to leave you traumatized like that but I just couldn't get this monster out of my head.

Dear Martha, you are closer than my BFF you are family. No really you're my cousin. I was really sad when you went to Europe and worse when you went to Florida but if its for your own good I'm all for it. Nothing will ever separate, not even death. And if you need someone to talk to I will always be there, because I know that I would never call you and I'm really sorry. Everything just built up in my head and I got so distraught that I stopped contacting you. You have helped me win battles with people who really hated me. You are sweet, smart, beautiful, and insanely kind to anyone. You will grow up to be more than the best as long as you don't quit. Never quit because even though I never came to enjoy the reward of the future, you will and you will live it up because that's all I ever cared. That you didn't turn out like me. You are my family and I love you.

To anyone that I didn't mention in this letter if I hated you then fuck you but thank you for helping me get stronger. If I love you then I am really sorry for flaking out on the world and never be a Jonathan because I am just a lonely loser who ragequit on life because he couldn't handle a little pain.

I love all of you guys. Thank you for caring. God bless all of you, goodbye

It is very clear that bullying pushed this adolescent over the edge. A number of this adolescent's friends had issues with depression, self-abusive behaviors, identity, and sexual identity concerns. The author of the letter is a gifted writer, and he was so recognized by his teacher and mentors.

Bullied children have difficulties keeping up with their grades. For many, grades worsen and behavior problems at school and absenteeism become common. Depression is associated with cyberbullying, and in some cases cyberbullying is associated with self-abusive behavior, suicidal ideation, and suicide attempts (Wagner 2016). Close to 25% of cyberbullying victims do not speak about this with anybody. The frequency of bullying is correlated with the development of depression: 14.8% of youths who were frequently bullied developed depression by age 18; 7.1% became depressed if they were occasionally bullied, and only 5.5% became depressed even though they did not experience bullying. In other words, bullying increases the risk for the development of depression threefold; this is true for both sexes. Students who were bullied were significantly more likely to be sad (51%) or to report suicidal ideation (39.3%) and suicide attempts (18.3%) (Wagner 2016, p. 28). It is interesting that the students who exercise four or more times per week were less prone to depression and suicidal ideation even if they were bullied.

When a child or adolescent presents with new-onset depressive symptoms, anxiety symptoms, school avoidance, or disruptive behaviors (especially anger and aggression), the examiner should inquire about bullying. Bullying is likely a trigger or contributing factor to the development of new symptoms or the loss of adaptive behaviors. Other factors suggestive of bullying include worsening of mental health issues with the start of the school year and amelioration of symptoms during vacations, and sudden onset of symptoms at significant transitions (e.g., new school, start of a new grade, shifts to middle or high school). Bullying should also be ruled out in every case of "school phobia."

Bullying is often a trigger for the onset of mental health symptoms. but bullying may also result from perceptions of difference by peers. After disclosures of sexual orientation or gender confusion, issues of body image (weight or body flaws), unconventional dressing or makeup (including body piercings, visible tattoos, etc.), or rejection of treatment for medical or mental health issues, bullying should be suspected.

Although the majority of children and adolescents who present with bullying issues typically identify experiences as a victim, the interviewer should also assess the child or adolescent for experiences as a perpetrator. History that may shape perpetrator behaviors includes past trauma, family dysfunction, frequent school citations, and legal charges. These "bully victims" also experience higher rates of suicidal thoughts, self-harm, and suicide attempts in comparison with children who are classified only as victims (Espelage and Holt 2013) as in the example of Justin.

Case Example 1

Justin, a 10-year-old Caucasian male, was admitted to the acute inpatient unit for suicidal ideation and homicidal ideation directed toward his brother. During the initial interview, Justin reported that he, his mother, and 12-year-old brother had recently moved to a new town where Justin started a new school. At the new school, he stated peers were bullying him by calling him "fat" and ridiculing and shunning him for his visual impairment. As a result, he had become depressed, had stated that he did not want to attend school, and had voiced threats to shoot himself with a gun. He believed that his peers would continue to target him and disclosed having nightmares about being harmed by others. He reported that his homicidal ideation towards his brother was the result of bullying by his brother and neighborhood peers. He complained that his brother excluded him from play with the neighbors group and had punched him during a fight on the day of his admission.

Collateral information from Justin's mother indicated that he had instigated the fight with his brother and that Justin had, in fact, punched his brother hard enough to cause him to fall and hit his head on the ground. Mother confirmed that Justin frequently was excluded from play with neighbors because he would easily become assaultive towards them. Although Justin had reported that peers were bullying him at school, mother claimed that his principal and teachers had observed no changes in Justin's behaviors at school and that peers would often attempt to assist him and include him in their activities.

Justin's social history was significant for little to no current contact with his biological father. Justin's mother reported that she had divorced her husband when Justin was 5 because he was physically and emotionally abusive. During the course of his admission, Justin disclosed that during visits with his biological father, his father would often yell or deride Justin for his visual impairment; however, Justin's brother was usually the target for physical abuse. Justin reported nightmares and flashbacks consisting of the names his father would call him; he also reported dreams of being beaten up by his father.

Interventions to prevent and address bullying must include assessments for risks for perpetration as well as victimization. The most successful interventions incorporate strategies to decrease aggression and improve interpersonal skills (Lovegrove et al. 2012). Twemlow and Sacco (2012, p. 47) assert that successful interventions to prevent and address bullying involve synchronization among the family, school, and community and that the engagement of the family is crucial to the success of any intervention. Therapy to improve speech and language deficits or poor motor skills (Jansen et al. 2011) can improve a child's sense of competency in communication and engagement with same age peers in activities. The employment of *therapeutic mentoring* can help in the teaching of social skills to youth utilizing resources in the community and through building on a child's interests (Twemlow and Sacco 2012) (see Note 3 at the end of this chapter).

Evaluation of Symptoms of Abuse

In the United States, neglect is the most common form of maltreatment (75%), followed by physical abuse (17%), sexual abuse (8.3%), and medical neglect (2.2%) (Scheid 2016, p. 16). The clinical evaluation of abused children deals predominantly with the verification of the abusive acts perpetrated against children and the assessment of the psychological consequences of the abuse. Different branches of medicine deal with the physical assessment and treatment of sequelae of abuse. The psychiatric evaluation of abuse aims to ascertain the emotional impact of abuse—that is, the deleterious influences on the developmental process (developmental interference) and on the psychological and interpersonal functioning of the child and her family.

The examiner's first step in evaluating abused children is to clarify his or her role in the overall assessment process. The purpose of the evaluation will determine the examiner's approach and the information he or she will gather. The approach taken depends on whether the examiner is performing a forensic or a clinical examination. Because of legal implications, the examiner must pay careful attention to the facts and follow a strict protocol to gather evidence for a forensic assessment. Ascertaining the facts in allegations of sexual abuse is a delicate, difficult, and uncertain enterprise (Benedek and Schetky 1987a, 1987b). It requires a team approach and specialized expertise. Even the pelvic examination is fraught with uncertainties and controversy (Coleman 1989). Ascertaining facts in child abuse investigations is very difficult. Issues related to the reliability of children's complaints, and the particulars of conducting sexual abuse diagnostic evaluations will be discussed later in this chapter. One would think that the medical pelvic examination would be more effective as a fact-finding examination. That is not the case: findings are controversial. The use of anatomically correct dolls to elicit information regarding possible sexual abuse is a proscribed practice. Issues that need to be resolved in the validation of sexual abuse are listed in Table 11–2.

Benedek and Schetky (1987b, p. 916) warned that sexual abuse treatment should not be initiated without confirming that such abuse happened in the

Table 11–2. Questions representing issues that need to be resolved in validation of sexual abuse

1. Are there other plausible explanations?

2. Are the child's statements spontaneous?

3. Are the child's statements consistent?

4. Is the child's sexual knowledge incongruous with his or her developmental age?

   Examples:

   Does the child put the mouth on another's sexual part?

   Does the child request engagement in sexual acts?

   Does the child masturbate with an object?

   Does the child insert an object into the anus or the vagina?

   Does the child imitate intercourse?

   Does the child make sexual sounds?

   Does the child French kiss?

   Does the child talk about explicit sexual acts?

   Does the child undress others?

   Does the child invite others to watch explicit television or sexual movies?

   Does the child enact sexual acts with the dolls?

5. Does the child use appropriate developmental language?

6. Does the child indicate in play or by gestures that he or she was abused?

7. Does the child give personalized, experiential detail?

8. What is the content and context of the child's statements?

9. What is the child's manner and emotional display?

10. Does the child have motives or reasons to fabricate an allegation?

    Is this something that really happened, or is this make-believe?

    Are you saying this to get [the accused] in trouble?

    Are you saying this because you are mad at [the accused]?

    Does somebody else think this happened even though you don't?

    Are you saying this because you want to live with...?

Table 11-2.   Questions representing issues that need to be resolved in validation of sexual abuse *(continued)*

10. Does the child have motives or reasons to fabricate an allegation? (*continued*)

> *For older children:*
>
> Are you saying this to get out of the house?
>
> Are you saying this because [the accused] was not nice to you or was not paying enough attention to you?
>
> Are you saying this because you wanted to cover up the fact that you wanted to do it (to have sex)?
>
> Are you blaming the accused, after you had sex with your boyfriend?

11. Does the child correct the interviewer?

12. Does medical evidence exist?

13. Does forensic evidence exist?

14. What are the statements of the accused?

Source.   Mantell 2008. Modified from Cepeda 2010, pp. 297–298.

first place. These authors considered a comprehensive psychological evaluation an important part of the total assessment and emphasize the need for a comprehensive psychiatric evaluation of the child and the family, and for an extensive collateral corroboration from school, other families, and other relevant sources.

The clinician needs to focus his or her attention equally on the child's narrative and on the historical truths: Clinicians should not attempt to be detectives in search of historical truth, but neither should they blur narrative and historical truth (Allen 1995, p. 90).

Special Considerations in Interviewing Physically and Sexually Abused Children

Clinicians should always keep in mind their legal responsibilities when dealing with abusive situations: they are obligated to report abuse (even suspected abuse) to child protection services (CPS).

When interviewing children who may have been abused, the examiner must be particularly careful to avoid asking leading questions (Goodman and Saywitz 1994). Engagement is very important in assessments of this nature. Engagement helps to improve the child's sense of trust and comfort; good rapport decreases the degree of defensiveness and apprehensiveness the child may exhibit in communicating these sensitive, often secretive but traumatic events. The examiner should use the same vocabulary that the child uses, no matter how incorrect such terms may seem to the examiner. This is not the time to instruct the child on correct anatomic terminology or in correct English (see Case Example 2 below).

Questions like "Have you ever been physically or sexually abused?" are of uncertain value because the child may have been told not to tell or the child may feel a duty to protect his or her family. The examiner should begin the evaluation of physical abuse by exploring how the child is disciplined. The following questions may be helpful: "When you have done somethin' wrong, how do your parents discipline you?" "Have you ever been punished?" "Have you ever been spanked?" "Has your father or your mother ever lost control when disciplining you?" "Has anyone ever used a belt on you?" "Have you ever been whipped?" When asking these questions, the examiner needs to be sensitive to different cultural attitudes toward physical discipline.

The sensitive exploration of the topic of sexual abuse may begin with the following questions: "Has anyone ever touched you where they shouldn't?" "Where?" "When did that happen?" "Did you tell anyone?" "Did you tell your mom?" If the child answers "no" to this question, the examiner should ask whether there was a reason why the child couldn't tell the parent. If the child reports that "nasty" acts were done to him or her, the examiner should encourage the child to provide details of what happened, but the examiner must be careful not to suggest answers or to ask leading questions.

The examiner must note the events narrated by the child in the child's own words (i.e., using the child's own language and expressions).

Most sexually abused children have been threatened by the perpetrators of the abuse and have been told not to talk about it. Often these children have been told that horrible things, including death, will happen to them or their family if they disclose the abuse. The examiner should remember that the child is aware of the possible repercussions of disclosure at all times. The examiner's empathic understanding of the child's fear should reassure the child. When a child reveals sexual abuse, the examiner may tell the child that he knows that when children are abused, the abusers tell children not to tell anyone about the abuse. The examiner can then ask the child to tell him about any threats the perpetrator may have made. The examiner should explore the nature of the threats and reassure the child about the consequences and about any retaliation she may anticipate. If the child has active symptoms of posttraumatic stress disorder (PTSD), the fear of retaliation may reach psychotic proportions. When it is necessary to do so, the examiner should reassure the child that she will be safe and protected and that the examiner will make every possible effort to avoid any negative consequences for making the disclosure. If the examiner concludes that the child's safety cannot be guaranteed or that the traumatization is likely to continue, he should make arrangements with CPS to place the child, temporarily, in a safe environment until the concerns with safety are resolved.

All forms of psychological manipulation on the child and any form of cajoling or pressuring of the child are absolutely proscribed. Pressure from the examiner to remember traumatic events may promote confabulation (Allen 1995, p. 86). Confabulation is discussed in more detail in the last section of this chapter.

A child's ability to remember traumatic events may vary. Some memories may be clear, and some may be clouded; some memories may be corroborated and others may not. Four of the categories in Allen's (1995, p. 89) classification of memories regarding sexual abuse are of particular clinical and legal relevance. Category 4 includes clouded memories for which corroborating evidence is lacking; category 5 includes memories of trauma that are highly exaggerated or distorted, and categories 6 and 7 include memories of trauma that may or may not have occurred in individuals who believe they were abused. Memory distortion may occur if the patient has been exposed to suggestive techniques or has experience with therapists who erroneously believed that the patient's symptoms were the result of childhood sexual abuse.

Examiners should remember the moral and legal implications of accepting the patient's disclosures at face value. They must exercise caution and attempt to substantiate the truthfulness of the patient's revelations. Frankel (1996) stresses this point: "Those therapists who emphasize that what is recalled is a previously disconnected and accurate memory of a childhood event that has never before been recognized might be correct in some instances; however, these therapists should not underestimate the consequences of such material, which has been regarded as truth but is actually the product of imagination, becoming the basis of either accusations, within the family or litigation" (p. 69). Children may "remember" things that they have not experienced. In a discussion of Ceci's research on memory retrieval in small children, Terr et al. (1996) commented, "If children are coached…the incorrect suggestion that they have heard may turn up as memories. Using strong and repeated suggestions, Ceci's group was able to impart episodes that never took place into some preschoolers' minds" (p. 619). The examiner should also be aware that the act of reporting previous experiences modifies the nature of the child's narrative memory (Allen 1995; Lewis 1995). These issues are described in further detail in the last section of this chapter.

How reliable are children's report regarding abuse? Bruck and Ceci (2015) discuss this transcendental topic. They state that research provides a scientific basis for evaluating children allegations of abuse.

1. On average, a 6-year-old can recall information from more than 2 years previously. The same memories are not available if the child is asked to retrieve same memories a few years later. However, children can accurately recall stressful events many years after their occurrence. This is true if

the interviewer is neutral, questions are nonsuggestive, and the examiner has no motive to influence the child's testimony.

2. Biased interviewers can taint the child's report, rendering it unreliable. *Interviewer bias* relates to evaluators who hold a priori belief about the occurrence of an event and conduct the interview to obtain confirmatory evidence. Biased interviewers use a range of suggestive techniques that are associated with elicitation of false reports; these interviewers do not test plausible alternative hypotheses. The concept of biased interviewers is not limited to forensic interviewers but includes therapists, teachers, and parents (Bruck and Ceci 2015, p. 252).

3. Example of suggestive interviews include the following:

   a. *"Yes" or "no" questions; choice questions, such as, "Did he do A, B or C?"* "Loaded" and leading questions, such as, "Her mom told me what happened to her, did it happen to you?" This line of question forces the child to give an answer and provide indirect information about the suspected event, making it a suggestive technique. Young children do not say "I don't know" when they are presented with nonsensical or misleading statements; this is true even when children have been told that they can answer, "I don't know." A golden guideline to interviewing children emphasizes the need to ask open-ended questions to allow children to describe their experiences in their own words.

   b. *Repeated specific questions within interviews.* When children first deny the occurrence of an event, they frequently change the answer if the questions are repeated. Repetition of questions not only may provide the child additional misinformation but can also result in making the child shift from an accurate response to a false or inaccurate one.

   c. *Repeated suggestive interviews.* With each repeated suggested interview, children are more likely to assent to previously denied nonexperienced events, and these reports persist when the child is interviewed later by a neutral interviewer. With repeated suggestive interviewing, if the child presents new information, it is likely to be false. When the interviewer urges the child to tell him or her more, such a request may promote false reporting to comply with the interviewer's expectations. Often, these reports are highly detailed, even more so than the accurate ones.

   d. *Stereotyped induction (vilification).* A variety of studies have shown that when children are provided with information that a person does "bad things," they will creatively incorporate this content into the own reports of wrongdoing. For instance, when children were told that a man who visited the school was "clumsy," they often later claimed to have observed him doing "clumsy" things like breaking toys.

e. *Peer contamination (co-witness contamination).* Children will pick up information about an event from peers and, even though they have never experienced it, will elaborate on it and later claim it also happened to them. False claims are indistinguishable from true claims made by other children.

f. *Nonverbal props.* The use of props (e.g., toys, dolls) can be suggestive, particularly for younger children, and can result in false report about touching. Children use the props as toys to play with and to explore rather than to demonstrate experienced actions or events (Bruck and Ceci 2015, p. 253). The risk for false statement is greatly increased when the interview contains a variety of suggestive techniques, such as leading questions, peer pressure, and vilification through stereotyped induction, increasing the salience of the interviewer's bias (Bruck and Ceci 2015, p. 254).

4. The first interview with the child provides the most reliable testimony. However, if there is suggestion in the first interview or in conversations prior to it, the child's initial statements may be tainted and therefore unreliable. In documenting the evolution of the children's allegations, it is important to determine if the child's first statement is a) spontaneous, unprompted, and made in the absence of suggestive elements, or b) associated with previous or concurrent suggestive interviewing techniques.

5. Suggestive interviewing techniques can result in false beliefs that are longlasting. Children may come to believe that they actually experienced false suggested events, and once a child's testimony is tainted, it may be impossible to "un-taint" it in subsequent interviews even if the interviews are performed by the field's best experts. No amount of probing and deprogramming can unearth the original untainted memory because it may have been irrevocably modified by the prior suggestive questions, evolving into a false belief and becoming now part of the autobiographical memory.

Children's false reports seem credible. In fact, in some studies, children's narratives of false events contain more embellishments (descriptive and emotional) and have more detail than narrations of true events. False reports often contain more spontaneous statements than true narratives; they contain more bizarre statements than real events. A word of caution: we need to be cognizant that subjective rating of children's reports after suggestive interviewing reveals that such reports appear highly credible to prospective jurors or trained professionals in the field of child development, mental health and forensic. There are not scientifically acceptable markers for judging the child's truthfulness in interviews that have been preceded by suggestive interviews (Bruck and Ceci 2015, p. 254).

Developmental Consequences of Abuse

Abused children are prone to future psychopathology, and they are prone to repeat abusive behavior with peers and, later, with spouses and their own children. The idea that physical abuse may be repeated is commonly accepted, but the tendency of abused children to act out the experience of sexual abuse with other children should also be explored (see Carlos's case [Case Example 1] in Chapter 15, "Diagnostic Obstacles [Resistances]"). Children who have experienced sexual abuse should be asked whether they have done or have attempted to do the same thing to other children. Sexual abuse by children and adolescents, mostly boys, has become widely recognized and is no longer considered a variant of childhood or adolescent sexual development. A significant proportion of adolescent abusers are of low intellectual abilities and show heterogeneous maladaptive mental schemata regarding social interaction and abuse. Children and adolescent abusers have experienced psychosocial adversity, including, neglect, lack of supervision, sexual abuse by a female person, and exposure to domestic violence. Many adult abusers report the onset of their abusive behavior in adolescence, and abuse by an adolescent cannot necessarily be considered safely to "burn out" in adulthood (Glaser 2015, p. 378).

Not all children who have been sexually abused will develop behavioral or emotional difficulties; it is estimated that about one-third of individuals who have experienced sexual abuse will not exhibit adult psychiatric problems. Their resilience is related to perceived parental care, positive adolescent peer relationship, the quality of adult love relationships, and personality style (Heim et al. 2010, p. 6). Considering sensitive periods, there is evidence the trauma effects on the brain depend on the age at which the abuse occurred: hippocampal volume was reduced when child sexual abuse experience occurred between ages 3 and 5 and between ages 11 and 13; frontal cortex was attenuated in subjects with history of sexual abuse between ages 14 and 16 years. It is proposed that in victims of abuse there is an altered cytosine-methylation of the neuron-specific promoter region of the glucocorticoid gene in the hippocampal tissue. Such methylation silences the gene, resulting in decreased glucocorticoid receptor expression and, hence, potentially increased stress response (Heim et al. 2010, p. 12).

The examiner should attempt to identify any developmental deviations created by physical and sexual abuse. Cicchetti and Toth (1995, pp. 546–554) described specific mechanisms by which abusive experiences disrupt or interfere with the formation of fundamental functions or psychological structures (see Chapter 9, "Evaluation of Internalizing Symptoms"). These developmental deviations create or contribute to the development and maintenance of psychopathology (Table 11–3).

Table 11-3.   Developmental disruptions fostered by physical and sexual abuse experiences

Affect regulation (by promoting affect dysregulation [e.g., low tolerance for frustration; anger dyscontrol])

Normative attachment (by promoting atypical attachments [e.g., avoidant, resistant, and disorganized types])

Self-esteem (by promoting a defective self-concept and lower self-esteem, deficits in internal state language, and lower capacity for symbolic play)

Supportive peer relationships (by disrupting social competence and promoting a tendency to physical and verbal aggression in peer interactions)

Positive adaptation to school (by contributing to school maladaptation secondary to deficits in social cognitions and limited academic achievement)

Source.   Cicchetti and Toth 1995. Reprinted from Cepeda 2010, p. 298.

Examiners will encounter a variety of psychopathological syndromes in abused children. For example, van der Kolk et al. (1996, p. 89) suggested that PTSD does not occur in isolation. Frequently, it is associated with dissociation, somatization, and dysregulation of affect, including difficulties with anger modulation, sexual involvement, and aggression against the self and others (see Note 4 at the end of this chapter). These symptoms are found together in the same individuals, and their co-occurrence is at least in part a function of the age at which the trauma occurred and the nature of the traumatic experience. Table 11–4 lists psychiatric disturbances commonly found in sexually abused children and adults. According to Green (1993), these disturbances may represent sequelae of the abusive experiences.

Dissociative Symptoms

Dissociative disorders, including dissociative psychoses, are frequent complications of severe childhood abuse; unfortunately, these disorders are often incorrectly diagnosed. Dissociative psychoses are frequently misdiagnosed as schizophrenia (Hornstein and Putnam 1992; Putnam 1991). Otnow Lewis (1996) corroborated this point:

> Command auditory hallucinations, the experience of hearing voices speaking to each other in one's head, the sense of being controlled by these voices, the delusional system of hierarchies of imaginary companions, the blocking, and the illogical thinking of children with DID/MPD [dissociative identity disorder/multiple personality disorder] often lead to a misdiagnosis of schizophrenia. (p. 307).

Table 11–4. Psychiatric disturbances commonly observed in sexually abused individuals

Disturbances in children

Anxiety disorders, including posttraumatic stress disorder

Depression and suicidal behavior

Dissociative and hysterical symptoms

Disturbances in sexual behavior

Anger control difficulties

Promiscuous behavior

Conduct problems

Eating disturbances

Self-esteem and self-image conflicts

Disturbances in adults

Anxiety disorders, including posttraumatic stress disorder

Substance abuse

Borderline personality disorder

Dissociative identity disorder (multiple personality disorder)

Revictimization

Sexual dysfunction

Sexual offending

Source. Modified from Cepeda 2010, p. 299.

Otnow Lewis reviewed complex dissociative symptomatology (dissociative identity disorder/multiple personality disorder) and the difficulties of differentiating it from normal fantasy life, schizophrenia, mood disorder, seizure disorder or narcolepsy, borderline personality disorder, conduct disorder, or antisocial personality disorder.

In the evaluation of children suspected of having dissociative disorders, it is important to recognize that a number of symptoms are secretive and that children invariably are unaware of these disorders or of the switches from one state of mind to another that occur in association with them. The examiner should explore the presence of behaviors such as getting lost in fantasy, spacing out, losing track of time, or disconnecting from what is going on in the real world. The examiner may ask the child the following questions: "Are you able to go into a world of your own?" "Do you have a pretend world of your own?" "Is there any special place in your mind or in your imagination where you go when things get too painful, or a place where you go to seek comfort?" The examiner should ask about the presence of depersonalization, out-of-body experiences, premonitions, or feelings of being controlled from outside.

Another important part of the evaluation of dissociation is the examination of memory disturbances, gaps in time, lack of recollection of important personal or family events, and fugue state experiences. Recurrent somatization, pseudoseizures, and self-abusive or self-mutilating behaviors may be indicators of dissociative states. The same could be said about precocious sexual behaviors. More obvious and more suggestive of the presence of these states are behaviors indicating that the child uses different names; that the child has subjective experiences of being like two or more people; or that he or she experiences a sense of being possessed or a sense of unfamiliarity with the self.

Other issues that need to be explored in abused children with dissociative symptoms are the presence of imaginary companions and the presence of auditory hallucinations. In these hallucinations, the voices are of a variable nature: some console, some counsel, some give orders, and some intimidate. The differentiation of these perceptual experiences from other psychotic states, from fantasy play, or from malingering may be a great challenge for the examiner. The only way the examiner can differentiate these experiences is through extended and sensitive questioning, the gathering of collateral information, and the use of other techniques (e.g., writing and drawing) or by specific procedures such as psychological testing.

Other Symptoms of Abuse

Pervasive Refusal

Lask et al. (1991, pp. 868–869) described a potentially life-threatening, extreme form of PTSD, which they named *pervasive refusal*. This avoidance variant is characterized by a refusal to eat, drink, walk, talk, or care for oneself. Children with this disorder demonstrate willfulness in their symptoms and show great fear of disclosing the nature and extent of their trauma. Children adopt this behavior as a way of escaping an intolerable situation.

Self-Abusive Behavior

Calof (1995a, 1995b) described chronic self-injury in adult survivors of childhood abuse. Similar symptomatology is often observed in children and adolescents with abusive backgrounds. When a child exhibits self-abusive behavior, the examiner should ask about prior sexual or physical trauma.

Evaluation of Regressive Behavior

During the initial psychiatric examination, the examiner may be confronted with the emergence of regressive behaviors in a patient. See Chapter 3, "Special Interviewing Techniques," for a description of behaviors associated with regressive behaviors and for an approach to deal with them.

Assessment of Truthfulness in Abused Children

When there are concerns about the patient's truthfulness, the examiner should be particularly careful about the types of questions he or she asks. Leading questions must be avoided at all times. As discussed earlier in this chapter, the examiner should use the same language that the patient uses: the examiner must use the patient's words and expressions, no matter how incorrect or inappropriate they may sound. The introduction of different words or expressions may change the patient's intended meaning. These recommendations are even more important in forensic interviews, regarding allegations of physical or sexual abuse. The following case example illustrates a situation in which the examiner respected these principles.

Case Example 2

Mary, a 14-year-old Caucasian female, claimed she was raped by a 21-year-old man. When describing what the man had done to her, she said that the man had "perpetrated" her. When Mary was asked to explain, she said that the man had "gone all the way." She added that he had put his "thing" inside of her. Mary reported her story consistently when she was asked about the incident. This was compatible with a truthful/factual story.

The examiner understood that Mary wanted to say "penetrated" but did not correct her. The examiner also understood that "thing" meant "penis," but he did not correct her word either. Instead the examiner asked Mary to explain what "perpetrated" and "thing" meant.

Bernet (1993) has clarified many important concepts in the identification of false statements of sexual abuse. Allegations of sexual abuse are true in about 90% of the complaints. As a result, the first assumption should be that the allegations could be true. Bernet organizes the mechanisms of false statements of sexual abuse into three groups:

1. The false statement arises in the mind of the parent or other adults and is imposed on the mind of the child. This may be due to

    a. *Parental misinterpretation and suggestion.* The parent takes an innocent remark or a neutral piece of behavior and inflates it into something worse and inadvertently induces the child to endorse his or her interpretation.

b. *Misinterpreted physical condition.* A vindictive or anxious parent or a health professional may jump to the conclusion that the child's injury or illness is due to sexual abuse rather than accepting a more benign explanation.

c. *Parental delusion.* The parent is paranoid and very disturbed and shares the distorted view of the world with the child, who comes to share the same delusion. There may be a shared delusion, or the child may give in to the parent's contention that abuse occurred.

d. *Parental indoctrination.* This occurs when the parent fabricates the allegation and instructs the child in what to say.

e. *Interviewer suggestion.* Previous interviewers may have contaminated the evidence by asking leading or suggestive questions.

f. *Overstimulation.* The parent lacks modesty or discretion and exposes the child to nudity or sexual activity.

g. *Group contagion.* The child and parents fall victim to epidemic hysteria.

2. The false statement is caused primarily by mental mechanisms in the child that are not conscious or not purposeful.

a. *Fantasy.* The child may confuse fantasy with reality.

b. *Delusion.* Delusions about sexual activities may occur in children and adolescents in the context of psychotic illness.

c. *Misinterpretation.* The false belief is based on an actual happening.

d. *Miscommunication.* The false allegation arises out of simple verbal misunderstanding.

e. *Confabulation.* The person fabricates statements or stories in response to questions about events that the person does not actually recall.

3. The false statement is caused primarily by mental mechanisms in the child that are usually considered conscious and purposeful.

a. *Pseudologia phantastica* (also called *fantasy lying* and *pathological lying*). The person tells stories without discernible motive and with such zeal that the subject may become convinced of their truth.

b. *Innocent lying.* Young children frequently make false statements because doing so seems to be the best way to handle the situation they are in.

c. *Deliberate lying.* This refers to self-serving, intentional fabrications that are common among children and adolescents.

Bernet (1993, p. 908) makes clear the distinction between confabulation and pseudologia phantastica:

1. *The social context is different.* Confabulation is evoked by questions raised by another person. Pseudologia phantastica is created to impress and influence others.
2. *The form of the statement is different.* Whereas confabulation is usually a short statement in response to a specific question when the person has no real memory for the answer, in pseudologia phantastica there is a lengthy, complex story that goes beyond the question raised and that is delivered with zest and in an engaging manner.
3. *Confabulation and pseudologia phantastica differ in the way the person responds when confronted with contradictory evidence.* The confabulator sticks to his or her story, whereas the individual with pseudologia drops the story and moves on to another one.

Bernet also distinguishes confabulation from misinterpretation: A misinterpretation may cause a false belief but is derived from something that actually happened. A child with a misinterpretation may say that two people were fighting when in reality they were having sexual intercourse. A confabulating child may say that two people were fighting when they were having an unremarkable conversation. Confabulation is also different from deliberate lying in that the child who is lying knows that he or she is trying to deceive. The confabulator does not realize what he or she is doing. Pseudologia is different from deliberate lying in that the delinquent liar intends to deceive and knows exactly what he or she is doing. In pseudologia phantastica, the fabulist, intending to enhance an interpersonal relationship or influence another person, embellishes the stories and may be so involved in the deception that he or she comes to believe it (Bernet 1993, p. 908).

The following case example is an intriguing illustration of pseudologia phantastica in a very disturbed adolescent.

Case Example 3

Victor, a 15-year-old Caucasian male, presented with a prolonged history of psychiatric problems, including a profound inability to establish and to maintain interpersonal relationships, lying, stealing, destructiveness with lack of remorse, severe enuresis, difficulties at school, sexually inappropriate behaviors, aggression toward his peers, and a lack of interest in participating in treatment. He had been in state custody for 8 years because his family had abandoned him. His natural mother had a history of a neurological disease and polysubstance abuse. Victor had a history of multiple placements and multiple psychiatric hospitalizations. At birth, Victor was thought to have fetal alcohol syndrome. On earlier testing, Victor was found to have a borderline level of intelligence.

Victor had been evaluated when he was readmitted to an acute psychiatric program for aggressive and inappropriate behaviors including the difficulties already mentioned. Victor exhibited involuntary movements of the mouth and jaw. These dystonic signs had been erroneously considered as the "bizarre mannerisms of an elderly man." When Victor was asked his name, he said, "I'm a third-degree Nijitsu." The examiner asked Victor what a Nijitsu was. He replied, "We're licensed to carry weapons. Nobody else carries weapons in America." The examiner asked, "What kinds of weapons?" Victor replied, "Swords, knives, stars, nunchakus, sticks, slingshots." He reported that his father was a Ninja and asserted that he was not an American. "I'm Japanese Indian, second generation of Americans." He stated that he had studied with a samurai who had been stabbed to death with a sword. He claimed that his father had died in combat, and he reasserted that he was not an American.

Victor's verbalizations could be considered megalomanic delusions. He did not strongly uphold any of his beliefs: when the examiner would challenge one confabulated idea, he would create a new one. What was intriguing about Victor was the lack of emotion he displayed when he presented his fantastic background.

A pediatric neurologist determined that Victor had tardive dystonia and other neurological problems. Neuropsychological testing was positive for multiple neuropsychological deficits, including bilateral fine motor deficits, receptive and expressive language disorder, poor verbal learning, memory and attention difficulties, and executive dysfunction.

Multiple factors, then, contributed to Victor's pseudologia phantastica.

Key Points

- Suicide could be a consequence of bullying or cyberbullying.
- The evaluation of abuse, and of sexual abuse in particular, should be performed by experts in this particular field. The examiner is basically walking through a minefield; each step needs to be carefully and deliberately taken.
- Inducing false memories is the greatest danger. There are profound implications for the child, the family, the alleged abuser, and the judicial system.
- The examiner needs to know, or to establish clearly, what his or her role is in the evaluation of children with an allegation or history of abuse.

Notes

1. High-profile cases of suicides involving bullying include the 2006 death of 13-year-old Megan Meier in Missouri (Steinhauer 2008), the 2012 death of 15-year-old Amanda Todd (BBCnewsbeat 2012) in British Columbia, and the 2013 death of 12-year-old Rebecca Ann Sedwick (Schneider and Kay 2013) in Florida. The 2014 stabbing death of Timothy Crump in New York allegedly resulted from a history of bullying his classmate, Noel Estevez (Mongelli et al. 2014).

2. The work of Dan Olweus in the 1970s provided the standard research definition of bullying that organizations such as the U.S. Centers for Disease Control and Prevention, the American Psychological Association, and the National Association of School Psychologists continue to espouse (Hymel and Swearer 2015).

3. Therapeutic mentors work with supervising mental health professionals in developing strategies for engagement and the teaching of social skills. They utilize a variety of strategies (e.g., role modeling, structured activities, problem solving) to strengthen social skills. They may also coordinate with schools and the family in reinforcing these social skills in multiple environments and situations (Twemlow and Sacco 2012).

4. Dissociation is considered a parasympathetically mediated response that occurs after exhaustion of sympathetically mediated defenses or coping mechanisms. Change in vagal tone, a well-documented parasympathetic marker, is associated with PTSD. Situations of extreme threat may lead to the parasympathetically mediated shutting down of emotions phenotypically observed as dissociative symptoms and prospectively related to PTSD (Saxe et al. 2005).

CHAPTER 12

Neuropsychiatric Interview and Examination

In this chapter, we offer a practical and clinically oriented approach to the complex aspects of the neuropsychiatric interview and examination of children and adolescents. In addition to discussing the various parts of the examination, we describe the most common symptoms that merit a neuropsychiatric conceptualization in children and adolescents.

The patient's history is the cornerstone of neurological or neuropsychiatric diagnosis. The patient's history often suggests whether the condition is static or progressive and whether it has an organic cause. The first part of the examination requires the physician to look, listen, and observe. More can be learned about the child's neurological status by an initial hands-off careful observation than by forcing the child to conform to the physician's set of patterns of performing the neurological examination (Larsen 2006, p. 54).

For most of the neuropsychiatric disorders of childhood, the labeling of "brain damage" is incorrect. Instead, the examiner should refer to these conditions as "brain dysfunctions" or "brain impairments." The concept of brain damage is associated with two erroneous assumptions: 1) that the brain was developing well until something damaged it, and 2) that brain damage is irreversible. The first assumption is true in certain situations, such as when hydrocephalus follows tuberculous meningitis or when epilepsy follows a penetrating head injury. Most commonly, brain development is probably abnormal from the very beginning, perhaps as a result of an inherited disorder, chromosomal abnormality, environmental insults, or chromosomal mutation. Also, intrauterine insults (viral, vascular, or toxic) may negatively affect brain development (Laplante et al. 2008). The second assumption is not entirely true; some children do grow out of disorders such as epilepsy and even cerebral palsy (Goodman 1994).

A complete and accurate history and the neurological examination are the clinician's window to the brain, and they have not been replaced by laboratory or other diagnostic tests. For neuropsychiatric problems, an expanded mental status evaluation is particularly important (Larsen 2006, p. 72).

The neuropsychiatric evaluation is a structured, specialized, and orderly examination of a number of specific functions that is aimed at determining or ruling out brain dysfunction or impairment that may underlie behavioral, emotional, cognitive, or interpersonal disturbances. The field of neuropsychiatry correlates performance on specific tasks with certain neuroanatomical areas; the same is true of certain specific neurophysiological and neuropsychological events. The neuropsychiatric evaluation probes the integrity of neuropsychological functioning of many cortical association areas and of certain subcortical functions. This evaluation includes the assessment of attention, language, cognition, memory, visuospatial skills, motor function, sensory functioning, and executive functions. More specifically, the neuropsychiatric examination assesses functioning of the frontal, temporal, parietal, and occipital lobes and of subcortical regions. It also explores so-called soft neurological signs.

In general, neuropsychiatric syndromes are not associated with focal, or precise, anatomical lesions. In these syndromes, the lesion must be present in the appropriate location for the disorder to occur; that is, the existence of the lesion by itself is often insufficient to produce the disorder. Other factors need to contribute to the expression of the disorders, such as age, development, toxicity, and trauma, and other considerations are important as well: laterality of the lesion (unilateral or bilateral), genetic factors, comorbidity, gender, premorbid personality, environmental stress, coping skills, and social supports (Cummings 1995b) (see Note 1 at the end of this chapter).

In contrast to adult conditions, neurodevelopmental disorders, in children and adolescents, encompass a group of complex disorders that result from abnormal development of the central nervous system (CNS). This abnormal development results in delays, deviations, or a lack of emergence (acquisition) or progression of certain capacities or skills.

The field of pediatric neuropsychiatry is in its early stages but is making steady and rapid progress. The field has borrowed a significant body of knowledge from the field of adult neuropsychiatry, but generalizations from one field to the other may not be warranted. Pediatric neuropsychiatry is starting to rely on its own body of knowledge, experience, and research methodology with pediatric subjects. Longitudinal developmental observations have been crucial in elucidating the nature of skill emergence and to determine atypical developmental pathways. In addition, these studies also trace the vicissitudes of traits, symptoms, or other observations over time. These studies are also needed to make adequate prognostications regarding a variety of neurodevelopmental disorders (see Note 2 at the end of this chapter).

Broadly conceived, the pediatric neuropsychiatric examination is based on a multidisciplinary approach that involves developmental pediatricians, pediatric neurologists, speech pathologists, developmental psychologists, geneticists, neuropsychologists, neuroradiologists, electrophysiologists, neurosurgeons, educators, and other specialists. The field of behavioral neurogenetics studies etiologically defined and relatively homogeneous genetic syndromes (e.g., fragile X syndrome, Williams syndrome, Prader-Willi syndrome, Rett syndrome, Turner syndrome; see Chapter 6, "Evaluation of Special Populations"). These syndromes have identified genetic alterations and neural mechanisms underlying maladaptive cognition, psychiatric symptoms, and abnormal behaviors that can be systematically investigated (Gothelf 2007). Many neuropsychiatric syndromes that occur in childhood or in adolescence require timely diagnosis and treatment. Complete pediatric physical and neurological examinations are essential components of the neuropsychiatric evaluation of children.

In general, adult clinical neuropsychiatry focuses on the loss of neurological function and the process of its recovery (rehabilitation). In contrast, pediatric clinical neuropsychiatry focuses on the emergence of function (skill acquisition), and developmental deviations from that process, and functional habilitation, as well as the psychological and psychosocial consequences of neurodevelopmental disorders. Kim et al. (2008) presented a relevant and comprehensive review of the use of laboratory, imaging, and other testing in adult psychiatry; the discussion has obvious relevance for the child and adolescent psychiatrist.

There has been a shift in the field of neurosychiatry from the "what" and "where" of brain regions implicated in the neuropsychiatric disorders to an effort to understand the neural basis of clinical symptoms or "how" abnormal brain regions produce the clinical picture of disorders such as depression, autism, or schizophrenia (Shenton and Turetsky 2011, p. xiii) (see Note 3 at the end of this chapter).

Elements of the Neuropsychiatric History

The neuropsychiatric assessment involves a comprehensive maturational and developmental history; the emphasis is on systematic data gathering. If it is

Table 12-1. Comprehensive neuropsychiatric history

Family history of neurological or psychiatric illnesses

Parental age at the time of conception

Gestational history

    Mother's alcohol or drug consumption (including tobacco use) during pregnancy

    Mother's viral infections or other illnesses during early pregnancy

Prenatal, neonatal, and perinatal histories

History of exposure to heavy metals and other toxins

History of medical or surgical conditions

History of neurological disorders: seizures, loss of consciousness, and head trauma

Maturational history

    Developmental milestones

    Attachment history

History of language acquisition

History of motor coordination competence

History of attention-concentration development

History of consistent impulse control

History of control of aggressive behavior

History of control of sexual behavior

History of observance of rules and expectations

History of academic performance and learning competence

History of social and interpersonal functioning

History of psychiatric behavioral problems

History of drug abuse and intravenous drug use

History of practice of protected sex (sexual contact with HIV-positive individuals or with individuals who have sexually transmitted diseases)

Source.   Modified from Cepeda 2010, p. 313.

appropriate to do so, the examiner should obtain the history from the child, even from young children, before obtaining historical data from the parents. This approach may generate information that is free of parental bias, which is often invaluable in making a diagnosis and in determining how the condition affects the child. A comprehensive neuropsychiatric history includes a systematic exploration and evaluation of the areas listed in Table 12–1.

Table 12–2. Conditions indicating need for neuropsychiatric investigation

Developmental delays

Language delays

Learning problems

History of cerebral palsy

Presence of movement disorders

History of perinatal insult

History of meningitis, meningoencephalitis, or seizures

Dementing conditions

Head trauma accompanied with loss of consciousness

Sensorium impairment

Recent onset of neurocognitive signs

Loss of intellectual capacity or acquired skills

Sudden onset of regressive behavior

Developmental arrests or regression

Delirium

Psychotic conditions or visual, olfactory, gustatory, or other perceptual disorders

Catatonic features

Recurrent impulsive behavior

Psychiatric symptomatology that does not fit specific categories

Lack of progress in the treatment of a disorder

Chronic exposure to antipsychotics and other psychotropic medications

Note. This is not an exhaustive list of conditions in which neuropsychiatric factors need to be investigated.
Source. Modified from Cepeda 2010, p. 314.

Beyond the so-called hard neurological signs, such as seizures and paralysis, the most frequent complaints of neuropsychiatric patients are attention-concentration difficulties, cognitive impairments, impulse-control problems, impairments of judgment, affect dysregulation, language disorders, learning difficulties, memory impairments, interpersonal difficulties, and regressive behavior. Table 12–2 lists conditions for which a neuropsychiatric investigation should be indicated.

Neuropsychiatry and Psychosocial Factors

Neuropsychiatric conditions are susceptible to environmental influence. Favorable conditions facilitate early detection and prompt habilitation or rehabilitation of emerging deviations, developmental arrests, or loss of function. Symptoms may unfold unaltered, or they may be maintained or worsened by adverse psychosocial circumstances (e.g., infantilism, inappropriate parenting such as neglect or abuse). Cook and Leventhal (1992) described two key findings related to the increased morbidity associated with neuropsychiatric disorders in childhood and adolescence. First, children with neuropsychiatric disorders affect their parents and siblings substantially. Second, children with these disorders are often disabled for a long time. Frequently, the parents' response to the child's problems creates additional handicaps for the child. Williams et al. (1987) articulated this concern:

> Another common and more clearly psychological theme occurring throughout the spectrum of neuropsychiatric disorders in childhood and adolescence is the problem of dependency and its many permutations. While some degree of augmented parental solicitude and support is a natural and, indeed, healthy response to the sequelae of a chronic neurological dysfunction in a child, frequently this pattern becomes exaggerated as a by-product of features of anxiety, guilt, or demoralization in the patient, the parents or both. (p. 366)

Individuals with intellectual disability and other developmental disorders are at greater risk for psychiatric disorders due to CNS dysfunction, peer rejection, and decreased coping strategies (Cook and Leventhal 1992). The psychological disability associated with a neuropsychiatric condition can be worse than the handicap itself: "In effect, the patient can be tempted to exploit the sick role with its associated dependency gratifications when feeling overwhelmed by ongoing life stresses" (Williams et al. 1987, p. 366). In general, the secondary gain from the illness occurs because the parents become inconsistent with limit setting, usually because of parental guilt that interferes with appropriate and consistent discipline and the setting of appropriate consequences.

Mental Status Examination of a Child With a Neuropsychiatric Disorder

The neuropsychiatric examination starts as soon as the examiner greets the child in the waiting area (see Chapter 8, "Documenting the Examination"). The following observations are relevant in this regard: What is the child's appearance and overall complexion? What is the preliminary gestalt or impression? Are any dysmorphic features present? As the examiner guides and follows the child toward the office, he or she should observe the child's gait, movement of upper and lower extremities, balance, and coordination and the child's sense of space orientation. After the child enters the office, the examiner should complete the mental status examination, which includes a neurodevelopmental evaluation (described in the next section of this chapter) and a complete physical and neurological examination. A complete neuropsychiatric evaluation includes a thorough inspection of feet and hands. We agree with Gold (1992) regarding the importance of inspection: "Observations may be more rewarding than examination, encouraging the clinician to acquire and use observational skills that may result in a diagnosis by inspection. This is obviously preferred to the performance of diagnostic studies that can be anxiety producing, painful, invasive and expensive" (p. 4).

Elements of the Neurodevelopmental Evaluation

Areas that need to be assessed in the neurodevelopmental evaluation are listed in Table 12–3 and are described in more detail below.

Dysmorphic Features

The examiner should describe the child's stature (e.g., small or large), head size (e.g., microcephaly, macrocephaly), any abnormalities of the skull shape or structure, and any other dysmorphic features. Young et al. (1990) highlighted the importance of the identification of dysmorphic features: "The detection of minor congenital anomalies during the physical and neurologic examination may be clinically pertinent. These stigmata are correlated with a variety of behavioral and intellectual deviations, even in children with no major physical pathology who do not fall into the conventional diagnostic categories. They also may have value in suggesting a chromosomal abnormality or an insult to the fetus during the first trimester of pregnancy" (p. 455).

The examiner should note any signs of readily identifiable syndromes (e.g., Down syndrome, fragile X syndrome, fetal alcohol syndrome, Prader-Willi syndrome), neurocutaneous disorders (e.g., ataxia-telangiectasia, neurofibromatosis, tuberous sclerosis, or Sturge-Weber-Dimitri syndrome), or neurogenetic disorders.

Abnormal Posture and Involuntary Movements

The examiner should note the presence of tiptoeing, tics, chorea, athetosis, or any other involuntary movements and balance and coordination problems. He or she should also note whether the child stands or sits erect and whether the child displays stiffness, hypotonia, dystonia, or other unusual movements

Table 12–3. Elements of the neurodevelopmental evaluation

Dysmorphic features, including assessment of trajectory of head growth

Abnormal posture and involuntary movements

Gross motor skills

Fine motor skills

Sensory functioning

Midline behaviors

Laterality and dominance

Cerebellar function

Praxis

Receptive and expressive language function

Information

Orientation to time and place

Abstraction ability

Writing and reading

Calculating ability

Immediate, short-term, and long-term memory

Executive functions

Source. Modified from Cepeda 2010, p. 317.

or abnormal postures. The examiner should inspect and look for acute extrapyramidal symptoms (EPS) in children recently exposed to neuroleptic medications, and for chronic extrapyramidal symptoms, such as chronic akathisia or chronic dystonia (tardive dyskinesia), in children with extended exposure to these medications.

Gross Motor Skills

The examiner should pay attention to the child's motor function, considering whether it is smooth, spastic, choreic, dystonic, or athetoid. As the child walks, the examiner should observe the child's stance and gait. Is the child's standing base either broad or variable? The examiner should note associated involuntary movements. Does the child display a normal steppage? Does the child limp, waddle, or tiptoe? Is the child's gait stiff? When the examiner throws a ball to the child, is the child able to catch it? Is the child able to throw or roll the ball back?

In a child with a history of cerebral palsy, the examiner should explore for signs of spasticity, rigidity, paralysis, dystonia, athetosis, chorea, or tremor. Spasticity and athetosis are the most frequent neurological sequelae of cerebral palsy, followed by rigidity and ataxia. Any pronator drift indicates a cortico-spinal tract disease and has the same clinical significance as a Babinski sign (Larsen 2006, p. 66).

Fine Motor Skills

The examiner should observe how the child grasps an object and how he or she manipulates toys. After offering the child a pencil or a crayon, the examiner should observe how the child picks it up and should note whether the child's grasp is normal or atypical. Pencil grasp is an important indicator of motor control: this hard-to-change motor habit is acquired early and may represent a residual indicator of the state of maturation of the child's motor system at the time the child began to use a pencil. The quality of the grasp does not "stigmatize" the current motor repertoire but may be an early snapshot of past status during the period of motor skill learning (Denckla 1997). The examiner should ask the child to copy a circle, a cross, a square, a triangle, and a diamond. A 2-year-old child will be able to copy the circle, a 3-year-old child the cross, a 5-year-old child the square, a 6-year-old child the triangle, and a 7-year-old child the diamond. We once examined an adolescent who wrote with both hands!

Sensory Functioning

To assess sensory functioning, the examiner begins by asking the child to close his or her eyes. Then the examiner touches the child, first on one limb and then on another, each time asking the child to identify the body part and laterality of the area touched. After this, the examiner simultaneously touches either ipsilateral or contralateral limbs and again asks the child to identify where he or she has been touched. The examiner can test the child for graphesthesia (ability to recognize symbols drawn onto parts of the body) by tracing numbers or letters onto the back of each of the child's hands and asking the child to identify them (see Note 4 at the end of this chapter). To test for stereognosis (i.e., ability to recognize objects by touch), the examiner can ask the child to identify, without looking, items such as a coin, a paper clip, a key, or a stamp. The examiner should first ensure that the child has these items in his or her vocabulary. The child needs to identify these items with each hand. These tests explore parietal lobe functioning. Stereognosis is well developed in early childhood, and graphesthesia is well established by age 8 years (Swaiman 2006).

Midline Behaviors

The examiner should observe whether the child uses both hands coordinately and supportively, and whether the child transfers any given item from one hand to the other. The examiner should also note whether the child is able to cross the body's midline (e.g., the examiner should note the extent to which the child's right hand is able to cross the midline and operate on the left side of the body, and vice versa). These behaviors reflect the functional integrity of the corpus callosum (Spreen et al. 1995). One mother reported that her 8-year-old child, who had no evidence of motor difficulties, used only one hand, even when he combed his hair or when he put on his belt. He also had attention problems, difficulties with learning, and problems with impulse control.

Laterality and Dominance

Lewis (1996) clarified the concepts of laterality, preference, and dominance. *Laterality* is a measurable, specialized, central function of a paired faculty, such as eyes, ears, hands, and feet. *Preference* is the subjective, self-reported experience of an individual, as opposed to laterality, which may be objectively measured. *Dominance* is a term used for the concept of cerebral hemisphere specialization, such as language and speech. Clinically, the examiner may merely be testing preference, which depends more on a peripheral organ than on a central mechanism (Lewis 1996). Handedness is consolidated by age 5 years, footedness by about age 7, eye lateralization by age 7 or 8, and ear lateralization by about age 9. The examiner should observe which hand the child uses predominantly when manipulating objects and when asked to write or to draw. The examiner should also observe which foot the child uses when asked to kick a ball. The child's eye preference is tested by asking the child to look into a particular item in the office using a "telescope" (a rolled-up piece of paper).

A useful test to assess right-left discrimination consists of asking the child to follow some ipsilateral and contralateral commands. For example, for ipsilateral discrimination, the examiner tells the child, "With your right hand, touch your right ear" or "With your left hand, touch your left knee." For contralateral discrimination, the examiner says, "With your right hand, touch your left ear" or "With your left hand, touch your right knee." A child can identify right and left hands by age 5 years; ipsilateral double orientation (e.g., left hand on left ear) should be possible by age 6 years; contralateral orientation is achieved by age 7 years. Problems in these areas are common in children who have learning disorders. Confusion of laterality should be suspected when the examiner extends a hand for a handshake and the child does not seem to know which hand to respond with.

Cerebellar Function

To assess cerebellar functions, the examiner asks the child to stand up, to put his or her feet together, to put both hands out in front, and to close both eyes; the examiner should then observe whether the child sways to the sides (Romberg's sign). The child should be asked to walk in a straight line, and the examiner should observe the child's balance and coordination. Next, the child should be asked to stand on one foot and then on the other and then to hop on one foot and then on the other. The examiner should observe the child's sense of equilibrium and the smoothness and proficiency with which the child accomplishes these tasks. The examiner also should assess the child's muscle tone and determine whether the child's tone is hypotonic, normal, or hypertonic.

The finger-to-nose test is sensitive to cerebellar defects. The examiner asks the child to abduct one of the arms with the index finger of that hand extended. The child is asked to touch the tip of his or her nose with that finger three times. The examiner observes for precision and smoothness of movements (*metria*) or the presence of *dysmetria*, which is evident when the child hesitates before the finger reaches the tip of the nose or when the impact is brusque or unsmooth. The examiner then asks the child to do the same challenge with the other hand.

The role of the cerebellum in higher cortical functions, including language and attentional processes, has been recognized. The cerebellar circuits that modulate the prefrontal cortex close loops may also influence the coordination of nonmotor programs such as problem solving in a manner similar to the modulation of movement-related signals (Purves et al. 2012, p. 422).

A syndrome of mutism and subsequent dysarthria has been identified. This syndrome is not related to cerebellar ataxia and is characterized by a complete loss of speech that resolves into dysarthria. Dysarthria relates to a group of speech disorders resulting from disturbance in the muscular control of the speech mechanisms due to damage to the central or peripheral nervous system (Pryse-Phillips 2003).

Praxis

Ideokinetic praxis (or *ideomotor praxis*) is the ability to perform an action from memory on request without props or cues. The child could be asked to demonstrate, for instance, how he or she would use a key, a toothbrush, and a comb. The child's nonpreferred hand should be tested first. The examiner can test the child's kinesthetic praxis by asking him or her to mimic the examiner's finger and hand movements. Difficulties with finger sequencing correlate with graphomotor dyspraxia and with poor handwriting (Denckla 1997). To test for finger sequencing, the examiner raises his or her dominant hand and asks the child to imitate the following movements: touching the tip of thumb to tip of index finger, then to middle finger, then to fourth finger, then to little finger. The examiner then reverses the order (which is more challenging): touching the thumb to fifth finger, followed by the fourth finger, and so on. Then the examiner proceeds to test the other hand. The examiner may ask the child to perform more complex tasks, such as unbuttoning and buttoning the child's shirt and untying and then retying the child's shoelaces. The latter task involves complex functions, out of reach of children who have impairments in interhemispheric integration.

Receptive and Expressive Language Function

The examiner should attempt to differentiate among speech, language, and communication disorders. *Disorders in speech* refers to difficulties in the production of speech that relate to problems with output and the utterance of meaningful and communicative sounds. *Language* is the organized and retrievable view of the self and the world; phonemics, morphemics, syntactics, and semantics relate to different aspects of integrated language. *Communication* relates to the social use of language—to the transmission of meanings between and among persons. The process of communication is regulated by a number of norms, so-called communication pragmatics (e.g., eye contact, turn taking, topic continuity). Delays in language acquisition may be global or may appear in only selected aspects of language acquisition. The latter are the most common language disorders.

When evaluating the child's language, the examiner should observe the child's capacity to understand verbal communication and to utter verbalizations. When interviewing the child, the examiner will have multiple opportunities to observe the child's understanding of verbalizations. The examiner should note whether he or she has to repeat questions frequently, use redundant and simple language, or supplement utterances with gestures or with deliberate nonverbal language. The examiner should also observe whether the child is unable to understand even simple expressions. As the child speaks, the examiner should note the child's fluency and pronunciation; prosody and gesturing; vocabulary, grammar, and syntax; and capacity for abstract thinking (see Chapter 8, "Documenting the Examination").

The capacity to name objects may be tested by asking the child to name a number of body parts. The examiner should point to his or her own eyebrow, chin, wrist, or other body areas and ask the child to name the part. The examiner may also point to the child's own jacket, belt, collar, shoe, or tie and ask the child to name those items. In adults, dysnomia (i.e., a disturbance in the capacity to name objects) may result from dominant temporal or parietal lobe lesions. In children, the disturbance is related to significant developmental delays in language.

For example, a 6-year-old child with significant language delays was retained in kindergarten. During the language evaluation, the examiner asked the child to name some body parts. When the examiner pointed to his ear and asked the child to name it, the child said "head"; when the examiner pointed to the child's foot, she said "leg."

In another case, a 12-year-old Asian American male demonstrated difficulties with understanding of language as soon as the examiner came to the lobby and called him to the office. The examiner extended his hand to greet him, and the child showed the examiner a ribbon he had on his shirt. As soon as the child sat in his chair and the examiner started asking questions, the child looked puzzled and would talk about things unrelated to the questions. The examiner readily recognized the issue and indicated to the mother that the child had a receptive language problem. The mother responded, "No wonder he is not progressing at school."

In adults, disturbances of prosody and gesturing in which spontaneous gesturing and emotionality of speech are lacking could be related to frontal lesions; disturbances in the understanding of the prosody and gesturing of others could be related to temporal lesions. The neuropathology of developmental language disorders is poorly understood, but the disorders have been associated with mild neuronal migration disorders in the left inferior frontal cortex (Kinsbourne and Wood 2006).

Information

The child should be asked to narrate recent events. If the child demonstrates no awareness of or interest in recent news, he or she should be asked to talk about a favorite sport, favorite team, or favorite players. The following questions are commonly used in this part of the assessment: "What town do you live in?" "What state do you live in?" "What is the state capital?" "Name the biggest cities in your state." "Name the states that border your state." "What is the capital of the United States?" "Who was the first president of the United States?" "Who is the current president?" "Do you know the vice president's name?" Other factors to be considered when assessing this area are the child's level of intelligence and his or her cultural and socioeconomic background.

Orientation to Time and Place

The child should be asked to identify where he or she is, including the name of the place, the floor number, and so on. The examiner should ask the child to indicate on a map where north or south is. The examiner may also ask the child to point to directions on a wall picture; for example, "In this picture, where is north?" The examiner should ask the child to indicate the day of the week and the date, including the month and the year. The child may also be asked to identify the season and the most recent holiday. Children with non-verbal learning disabilities and children with cognitive deficits have difficulty with time tasks.

Abstraction Ability

The examiner should note the child's complexity of thought as the child responds to the examiner's questions during the interview. When assessing an adolescent or intelligent child, the examiner can test for abstraction ability by testing for similarities or by asking the child to interpret proverbs.

Writing and Reading

The child should be asked to write his or her name and the date. If the child is old enough, he or she should be asked to use cursive script because this type of writing is the most sensitive for detecting dysgraphia (difficulty in writing). (Note, though, that cursive writing will not be a learning objective in the very near future in the United States.) The child should be asked to read and to carry out a written command such as "Go to the table, pick up the pencil, and bring it back to me."

Calculating Ability

For the assessment of calculating ability, see Chapter 8, "Documenting the Examination." Acalculia is a common developmental disorder and is a frequent sequela of acute and progressive left posterior hemispheric lesions in children and adults (Grafman and Rickard 1997). Children with dominant inferior parietal lobe dysfunction will display elements of the developmental Gerstmann syndrome, such as right-left confusion, finger agnosia, dyscalculia, and dysgraphia. Finger naming, or its dysfunction (finger agnosia), is a predictor of arithmetic abilities (Larsen 2006, p. 62).

Immediate, Short-Term, and Long-Term Memory

As the examiner asks questions, he or she should observe the child's recall. Children who ask their parent (or other caregiver) either for assistance or to respond for them may have memory and language problems. Immediate memory can be tested by asking the child to repeat a number of digits forward and backward. By age 8 years, a normally developing child is expected to recall five digits forward and two or three digits backward; by age 10 years, the child should be able to recall six digits forward and four digits backward (Lewis 1996). Short-term memory can be tested by giving the child three words and asking the child 5 minutes later to recall the words. This challenge is increased when one of the words is abstract.

Executive Functions

Executive functions could be defined as a number of higher cognitive activities (in an information-processing model) involved in self-managing including, organization, planning, initiating and completing tasks on a timely basis, tracking and shifting tasks, self-monitoring, and self-inhibition (Solanto 2015, p. 256). Such functions are thought to be localized in the prefrontal cortex, an area that is not functionally mature until young adulthood (Spreen et al. 1995). Executive dysfunctions may be developmental in nature (e.g., because of attention-deficit/hyperactivity disorder [ADHD], autism spectrum disorder, Tourette's disorder) or acquired (e.g., due to traumatic brain injury). These dysfunctions may be manifested as problems with attention, impulse control, perseveration, apathy, and emotional dysregulation. Students with learning disabilities tend to display executive function difficulties, such as problems with initiation, inhibition, and shifting (Lajiness-O'Neil and Beaulieu 2006).

To assess executive functions, the examiner should ask the child to do a puzzle, for instance. The examiner should observe the child's behavioral organization and his or her capacity to maintain and to shift attention while performing the task. The examiner should also observe the child's degree of planning for and persistence with the given task and his approach to problem solving. The examiner should note the presence of impulsiveness, disinhibition, or perseverance.

Indications for Consultation and Testing

A variety of consultations may be useful in evaluating neuropsychiatric conditions. Pediatric neurological consultation may be requested to ascertain the presence of neurological deficits and to pursue, when indicated, further neurological workup, including neuroimaging studies (e.g., computed tomography [CT] scan, magnetic resonance imaging [MRI]) (see Note 5 at the end of this chapter) or electrophysiological studies (e.g., electroencephalogram [EEG], evoked potentials). Consultation with a speech-language pathologist is mandatory when a child demonstrates language and communication deficits. This evaluation helps the clinician to diagnose the nature of the language pathology and to determine an appropriate treatment. A geneticist should be consulted when chromosomal or genetic factors are suspected.

Assistance from psychologists and neuropsychologists is indispensable for both the evaluation and the treatment of neuropsychiatric conditions. The psychologist provides invaluable assistance in determining the child's intellectual abilities and achievement levels. Intellectual assessment scales, such as the Wechsler Intelligence Scale for Children—4th Edition (WISC-IV; Wechsler 2003), indicate the child's Verbal IQ, which measures language-based reasoning abilities, and the child's nonverbal Performance IQ, which measures visuospatial abilities. Test results may also suggest deficits that need further exploration through neuropsychological testing or speech and language assessment. When a discrepancy exists between the child's achievement level (i.e., grade placement in reading, spelling, or math) and the child's level of intelligence, the determination of learning disabilities, for purposes of psychoeducational programming, should be made. This general determination does not address the specific factors that contribute to the child's underachievement; elucidation of such factors requires neuropsychological testing.

The psychologist also assists in the determination of subjective and interpersonal issues that are associated with neuropsychiatric disorders. These issues may precede, follow, or be concomitant with the evolution of neuropsychiatric pathology. Projective testing (e.g., Thematic Apperception Test, Rorschach Inkblot Test, Sentence Completion Test) helps the examiner to understand the child's ongoing psychological conflicts; to determine whether reality testing is intact; to establish the presence of thought disorder; to evaluate the child's relatedness (attachment or object relations), coping mechanisms, and psychological resources; and to establish the degree of the child's depression or anxiety or the nature of his or her impulse control. The psychologist could help the examiner to determine whether secondary gain is present as well.

Neuropsychological assessment, according to Berkelhammer (2008), is

> a hypothesis-driven assessment of higher brain functions resulting in an integrative analysis of findings in the context of a neurodevelopmental-systems approach and detailing recommendations for addressing the presenting problems as well as those that may be revealed in the course of the evaluation. At an individual level, neuropsychological testing samples multiple cognitive domains and contextualizes findings within a neurodevelopmental approach. Indeed, skilled clinicians are able to translate test results into meaningful relevance for parents and educators such that the feedback sessions serve as a therapeutic intervention. (p. 498)

Harris (1995a) states that neuropsychological testing has unique importance and relevance in the diagnosis and treatment of neuropsychiatric disorders. It is "particularly helpful in appreciating those mental status items that deal with speech/linguistic functions, memory, attention, executive functions (vigilance, set maintenance, planning, and inhibitory motor control), praxis (learned motor behavior), and visuomotor and visuospatial functions. In addition, the processing/production of social-emotional signals (including vocal tone, facial expression, and 'body language,' or gesture) [are also amenable to testing]" (p. 20). Harris emphasizes that "the linking of test findings to adaptive function is crucial because children may compensate for the brain dysfunction in a way that the overall functioning is 'better than they look' on the tests applied" (p. 20).

Neuropsychological findings assist psychiatrists in the process of devising optimal rehabilitation programs for children who are recovering from brain injury or brain disease. Such findings also help child psychiatrists to construct—with the assistance of experts in special education, speech-language pathology, and other specialties—optimal psychoeducational and remediation programs for children who develop neuropsychological deficits. Contemporary neuropsychological testing is used to help understand the cognitive and behavioral phenotypes of a multitude of neuropsychiatric disorders, with the goal of aiding in diagnosis and treatment, and of deepening the neurobiological knowledge of these disorders. The data obtained from such testing provides the clinician with a profile or pattern of strengths and weaknesses from which to generate diagnoses, as well as compensatory, remedial, therapeutic, and rehabilitation recommendations (Lajiness-O'Neill and Beaulieu 2006).

Indications for Neuropsychological Testing

Neuropsychological testing is not a uniform examination. Testing varies in scope and depth, and there are many schools and methods of neuropsychological assessment. Pendleton Jones and Butters (1991, p. 413) explained one major difference: A major dichotomy in the field of neuropsychological assessment is characterized by the use of either a uniform battery for all patients or an individualized approach. Practitioners of an individualized approach usually administer a small, core group of tests to all patients, and then select further tests for the optimal elucidation of the referral questions or issues that may have been arisen during testing. Batteries undoubtedly have some advantages. These include comprehensiveness in the range of functions they sample. They greatly facilitate the combination of research with clinical objectives in that the same database will automatically be compiled for all patients. A serious disadvantage of batteries is that they may be providing redundancy of information in some areas of functioning while achieving insufficient exploration of others.

Despite variations, a comprehensive neuropsychological evaluation attempts to measure all domains of neuropsychological functioning believed to be important for supporting the child's abilities for a successful interaction with environmental demands (Lajiness-O'Neill and Beaulieu 2006).

A number of indications for neuropsychological testing are listed in Table 12–4. In general, neuropsychological batteries are reliable for children age 6 years and older. For younger children, neuropsychological testing involves combining a variety of age-appropriate motor, language, and cognitive tasks with various standardized assessments somewhat similar to those used in neuropsychological batteries administered to older individuals (Hartlage and Williams 1997). There are multiple misconceptions about neuropsychological testing (regarding the testing process or its interpretation) that may lead to inaccurate expectations of the testing results in real-world settings. These misconceptions are equally applicable to neuropsychological testing and its interpretation in children and adolescents (see Note 6 at the end of this chapter).

Table 12–5 summarizes the advantages and disadvantages of commonly used neuropsychological batteries and individualized approaches. One of the shortcomings of neuropsychological testing is the lack of ecological validity, meaning that the results do not predict how the patient will perform in the real world (Hartlage and Williams 1997).

Interviewing Children With Learning Disabilities and Other Neuropsychiatric Deficits

An *inner language* is necessary for the formation of self concept and for the understanding of self in relation to others. Inner language facilitates self-awareness and conceptualization of problem solving. It permits transmission of mental contents (e.g., thoughts, memories, emotions) in ways that can be understood in interpersonal communication. Inner language allows trial action and planning, a prerequisite for understanding psychological and interpersonal problems. *Verbalization*, or the capacity to communicate inner experience, is necessary for the process of psychological change.

Children with learning disabilities have problems processing information and difficulties in encoding or decoding emotions (affects). As a consequence, mood disorders in this population may have a different clinical outlook, in particular in their nonverbal display. This difference may mislead diagnosticians.

Children with language disorders or learning disabilities lack the capacity to use language as an efficient and reliable information-processing tool; they cannot use language for verbal or conceptual planning prior to action, and for this reason they are prone to impulsivity. These problems contribute to the child's sense of isolation, personal inhibition, diminished sense of competence, and poor self concept. Rarely are these children able to convey their inner lives satisfactorily. For children with language disorders, communicating (or attempting to communicate) with others demands great effort, generates anxiety, and brings disappointing results. For these children, putting thoughts together and organizing thinking—in a relevant and meaningful manner—is usually a difficult, laborious, and frustrating task.

Table 12–4. Indications for neuropsychological testing

Evaluating for neurodevelopmental disorders

Evaluating dysfunctional domains related to cognitive or behavioral disorders (nonverbal disabilities are the most challenging)

Detecting conditions not demonstrated on standard neurodiagnostic testing

Assessing for lack of academic progress

Defining specific learning disorders

Identifying subtle brain trauma

Monitoring neuropsychological status

Assessing baseline and measuring recovery associated with therapies/ interventions

Characterizing patient strengths for planning rehabilitation programs

Determining suitability for educational or vocational programs

Assisting in medico-legal situations

Determining responsibility in forensic examinations

Assisting in research

Source. Adapted from Harris 1995a and Tranel 1992. Modified from Cepeda 2010, p. 328.

The challenge in the diagnostic assessment of these children lies in the timely identification of their communication difficulties. The examiner must open communication channels that compensate for the child's language limitations. By creating such pathways, the examiner facilitates the child's expression of his or her psychological and interpersonal problems. Although verbalization is the most efficient modality for self-revelation, the diagnostic assessment of children with language impairments must be aided by a variety of expressive, nonverbal techniques (e.g., drawing, playing, puppetry, kinetic or mimetic enactments).

In cases of receptive language deficits, the examiner has the added challenge of ensuring that the child understands what the examiner says or wants to convey. The examiner must use simple, deliberate, and redundant language. The examiner also needs to verify on an ongoing basis that he or she is being understood by asking the child, "What did I say?" or "What did I ask you?"

Many children with language difficulties use pragmatic adaptational behaviors (e.g., nodding to imply assent) to please others and to secure acceptance. The naive interviewer may misunderstand this adaptive nonverbal body language. For example, when the examiner is talking, the child may be nodding as if conveying that he or she understands. The nodding misleads

Table 12–5.   Advantages and disadvantages of commonly used neuropsychological batteries and individualized approaches

	Advantages	Disadvantages
Batteries		
Halstead-Reitan Neuropsychological Battery	Has been adapted for use with children: the Reitan-Indiana Test Battery for Children may be used with children ages 5–8 years; the Halstead-Reitan Neuropsychological Test Battery for Children is used with children ages 9–15 years. Samples a wide range of functions. Can be used to make inferences as to lesion localization and chronicity.	As with other batteries, the accuracy of detecting structural brain damage declines when applied to psychiatric patients. Lacks measures of memory assessment. Is lengthy and costly to administer. Contains a large element of subjective evaluation. Does not reflect progress in neuropsychological assessment during the past 40+ years.
Luria-Nebraska Neuropsychological Battery	Brief and comprehensive. Complex functions are divided into simple components so that more information is gleaned about the precise nature of the deficits. Can discriminate between brain-injured and control subjects and between brain-damaged patients and schizophrenia patients.	Serious questions exist regarding standardization, validity, and reliability. It has been questioned whether the assessment method developed by Luria can be operationalized as a fixed battery.
Individualized approaches		
Boston process approach	Emphasizes higher cortical assessment and is flexible. Focuses on the patient's successes and failures. Emphasizes process and strategy; similar deficits may reflect very different underlying processes. Is comprehensive in the areas of language and memory. Is useful and sensitive in rehabilitation planning.	Standardization and validation are incomplete. Testing requires a high level of training and experience.

Table 12–5. **Advantages and disadvantages of commonly used neuropsychological batteries and individualized approaches *(continued)***

	Advantages	Disadvantages
Individualized approaches *(continued)*		
Muriel D. Lezak approach	An individualized approach that emphasizes patient's successes and failures. Contains the most comprehensive list of individual tests.	Test selection is critical. May require 6–9 hours of administration time.
Arthur Benton approach	An individualized and patient-oriented approach. Sequential process leads to a diagnostic decision. In 80% of cases, experienced neuropsychologists may complete testing in 60–90 minutes.	Tester requires a high level of training and experience.

Source. Reprinted from Cepeda 2010, pp. 329–330.

the examiner because it is a learned behavior the child has incorporated to fit into the social milieu; nodding does not guarantee that the child understands. The examiner needs to break through this adaptive facade by repeatedly asking for feedback until he or she is certain that the child is processing or understanding what is being communicated. We have evaluated children who have been referred because of apparent psychotic features. These children were said to "talk to themselves" and so on. Careful observations revealed that these children were thinking aloud or trying out ideas they wanted to express. This self-talk was a trial speech.

The following case example involves a child with aphasia, profound neuropsychological problems, and global cognitive deficits whose interpersonal behavior baffled her teachers.

Case Example 1

Frances, an 11-year-old Caucasian female, was referred by the school district for assessment of "psychotic behavior," specifically, because "the child talks to herself frequently…she talks to imaginary friends..she laughs inappropriately." Frances had been diagnosed with global aphasia and was known to have global cognitive deficits. She attended a special education program because of demonstrated serious learning difficulties.

Frances's mother alleged that Frances had developed satisfactorily until age 2 years, at which time she sustained a severe head injury when her father, who had been holding Frances on his back, lost his grip, and she fell on her head. Frances forgot how to speak after the accident. Her mother spent a great deal of time and effort teaching her to speak again and, later, to read.

Frances was born at full term but was delivered by forceps and may have been oxygen deprived at birth. Frances's mother described her as an easy-tempered baby. She indicated that early developmental milestones had emerged at the expected times. She reported that developmental delays began after her fall. She had no history of seizures or of any other medical problems, and she had no psychiatric history.

At the time of the evaluation, Frances's parents were separated. Frances's father had abandoned the family some time earlier. Frances's mother alleged that her husband was mentally ill and that there was significant mental illness on the side of his family. The family was experiencing significant economic stress and received assistance from charity organizations.

The mental status examination revealed an attractive and engaging preadolescent female who appeared her chronological age. Frances was appropriately dressed and well groomed. She exhibited a significant degree of anxiety, and although she appeared euthymic, she demonstrated some social-adaptive but inappropriate smiling. Her affect was increased in range and in intensity.

As Frances began to talk, her dysprosody became apparent. Her voice was hoarse and rasping, like that of an old woman. She had difficulties initiating speech and frequently showed hesitancy and significant problems in the flow of expressive language. Frances tended to perseverate, and the examiner frequently needed to repeat questions because Frances seemed to have problems understanding speech, too. Frances's sentences were short and simple, and she had frequent problems with grammar and syntax, including improper use of prepositions and conjunctions. The examiner noted that Frances had recent and remote memory problems. Although she was coherent, she also displayed dysnomia and some illogical thoughts. The examiner found no evidence of a mood disorder, suicidal or homicidal ideation, or psychosis.

Summary of Positive Findings

Physical examination. Findings were unremarkable.

Neurological screening. Frances showed evidence of receptive and expressive language disorders; she also exhibited some ataxia and frontal release signs.

Neurological consultation. Frances's left ear was mildly malformed, and mild facial asymmetry was observed. There was no evidence of dysarthria, but word usage and syntax problems were noted. Frances could not read at her grade level, and her reading comprehension was poor. Visual perceptual deficits were also observed. When she was challenged with commands of medium complexity, Frances's speech comprehension was below the expected level. The diagnostic impression was of dysphasia (expressive-receptive speech deficits). A tic disorder was also suspected. The examiner recommended a speech evaluation and a sleep-deprived EEG.

Cognitive testing. Frances obtained a Full Scale IQ of 75, a Verbal IQ of 66, and a Performance IQ of 87. Frances's scores on tasks requiring elaborate explanations were quite impaired, reflecting her significant aphasic deficits. Her scores on subtests associated with perceptual organization showed scatter (i.e., a large spread in subtest score values). She had borderline scores for the arrangement of pictures to tell a story and the reproduction of designs using patterned blocks. She exhibited an average ability to scan for visual incongruities and a high-average ability to assemble puzzles. Her scores associated with attention and freedom from distractibility were average (repetition of digit strings) and borderline (mental arithmetic). Processing speed scores were average (visual target detection) and borderline (copying of symbols from a key). The pattern was consistent with a significant language deficit in the presence of better-developed visuoperceptual abilities.

Projective testing. Findings were consistent with the diagnosis of schizotypal personality disorder. Frances exhibited significant evidence of deficits in perceptual accuracy but no evidence of a thought disorder. Frances's behavior during the evaluation aptly depicted her internal confusion: she had difficulties interpreting the actions of others in a positive and caring way, and she was uneasy in interpersonal relationships, expecting that she would be misunderstood or that she would misunderstand others. Although she said that she was unwilling to participate in the evaluation, Frances's behavior was generally cooperative and pleasant, but she had a tendency to become disorganized under stress.

Neuropsychological testing. The neuropsychologist reported that Frances was an attractive, slim girl who was somewhat small for her age. She was adequately groomed and appropriately dressed. Her speech and language were unusual in several regards. Frances's word usage was quite concrete; she frequently used the word "thing" to refer to objects or made paraphasic errors (e.g., "eyelashes" for eyebrows). Frances talked almost continuously and at a rapid rate. Her spontaneous comments and questions appeared to reflect her personal concerns and anxiety (e.g., she frequently expressed fear of punishment) and were frequently off topic. Frances tended to ask repetitive questions, such as asking what time it was every few minutes. Her receptive language appeared impaired; she often had difficulty understanding spoken instructions and needed more explanation and demonstration than expected based on her age.

Frances's motor activity and energy level were significantly increased. She fidgeted, squirmed, and attempted to get out of her chair and explore the room. Her motor activity increased every time she was faced with a task she found difficult. She had significant problems maintaining attention. Frances got off task frequently and required a great deal of redirection. Her approach to various tasks was inefficient; for example, she often indicated that she was finished with a task without checking it for accuracy. Her mood was anxious and her affect incongruent. For example, even when obviously frustrated and having protested that a task was too difficult, Frances continued smiling. Her cooperation fluctuated. She was most cooperative on tasks she enjoyed, and she appeared quite responsive to praise and encouragement. On tasks she found difficult, she protested verbally or responded in a random or silly manner until redirected. On one task, she simply refused to continue.

Visuospatial skills. Right-left confusion and poor visuospatial construction skills were revealed.

Language. Frances exhibited mild impairment in all aspects of language. Her receptive vocabulary was in the first percentile: Frances had problems understanding spoken questions and directions. Her expressive vocabulary was in the impaired range, and her abstraction skills were in the borderline range. Findings were consistent with a significant aphasic disorder.

Memory. Frances exhibited impairments in immediate memory recall and learning. Her pattern of performance indicated poor initial encoding. On a task of learning and recall for a set of spatial coordinates, Frances became extremely frustrated, responded randomly, and refused to complete the task. The pattern of errors suggested inconsistent attention.

Executive functions. Frances exhibited severe deficits in executive functions.

Diagnostic impression. Tests were consistent with multiple neurological deficits, most notably in receptive and expressive language, psychomotor coordination, and executive functions. These deficits significantly impeded Frances's ability to problem solve verbally or organize novel information, leading to a reliance on repetitive and often inappropriate behavior. Frances's neurocognitive problems were exacerbated by anxiety. Frances was not considered intellectually disabled. Her symptoms were consistent with pervasive developmental disorder and appeared to be secondary to her neurocognitive deficits. For more findings in Frances' evaluation, see Note 7 at the end of this chapter.

Regarding localizing principles of aphasia in children, Cummings (1995b) pointed out, "Children often exhibit nonfluent aphasia regardless of the lesion localization in the left hemisphere" (p. 181). Severe linguistic deficits are rarely isolated. These deficits are frequently associated with other neurocognitive and neuropsychological deficits. Understandably, depression, anxiety, and psychotic disorders are frequent comorbid conditions in children with language disorders and neuropsychological deficits. Receptive language disorders are frequently misdiagnosed as oppositional defiant disorders. In reality, children with these disorders do not understand the oral commands they are given and on the surface it appears that they are being oppositional. Impulse-control difficulties are common in these children.

Children with severe expressive language disorders display surface thought disorders that are similar to those of individuals with schizophrenia (e.g., looseness of associations, incoherence, circumstantiality, neologisms). The main differences are in the areas of relatedness and affective expression. In general, children with language disorders are likable, have a strong interest in people, and frequently display broad and congruent affect, as well as an interest in communicating. Children with schizophrenia usually have schizoid behaviors and display blunt or inappropriate affect. Elaborate delusions and multisensory hallucinations are characteristic.

Both Frances and Ruben (whose case is discussed later in this chapter) demonstrated significant mixed language impairment and moderate to severe memory deficits, reflecting the close connection between language and memory functions. Surprisingly, parents and even teachers failed to recognize these language problems.

Patients with severe neuropsychiatric problems often grow up with deep-seated doubts about their competence and intellectual capacity. Because of their communication difficulties, they develop a sense of defectiveness and a poor self-concept. They may be demoralized or chronically depressed. Language limitations also interfere with their social relationships. These children have problems making friends and gaining acceptance from their peer groups; usually they are isolated and insecure. Neuropsychiatric impairments interfere with school and vocational achievement. Lack of achievement further interferes with these children's overall adaptation (i.e., sense of competence, self-esteem, and attitude toward life problems). Serious behavioral and attitudinal difficulties develop in children in whom these disorders are not properly diagnosed and treated.

In general, learning disabilities and related neuropsychological impairments represent cortical association disconnections or cortical-subcortical disconnections caused by a variety of noxae, and even correlated with socioeconomic status (SES). Singh (2012, p. 854) reported that higher socioeconomic status correlated with larger hippocampus volume and that higher amygdala volumes correlated with lower SES. Furthermore, left temporal lobe and left frontal gyrus size correlated with SES, and lower specialization of left hemisphere correlated with low SES.

Specific Neuropsychiatric Symptoms

Attention and Concentration Deficits

According to Barkley (2015), ADHD is neurodevelopmental disorder and is classified as such in DSM-5 (American Psychiatric Association 2013). Although there are multiple etiologies that contribute to ADHD, the greatest contributors to the expression of the disorder are a) genetics, b) neurological factors, and c) environmental factors (biohazards). Some issues with cellular migration—termination and support (neuroglia) may also be implicated. There is no credible evidence that ADHD can be caused by social factors alone. Among the biohazards, prematurity, prenatal toxins and infections, and postnatal events such as lead poisoning, traumatic brain injury, and other injuries that interfere with brain development or that transact with genetic propensities need to be considered (Barkley 2015b, p. 356–363) (see Note 8 at the end of this chapter).

ADHD diagnosis assumes a developmental delay or an acquired impairment of the behavioral inhibition networks of the brain that control self-regulation; this theory links behavioral inhibition and executive functions. Behavioral inhibition is the foundation of the relationship of self-control and executive functions (discussed below). *Self-regulation* is defined as self-directed action to change one's own behavior to alter the probability of a delayed (future) consequence; *executive functions* are forms of self-behavior, that is, the actions one uses to change oneself so as to change the future (Smith et al. 2007).

The four executive functions (forms of self-directed actions) are as follows (Smith et al. 2007):

1. *Nonverbal working memory* (covert self-directed sensing) represents hindsight of the retrospective function of working memory; this contributes to the subjective estimation of psychological time involved in forethought or prospective function of working memory.
2. *Verbal working memory* (internalized self-directed speech) is involved in self-control, planning, and goal-directed behavior.
3. *Self-regulation of affect-motivation-arousal* (self-directed emotion) is inner speech that is important in managing motivational states. (By privately manipulating and modulating emotional and motivational states, the child can induce drive or motivational states that may be required for initiating and maintaining goal-directed behavior.)
4. *Planning and reconstitution* (self-directed play) involves inner speech and imagery that permit analysis (deconstruction) and synthesis (recombination) of the world. Action-to-the-self is based on play in childhood that progresses from manual-verbal play to private mental manipulations

of images and words that generate new ideas and related behaviors to use in goal-directed problem solving.

Attention processes are fundamental executive and neurocognitive functions that entail a variety of capacities, including sustained attention, selective attention, intensity of attention, and inhibitory control. Alertness, target detection, and vigilance are major components of the attention processes. *Alertness* refers to the readiness to process information and depends on the intactness of the right hemisphere. *Target detection*, or *selection*, depends on parietal lobe functioning and involves selective attention of a specific stimulus. The disengagement of attention from a given stimulus seems to be even more specific for intact parietal functions. *Vigilance* refers to the mental effort needed to maintain attention. This higher aspect of attention involves effortless problem solving, motivation, and commitment to memory.

Up to 20% of children with ADHD may also have a severe social disability (i.e., profound deficits in interpersonal and social functioning). Although ADHD as a primary disorder can occur without other psychopathology, the disorder may accompany many neurological, psychiatric, and psychosocial conditions. Although distractibility and hyperactivity are the predominant features of ADHD, these symptoms are also found in many medical and neurological conditions.

According to Criterion B of the DSM-5 criteria for ADHD, several inattentive or hyperactive-impulsive symptoms should be present prior to age 12 years (American Psychiatric Association 2013, p. 60). Findings by Moffitt et al. (2015), in the Dunedin, New Zealand, longitudinal cohort study, question the dictum that ADHD starts in childhood. They found a small group of adults with ADHD—representing de novo cases—that had not had ADHD as children. These group of patients had IQ scores comparable to those of controls and showed negligible neuropsychological impairment (the opposite being markers of ADHD beginning in childhood). The authors suggested that their ADHD adult sample may have suffered from a different disorder (Moffitt et al. 2015, pp. 972, 975).

For many decades, it has been known that overcorrection of hyperactivity with stimulants brings a decrement of concentration and other cognitive dysfunctions. In this vein, Sarver et al. (2015) demonstrated that for children with ADHD, hyperactivity is a compensatory adjustment that props up phonological neurocognitive function. High rates of gross motor behavior positively predicted phonological working memory performance for children with ADHD but not for the control children. This association was robust. The higher rates of gross motor behavior were associated with improvement in phonological neurocognitive function but not with its normalization. It is well known that children with ADHD display hypoactivation of the frontal and prefrontal regions when they engage in cognitive activities. It is likely that the increased psychomotor activity increases the level of arousal of these areas, resulting in an improvement in the neurocognitive function. Hyperactivity in ADHD children do not improve visuospatial functioning. These observations have important clinical and pedagogic implications.

Delirium

Delirium is usually a transient and reversible dysfunction in cerebral activity that has an acute or subacute onset and is clinically manifested by a wide range of neuropsychiatric abnormalities causing a confusional state. Intrinsic predisposing factors for delirium include a previous delirium episode, a preexisting cognitive impairment, a CNS disorder, blood-brain barrier permeability, and the following environmental factors: social isolation, sensory extremes (sleep and sensory deprivation and sensory overload), visual and hearing deficits, immobility, and environmental novelty or stress (Williams 2007). In an analogy with other organ failures, delirium has been recently considered as an indicator of brain failure. Although delirium occurs in children, it is seldom identified. Delirium is potentially life threatening and requires immediate medical attention. Patients are inattentive and disoriented and display incoherent or rambling speech. They may appear to be in a stupor or a state of restless agitation. Perceptual disturbances (e.g., illusions and visual, auditory, or haptic hallucinations) are common. In addition, sleep-wake cycle disturbances or memory impairments may occur. Characteristically, the patient's level of alertness waxes and wanes: the patient may by oriented and alert at one moment and become disoriented and confused the next; symptoms tend to worsen as the day progresses and sunlight wanes (the so-called sundowning effect). Autonomic instability (changes in heart rate and blood pressure, sweating, and pupillary changes), as well as mood and emotional alterations are common in delirium. Delirium should be suspected in patients who are taking psychotropic medications. Neuroleptic malignant syndrome and serotonin syndrome are life-threatening complications of psychotropic use that must be timely identified.

The DSM-5 guidelines for the diagnosis of delirium (American Psychiatric Association 2013, p. 596) include the following criteria:

A. A disturbance in attention (i.e., reduced ability to direct, focus, sustain, and shift attention) and awareness (reduced orientation to the environment).

B. The disturbance develops over a short period of time (usually hours to a few days), represents a change from baseline attention and awareness, and tends to fluctuate in severity during the course of a day.

C. An additional disturbance in cognition (e.g., memory deficit, disorientation, language, visuospatial ability, or perception).

D. The disturbances in Criteria A and C are not better explained by another preexisting, established, or evolving neurocognitive disorder and do not occur in the context of a severely reduced level of arousal, such as coma.

E. There is evidence from the history, physical examination, or laboratory findings that the disturbance is a direct physiological consequence of another medical condition, substance intoxication or withdrawal (i.e., due to a drug of abuse or to a medication), or exposure to a toxin, or is due to multiple etiologies.

A number of mnemonics have been used to aid in the recollection of the multiplicity of conditions that cause delirium. I WATCH DEATH (Infectious, Withdrawal, Acute metabolic, Trauma, CNS pathology, Hypoxia, Deficiencies, Endocrinopathies, Acute vascular, Toxins or drugs, Heavy metals) is one such mnemonic for delirium. Williams (2007, p. 649) proposed PLASTRD for the signs and symptoms of delirium:

- **P**sychosis: Perceptual disorders, visual illusions, hallucinations, metamorphopsias. Poorly formed paranoid delusions. Thought disorder: circumstantiality, tangentiality, loose associations.
- **L**anguage impairment: Word-finding difficulties, dysnomias, paraphasia, dysgraphia. Altered semantic content; severe forms may mimic expressive or receptive aphasia.
- **A**ltered labile affect: Moods incongruous to context or mood lability. Hypoactive delirium may be confused with depression.
- **S**leep-wake disturbance: Fragmented throughout 24-hour period; reversal of normal diurnal cycle. Sleeplessness.
- **T**emporal course: Acute, abrupt onset; fluctuation of symptom severity during 24-hour period. Usually reversible. Subclinical syndrome may precede or follow the episode.
- **R**eactivity altered: Hyperactivity, hypoactivity, mixed.
- **D**iffused cognitive deficits: Inattention, disorientation (time, place, person); amnesia (short and long term), verbal and visual. Impairment of visuoconstructional ability; executive function deficits.

We suggest the mnemonic TRACK CHAOS as a probably easier-to-remember alternative:

- **T**hought disorder: circumstantiality, loose associations.
- **R**eversible, usually affect lability, incongruous mood, depression-like signs.
- **C**ourse: acute/abrupt onset, fluctuating signs and symptom during the day.

- Kinetics: hyperactivity, hypoactivity, mixed.
- Cognitive disturbances, inattention, disorientation, memory impairments.
- Hallucinations multisensory, paranoia, illusions, psychosis.
- Aphasia: language impairment, dysnomias, paraphasias, word-finding. difficulties, receptive language difficulties.
- Orientation difficulties, confusion.
- Sleep disturbances, reversal of diurnal cycle.

See Table 12–6 for the differential diagnosis of delirium/psychosis.

The most common causes of delirium in children are head trauma, CNS infections, and intoxication. In adolescents, the most common culprits are CNS injuries caused by serious suicide attempts (e.g., from hanging, carbon monoxide poisoning, psychotropic drug overdoses), and side effects associated with abuse of hallucinogenic drugs and medications (including psychotropic medication side effects). Mortality from delirium in childhood could be as high as 20% (Williams 2007).

Soft Neurological Signs

Soft neurological signs have nonspecific neuropsychiatric significance. They are not localizing and are not invariably associated with specific structural lesions. Their clinical significance has been variably interpreted by different clinicians, and arbitrary hierarchical attributions have been assigned. They are closely related to the child's developmental status, because many of these signs are present at an early age. Soft neurological signs are often considered as evidence of developmental immaturity or of a developmental lag as they persist in older children. Soft signs are slightly more common in children who have several different types of psychiatric disorders. Attaching a well-defined clinical significance to soft signs is impossible. Within a specific diagnostic group, soft signs may have some predictive value. Soft signs are more prevalent in psychiatric patients. The Physical and Neurological Examination for Soft Signs (PANESS; Guy 1976) is the preferred assessment instrument for soft neurological signs.

Patankar et al. (2012, p. 2) studied the prevalence of *soft neurological signs* in ADHD children. According to them soft neurological signs include poor coordination; poor speed or accuracy of limb or axial movements, including those required to keep balance; dysrhythmias; and overflow. Of the timed motor movements, speed of movement and dysrhythmias are the most reliable findings. *Synkinesias*, or movement overflow, are indicators of a developmental delay of motor inhibition. Dysrhythmias and slow speed are an indication of functional deficits of the cerebellum and the basal ganglia (see Note 9 at the end of this chapter).

Table 12–6. Differential diagnosis of delirium/psychosis

1. Toxic conditions

    a. Alcohol intoxication and withdrawal

    b. Substances of abuse: cocaine, amphetamine, MDMA, hallucinogens

    c. LSD, mescaline, psilocybin, PCP, dextromethorphan

    d. Acute lead encephalopathy

    e. Neuroleptic malignant syndrome, serotonin syndrome

    f. Drug-induced delirium

    g. Lead, mercury, bath salts

2. Metabolic disorders

    a. Electrolyte imbalances

    b. Adrenoleukodystrophy

    c. GM2 gangliosidoses

    d. Niemann-Pick disease

    e. Beta mannosidoses

    f. Acute intermittent porphyria

    g. Hemocysteinuria

    h. Porphyria

    i. Hypoxia

3. Endocrinological disorders

    a. Thyrotoxicosis

    b. Hypothyroidism

    c. Addison's disease

    d. Cushing's syndrome

    e. Hyperparathyroidism

4. Infectious diseases

    a. Viral encephalitis (HIV, herpes, rabies, measles)

    b. PANDAS

    c. Bacterial encephalitis

    d. Post-infectious encephalitis

    e. Fungal encephalitis (cryptococcosis)

Table 12-6. Differential diagnosis of delirium/psychosis *(continued)*

4. Infectious diseases (*continued*)

    f. Prion diseases

    g. Spirochetal infections (syphilis, leptospirosis, Lyme disease)

    h. Parasitic conditions: malaria

5. Structural and neurological lesions

    a. Temporal lobe glioma

    b. CTE

    c. Subdural hematomas

6. Autoimmune disorders

    a. Systemic lupus erythematosus

    b. Multiple sclerosis, sarcoidosis

    c. Limbic, anti-NMDA, anti-VGKC, ASL progressive multifocal leukoencephalopathy

    d. Paraneoplastic conditions

7. Paroxysmal disorder

    a. Temporal lobe epilepsy (complex partial symptomatology)

    b. Partial complex status epilepticus

    c. Post-ictal psychosis

8. Specific genetic disorders

    a. Huntington's disease

    b. Wilson's disease

    c. Parkinson's disease

    d. Fahr's disease

Note.   ASL=acute sclerosing leukoencephalitis; CTE=chronic traumatic encephalopathy; LSD=lysergic acid diethylamide; MDMA=3,4,-methylenedioxy-N-methylamphetamine; NMDA=*N*-methyl-ᴅ-aspartate; PANDAS=pediatric autoimmune neuropsychiatric disorders associated with streptococcal infections; PCP=phencyclidine; VGKC=voltage-gated potassium channel.

Source.   Modified from Towbin 2015, p. 458, and Sher et al. 2016, pp. 41–46.

Seizure Disorders

The psychopathology related to seizure disorders has multiple causes. Psychiatric morbidity related to seizure disorders is determined by several factors, including underlying neuropathology, neural effects of ictal and interictal states, psychological effect of loss of consciousness or altered consciousness, family reaction to epilepsy, and psychotropic effects of anticonvulsant treatment. According to Sankar et al. (2006, p. 872), mesial temporal sclerosis is the predominant cause of complex partial symptomatology. This entails damage to the hippocampus areas CA1, CA2, CA3 subfields and the granular dentate cells (p. 863). In a significant proportion of patients with complex partial symptomatology focal abnormalities are found outside the hippocampus: in the limbic system of the frontal lobes and lateral temporal lobes, and in the nonlimbic areas of the temporal lobe. As many as 85% of children with temporal lobe epilepsy had psychiatric disorders, including mental retardation (25%) and disruptive behaviors (including "hyperkinetic syndrome" and catastrophic rage), but only 30% had psychiatric disorders when followed to adulthood (Cook and Leventhal 1992, p. 652). Epilepsy in childhood is a powerful risk factor for emotional and behavioral disorders. Children with epilepsy have a three to four times higher rate of psychiatric disorders than children in non-epileptic samples (Heyman et al. 2015, p. 396). (Memory and attention are especially disturbed in patients with complex partial seizures, even in those with subclinical epileptiform discharges, particularly if the left hemisphere is affected (Spreen et al. 1995).

Aggressive behavior, mood disturbances, intolerance to frustration, poor integration into social groups, and marked dependency are common in children with seizures. Psychoses are more prevalent in children with left-hemispheric seizure foci. The following case example illustrates psychiatric consequences (i.e., aggressive behaviors and psychosis) in a child with poorly controlled seizures (see also Ralph's case [Case Example 8] in Chapter 8, "Documenting the Examination").

Case Example 2

Ricardo, a 6-year-old Hispanic male, was evaluated for oppositional and aggressive behaviors at home and at school. His mixed seizure disorder (grand mal and complex partial) was poorly controlled, primarily because of poor compliance with the neurologist's recommendations. Ricardo was in the care of his maternal grandmother, who was frail, forgetful, and psychiatrically ill. The school had reported Ricardo's grandmother to the department of social services because Ricardo had gone to school overmedicated on several occasions. When the school nurse checked on how much medication the grandmother had given Ricardo, it did not match the doctor's prescription.

The grandmother reported that Ricardo often stared into space and appeared confused. He would become unresponsive, his mouth would foam, and his skin would become discolored. The grandmother was more alarmed than the child; he often expressed fears that somebody was going to harm him. He had plucked out his teddy bear's eyes because, as Ricardo described it, the teddy "was staring at me funny." Ricardo's sleep-deprived electroencephalogram (EEG) confirmed the diagnosis of partial seizure symptomatology. Appropriate anticonvulsant medications and close monitoring ensured seizure control and produced marked improvement in Ricardo's aggressive behavior, paranoid symptoms, and overall symptomatology.

Most paroxysmal events (i.e., seizures) are diagnosed by history and not by laboratory studies (Larsen 2006, p. 70). Neurologists use anti-epileptic medications in cases in which the history is very suggestive of seizures, even though the EEG is not confirmatory of seizures. Normal EEG findings are common, however, during a single partial seizure and do not exclude the diagnosis (Fenichel 2005, p. 30).

Regressive Behavior

The loss of cognitive abilities or of acquired personal, social, or behavioral skills should call into question the integrity of the child's CNS. Clinicians should be cautious in making diagnostic closures in the assessment of regressive behavior. The following case example is illustrative.

Case Example 3

Roger, a 7-year-old Caucasian male, was referred for a psychiatric evaluation for regressive behavior. He had stopped talking and had problems eating. At school, he seemed listless and had limited academic progress. Roger also had problems with "enuresis and encopresis." When Roger's mother was asked about a history of similar problems in the family, she casually commented that many boys in her family had died at a very early age. Because the neurological examination was positive for equivocal Babinski's signs bilaterally, and given that Roger had difficulties in feeding, he was referred to a university pediatric neurology clinic.

At first, a pediatric neurologist found no reason to consider a neurological disorder; she suspected a functional disorder. A pediatric psychiatric consultation established that Roger had a psychotic disorder. Serendipitously, another neurologist noticed hyperpigmented creases in Roger's hands, after which adrenal gland involvement (Addison's disease) was confirmed. A brain CT scan showed extensive demyelination in the frontal and temporoparietal areas. A diagnosis of adrenoleukodystrophy was made. The dementing and deteriorating course of the illness continued unremittingly until Roger became bedridden a few years later.

What was initially interpreted as a lack of academic progress was early evidence of a progressive loss of cognitive faculties (dementia), and what was initially called "enuresis and encopresis" was a loss of voluntary sphincter control, a sign of frontal lobe dysfunction.

Investigations to detect organicity and appropriate referrals are indicated if 1) the child loses well-established linguistic, academic, or self-help skills and performs below previous levels; 2) features emerge that are suggestive of brain disorder; or 3) risk factors for genetic or infectious disease are present. The most common disorders that may manifest with dementing symptoms in child psychiatric practice are Batten disease, Wilson's disease, Huntington's disease, adrenoleukodystrophy, juvenile-onset meta-chromatic leukodystrophy, subacute sclerosing panencephalitis, HIV encephalopathy, Rett syndrome, convulsive disorders (e.g., Lennox-Gastaut syndrome, Landau-Kleffner syndrome), cerebral palsy, and head injury (see subsection "Chronic Traumatic Encephalopathy" later in this section).

Child psychiatrists have a key role in the identification of dementing disorders of childhood. Some of these disorders, like Wilson's disease, are potentially treatable. Prompt identification is important for timely clinical management.

Some severely regressed patients may exhibit complex and confusing clinical pictures that mimic neurodegenerative disorders. An 11-year-old preadolescent developed progressive speech difficulties and stopped eating. He also had displayed extensive catatonic symptoms. He was referred to a university hospital. The neurological workup (including neuroimaging) was negative. Under Amytal sodium, he talked about his history of severe physical abuse. Acute regressive pictures with complex psychiatric symptomatology have been observed in children with complex partial seizures who did not have a history of seizures.

Traumatic Brain Injury

Birmaher and Williams (1996) have highlighted risk-taking behavior as one of the causes of traumatic brain injury. Risk-taking behavior is an etiologic contributor to traumatic brain injury among children and adolescents. A number of studies point to the elevated incidence of documented alcohol use, preexisting cognitive deficits, preexistent deviant behavior, and diminished parental emotional stability among youths who sustain a traumatic brain injury. Children with head injuries have tended to be impulsive, aggressive, attention-seeking, and behaviorally disturbed, engendering a greater probability of being in dangerous situations likely to result in accidents. Frequently these children are in the wrong place at the wrong time. Families of children experiencing accidents show more parental illness and mental disorders, more social disadvantages of various kinds, and less adequate supervision of children's activities than is found in the general population (Birmaher and Williams 1996, pp. 370–371).

Table 12–7. Sequelae of traumatic brain injury

Major cognitive sequelae

Decrease in speed and efficiency of information processing

Difficulties with attention and concentration

Learning and memory problems

Perception difficulties

Language and communication problems

Problems with executive functions

Decrease in level of intelligence

Major affective and personality sequelae

Organic personality changes

Reactive personality changes

Noncognitive sequelae

Sensory complaints

Posttraumatic headaches

Posttraumatic epilepsy

Sleep disturbances

Psychotic features

Psychological reaction to the brain injury

Adjustment to adaptive impairments

Changes in self-concept and body image

Source.   Reprinted from Cepeda 2010, p. 345.

It is not a simple matter to disentangle the sequelae of traumatic brain injury from antecedent deficits. Bennet et al. (1997) classified the sequelae of traumatic brain injury into four categories, as shown in Table 12–7.

Many of the complications and sequelae of brain injury are illustrated in the following case example.

Case Example 4

Abe, a 13-year-old Caucasian male and the son of two physicians, was evaluated for depression, suicidal behavior, and increasingly aggressive dyscontrol. He had hit a child with a rock, and on another occasion he had to be separated from the same child. Eighteen months earlier, on the first day of a vacation, he was "accidentally hit" with a golf club in the left frontotemporal area. X rays demonstrated a depressed frontotemporoparietal skull fracture. Abe was comatose for 10 days. He sustained an intraparenchymal hematoma (bleeding within the brain) and lacerations of the frontal and temporal lobes. After neurosurgical intervention, Abe experienced expressive aphasia and right-side hemiplegia (paralysis). He also had difficulties swallowing and controlling his bowel functions. By the time of the psychiatric evaluation, Abe had achieved a "wonderful recovery:" most of the overt aphasia and hemiplegia had resolved. However, subtle impairments remained: he had difficulty writing due to loss of a fine motor coordination of the right hand, and he had episodic difficulties in word finding. Problems with concentration had also been observed.

Abe had been an honor student but was struggling to catch up at school and complained that the school's demands were harder to meet than before. Abe's parents noticed that he was painfully aware of his limitations and functional loss. They also noticed significant personality changes. Abe had become more irritable, and he was prone to angry outbursts and frequent confrontations with his father. On one occasion, he pushed his father and hit him on the chest. He also became destructive and self-abusive (he engaged in head banging). Abe became progressively more demoralized and began to show evidence of withdrawal and loss of motivation and interest.

The mental status examination showed a handsome teenager who was small for his age and was uncooperative and unfriendly during the interview. When Abe talked, he seemed to be making a deliberate effort to communicate. His difficulties with word finding and his loss of fluency of speech emerged intermittently. His sensorium was intact, and his intellectual function was assessed as above average. No disturbance in thought processes was detected. Abe endorsed auditory hallucinations in the form of voices that talked to him and put him down; he denied other hallucinatory experiences. Abe denied paranoid ideation and denied suicidal thinking at the time of the evaluation. His judgment and insight were considered fair. Abe tended to argue and disagree with most of his parents' concerns.

Eighteen months after the trauma, a new neuropsychological assessment, done before the psychiatric evaluation, showed a dramatic recovery from most of the cognitive, language, and motor deficits seen 15 months earlier. Abe demonstrated some speech hesitancies but none of the dysfluencies and paraphasias observed earlier. He had motor-related problems in writing, but his problems with spelling and reading (e.g., pronunciation) had resolved. Motor coordination in his right hand had improved to the point that he could write slowly and perform many fine motor tasks. His measured intelligence had increased to the superior range on subtests that did not require fine motor responses. The tactile response in Abe's right hand was mildly reduced. Abe was cooperative and easy to manage during a full day of testing, in contrast to problems seen earlier. Rapport with the tester was appropriate even though Abe had reported auditory hallucinations. The neuropsychologist suggested that the hallucinations could be related to the lesion of the temporal lobe and that the lack of motivation for reading could be related to residual language impairments.

Abe received the diagnosis of a mood disorder with psychotic features associated with a medical (neurological) condition. He was referred to a residential therapeutic program for him to learn to cope with anger and frustration in more adaptive ways, and to help him to deal with issues of chronic demoralization and ongoing problems with his parents.

Patients who have sustained severe traumatic brain injuries have demonstrated significant improvement in social, physical, and emotional functioning 2 years after an injury (Sbordone 1997). Recovery from brain injury does not stop after the first years of the injury. Patients have shown significant improvements in cognitive functioning even 5–10 years after the injury.

In the case examples of Frances and Abe, postnatal brain injuries involving neurocognitive and linguistic sequelae had a prominent role in each patient's dysfunction. In general, the prognosis after traumatic brain injury depends on the degree of intactness of the CNS (or on the degree of structural damage), as demonstrated by neuroimaging studies, and to a certain extent on the integrity and resources of the family environment.

Chronic Traumatic Encephalopathy

A new condition, chronic traumatic encephalopathy (CTE), initially identified in boxers, is now recognized as a chronic and cumulative brain injury in a variety of contact sports, including football and soccer. CTE causes a progressive cognitive deterioration and may occur years after retiring from the sport. The clinical features include parkinsonism, pyramidal signs, psychomotor slowing, memory difficulties, and attentional problems. Recent neuropathological studies associate this condition with a tau abnormality, and as such it is considered a progressive tauopathy (Flanagan 2015, p. 307). CTE is a controllable condition; there is an increasing awareness of this disorder, and incipient steps are being taken to decrease the prevalence and the progression of this disorder. Identifying a brain concussion and providing appropriate management of it is becoming a welcome practice in contact sports (see Note 10 at the end of this chapter).

Cognitive Impairments

Cognitive impairments are either congenital or acquired. Congenital impairments contribute to intellectual disabilities (previously, mental retardation). Children with congenital cognitive impairments exhibit delays in neuromuscular and postural milestones, and disturbances in attachment and social-relational behaviors, in language acquisition, and in communication competence. Children with congenital cognitive impairments demonstrate academic difficulties and problems in the rate of acquisition of new skills. A number of congenital, cognitively impairing syndromes are potentially treatable (e.g., phenylketonuria, fetal alcohol spectrum disorders); early identification is essential.

Ninety-five percent of genetic intellectual developmental disabilities are associated with the X chromosome. The most common causes of intellectual disability are Down syndrome, fragile X syndrome, and fetal alcohol syndrome. These conditions account for as many as 30% of the identified cases of intellectual disability (King et al. 1997).

Because of diagnostic overshadowing, many psychiatric disorders are unrecognized in children with intellectual disabilities. Psychiatric disorders that go unrecognized include psychotic, mood, and anxiety disorders, as well as ADHD and stereotyped habit disorders. Furthermore, gullibility and lack of awareness of risk may result in exploitation by others and possible victimization—fraud, unintentional criminal involvement, false confessions, and risk of physical and sexual abuse (see American Psychiatric Association 2013, p. 38).

Learning Difficulties

Learning difficulties are rarely the primary reason for initial consultation with a child psychiatrist; however, they are common comorbid conditions for a number of psychiatric disorders (e.g., autism, ADHD, Tourette's disorder, conduct disorder, mood disorders and anxiety disorders). Language disorders are commonly associated with learning problems; some experts believe that language deficits are the underlying cause of most learning disabilities.

Positron emission tomography studies in men with persistent developmental dyslexia demonstrated a failure to activate "the left temporoparietal cortex during a phonological task, and in the right temporal cortex during a rhyme-detection, non-language task" (Rumsey 1998, p. 12). These abnormalities are in contrast to a "robust activation of the left inferior frontal regions during a syntax task involving sentence comprehension" (p. 12). The posterior portion of the large-scale language networks may be affected in dyslexia. Convergent findings indicate that the posterior temporal and nearby occipital and parietal regions are involved in dyslexia and in phonological deficits (Rumsey 1998).

Language Disorders

Because language disorders have far-reaching implications for children's cognitive, social, and learning competencies, early identification and treatment are of the utmost importance (Bishop 2002). Speech apraxias, dysnomias, and other production or expressive disorders need proper and timely identification. Among the expressive disorders, the examiner must distinguish dysfunctions secondary to neuromuscular control and coordination (i.e., dysarthria), defects at the motor level of speech production (i.e., apraxias), and defects in the production of language at the semantic level (i.e., lexical and syntactic deficits; Spreen et al. 1995). There is a high degree of comorbidity between language disorders and a range of other psychiatric and learning disorders, including ADHD, learning disabilities, and conduct disorders. However, language impairments in children referred for psychiatric problems are frequently undiagnosed in as many as 40% of cases. For these reasons, school-age children referred for or suspected of having a psychiatric or learning disorder should be assessed for language disorder (Frazier Norbury and Paul 2015, p. 689). Receptive language disorders include a congenital word deafness (verbal auditory agnosia), which entails an inability to differentiate speech sounds from other environmental sounds (so-called auditory imperception). Neologisms and idioglossia (unintelligible verbal utterances) are common problems in individuals with receptive language disorders (Spreen et al. 1995). Receptive language disorders have the worst prognosis among the language disorders.

The diagnosis of aphasia needs special consideration. The consequences of childhood-acquired aphasia appear to be longlasting and extend in time far beyond the disappearance of aphasic symptoms. Even when clinical signs of aphasia abate, full and functional pragmatic language will not necessarily be acquired or restored. Academic achievement continues to be poor, and failure to accrue new knowledge may be more pronounced over time, perhaps because of the increasing demands in higher academic grades (Dennis 1997).

A close association exists between language disorders and psychopathology. At least 50% of children with language disorders have associated psychopathology. In a study by Cohen and Horodezky (1998), teachers and parents rated children with unsuspected language impairments as having more ADHD symptoms and more severe problems with aggression and delinquency than children with previously identified language impairments or children with normal language development. Parents of children with unsuspected language impairments rated their children as more delinquent than did the parents of children with previously identified language impairments across all ages. The parents of children with previously identified language impairments appeared to make accommodations for their children's communication difficulties, which apparently protected these children from being blamed unnecessarily for some of their behaviors (Cohen and Horodezky 1998). Early identification is important because it seems to improve the parents' level of empathy toward the child and may decrease the frequency of negative interactions. Language disorder diagnosed by 4 years of age is likely to become stable over time and typically persist into adulthood, although the particular profile of language strengths and deficits is likely to change over the course of development (American Psychiatric Association 2013, p. 43).

Memory Impairments (Amnesias)

Harris (1995b) stated that various forms of memory are mediated by separate brain systems. Conscious memory (declarative or explicit memory) and nonconscious memory (nondeclarative or implicit memory, which is involved in acquisition of skills, habits, and other procedures) involve different neuroanatomical systems. The hippocampus and its related structures are essential for declarative or explicit memory. Other structures are necessary for nondeclarative or implicit memory. The hippocampus and related structures are needed for the establishment of enduring memory, although long-term memory storage is believed to involve the neocortex. Nondeclarative memory appears to be stored in specific sensory and motor pathways. The cerebellum seems to be an important site for classical conditioning of skeletal musculature (Harris 1995a). The role of the hippocampal region (medial temporal lobe) in amnesia was defined by Zola (1997, p. 458). The findings show that circumscribed bilateral lesions limited to the hippocampal region are sufficient to produce amnesia. Additional findings indicate that the cortical regions adjacent to and anatomically linked to the hippocampal region—the perirhinal, entorhinal, and parahippocampal cortices—are also important for memory function.

Heindel and Salloway (1999) expanded on the above concepts: "Studies have convincingly demonstrated that memory should not be thought of as a single, homogeneous entity, but rather as being composed of several distinct yet mutually interacting memory systems that are mediated by specific neuroanatomical substrates" (p. 19). The authors integrate four memory systems: 1) *working memory* (involving information that is stored and manipulated for a very short period of time [20–30 seconds]), which is under central executive control and neuroanatomically based in the prefrontal cortex; 2) *episodic memory* (involving information that is remembered within a temporal or spatial context), which is mediated by the medial temporal lobe and the diencephalon; 3) *semantic memory* (involving the fund of general knowledge not dependent on contextual clues for retrieval), which is mediated by the temporoparietal association cortex; and 4) *procedural memory* (an unconscious way of remembering that is expressed through the performance of specific operations constituting a particular task), which is mediated by the basal ganglia (Heindel and Salloway 1999).

Children with static encephalopathies or with anomalies in brain embryogenesis may experience serious memory dysfunction. Learning or language disorders in some children may be the result of memory difficulties. These deficits can be demonstrated with careful testing and must be confirmed with pertinent neuropsychological testing. Memory difficulties are caused by encoding difficulties or by retrieval problems. The following case example illustrates a predominant encoding memory disturbance in a child who has multiple neuropsychiatric and neuropsychological problems.

Case Example 5

Ruben, a 12-year-old Hispanic male, was evaluated after his teacher overheard him saying that he had a person inside him who talked to him and told him to harm himself and others. During the evaluation, Ruben claimed he had had this person inside him since he was 4 years old. He claimed that the person had asked him not to tell anyone and had even threatened to throw him in front of cars or trains if he were to do so. Ruben's mother learned about the "person" 2 days before the psychiatric evaluation, when Ruben had been intercepted running toward railroad tracks, intending to kill himself. Apparently, he was responding to commanding hallucinations telling him to get run over by the train.

Ruben had a history of self-abusive behavior and had also displayed suicidal behavior. Three months earlier, Ruben's self-abusive behavior took a turn for the worse. He had a number of unexplained accidents over the previous months. These incidents included cutting his finger, burning his left forearm, and falling frequently.

Ruben revealed that he had hurt a baby and another boy and that he had sexually abused a 7-year-old boy. He also disclosed episodes in which he had sexually molested his 9-year-old brother, and had also displayed sexual behavior toward his babysitter.

According to Ruben's mother, he had been retained in school for 4 years in a row because "he didn't seem to be able to learn anything." He attended a special education program for second grade.

When Ruben was born, doctors discovered that he had a heart murmur and operated on him, after which he remained in an incubator for 3 months. He also had three eye surgeries. He had no history of seizures but had a history of significant neurodevelopmental delays: he sat at age 12–14 months, walked at age 3 years, and began talking between ages 3 and 4 years. He had been toilet trained by age 3 years and had no history of enuresis. When Ruben was asked to do a chore, such as taking the trash out, he repeatedly came back to ask what he was supposed to do. Any expectation of him had to be repeated many times.

Ruben's mother had attempted suicide in the past, had a history of psychiatric hospitalizations, and had ongoing problems with alcohol. Ruben's father had never cared for or provided for Ruben or his brother. During the family interview, Ruben and his mother related positively.

The mental status examination revealed a child who appeared his chronological age. Ruben wore glasses and displayed a serious countenance. He endorsed auditory and visual hallucinations, saying that he heard and saw Robert, or Robbie, the person inside him. He also acknowledged hearing voices telling him to do bad things to himself and to others. He said that 2 days earlier, he had seen Robbie: he was all red and had horns. Ruben also heard people other than Robbie; these people were with Robbie. Robbie was real to

Ruben, but Ruben acknowledged that at times his actions were the result of his own thoughts. He claimed that sometimes he was able to put Robbie away from his mind for a little while. Ruben disclosed sexual excitement and preoccupation. He was oriented to time, place, and person. As Ruben began to relax, he became more pleasant. Ruben also exhibited expressive and receptive language problems and a limited vocabulary. The examiner had to repeat many of the questions more than once before Ruben could attempt to answer them. Ruben's intelligence, insight, and judgment were considered impaired.

Summary of positive findings[1]:

Physical examination. Ruben exhibited synophrys (eyebrows meeting in the middle) and hypertelorism (eyes appreciably more separated than normal). A periscapular surgical scar, related to the neonatal heart surgery, was present. Heart auscultation was unremarkable.

Neurological consultation: Ruben exhibited dysmorphic features (e.g., hypertelorism, prominent ears, fragmented and abnormal palm creases).

He had global difficulties with reading, writing, and mathematics and had multiple perceptual deficits, including sequential memory deficits (auditory and visual) and right-left disorientation. His human drawing showed a lack of detail, consistent with important body-schema deficits. Cranial nerves, muscle power, tone, deep tendon reflexes, gait, and stance were all normal. Multiple scars were noted, as was a birthmark on the left side of the neck.

The diagnostic impression was of static encephalopathy (rule out chromosomal abnormalities, or a genetic disease) and possible fragile X syndrome. Chromosomal studies, a sleep-deprived EEG, and an MRI were recommended. The chromosomal analysis showed a normal chromosomal count (46XY) and no fragile X abnormality. The EEG showed no focal or paroxysmal abnormalities. The MRI showed evidence of striking cell migration deficits, a fissure in the right temporoparieto-occipital area, another milder cleft toward the central fissure, and evidence of pachygyria (abnormal clustering of gyri) and microgyria (gyri smaller than normal). The neuroradiological diagnosis was schizencephaly and cell migration defects.

Cognitive testing. Ruben's scores on the Wechsler Intelligence Scale for Children—3rd Edition (WISC-III) were as follows: Full Scale IQ 73, Verbal IQ 58 (intellectually deficient range), and Performance IQ 93 (average range).

Neuropsychological testing:

LANGUAGE: Ruben's language skills were generally impaired. His sentence construction was below average. His overall verbal abstraction and expressive skills were within the intellectually deficient range, and his receptive vocabulary was below expectations based on age.

ATTENTION AND MEMORY: Significant auditory and visuoperceptual deficits interfered with Ruben's concentration and encoding into memory. Ruben persisted at tasks but his distractibility score on the WISC-III was in the intellectually deficient range, reflecting his perceptual processing problems. Ruben's immediate recall of digits was substantially below average, and his immediate recall of sentences was in the second percentile. His delayed recall for a story

---

[1]For additional testing results and other findings, see Note 11 at the end of this chapter.

was below the first percentile; however, the difference between Ruben's immediate and delayed memory for the story was minimal, indicating a problem with encoding rather than with retrieval. Ruben's learning and recall for a word list was also below expectations; he did not appear to use organizational strategies to enhance learning. This pattern of performance further indicated encoding problems. In addition, Ruben's short-term memory for spatial coordinates was impaired. His visual reproduction memory, as assessed by drawing geometric designs, was in the ninth percentile for immediate reproduction.

EXECUTIVE FUNCTIONS: Ruben's executive functions were mildly impaired. He had some difficulty maintaining a cognitive set and generating new strategies when needed. His cognitive flexibility was mildly impaired. Diagnostic impressions of the neuropsychological testing: Ruben's memory difficulties were more related to encoding difficulties secondary to attention-concentration deficits. Ruben also had broad language and cognitive impairments. These deficits disorders were probably related to impairment of cell migration and other disturbances during cortical embryogenesis.

Although problems of retrieval are a common cause of memory difficulties, deficits of encoding need to be ruled out in children who demonstrate memory impairments. Ruben is a case in point (see also the case of Frances earlier in this chapter).

The DSM-5 criteria for mild neurocognitive disorder may be applicable to children and adolescent with losses in neurocognitive functioning—complex attention, executive function, learning and memory, language, perceptual motor, or social cognition (American Psychiatric Association 2013, p. 605).

Antisocial Behavior

The DSM-5 category of disruptive, impulse-control, and conduct disorders includes oppositional defiant disorder (ODD), conduct disorder, antisocial personality disorder, pyromania, kleptomania, among others. Of particular relevance for child psychiatrists are the specifiers for conduct disorder: childhood-onset type (when at least one symptom of conduct disorder is present prior to age 10 years) and adolescent-onset type (if symptoms of conduct disorder start after age 10). The examiner needs to ascertain the lack of prosocial emotions (American Psychiatric Association 2013, pp. 470–471):

1. The child has a lack of remorse or guilt: he or she shows no concerns for negative consequences of behavior.
2. The child is callous or lacks empathy: (disregarding or being unconcerned with the feelings of others; he or she and is considered cold and uncaring.
3. The child is unconcerned about performance: he or she does not show concern with poor/problematic performance at school, work, or in other important activities and blames other for poor performance.

4. The child is shallow or deficient in affect: he or she does not express feelings or emotions to others. The child is unable to make rapport and is insincere or superficial. He or she quickly turns emotion on and off and uses emotions to manipulate or to intimidate others.

Several studies have related antisocial behavior to low serotonin levels, high testosterone, and low epinephrine. Low arousal is related to antisocial behavior, and sensation seeking is conceived as a means of increasing arousal to a normal or optimal level (fearless individuals such as bomb disposal experts have particularly low heart rate levels and reactivity). Lack of fear punishment in early childhood may contribute to disturbed fear conditioning and lack of conscience development (Popma and Vermeiren 2008).

Low heart rate is the most frequently replicated biological correlate of antisocial behavior in children and adolescents. Low heart rate predicts antisocial behavior. Resting heart rate as early as age 3 years has been found to be related to aggressive behavior at age 11 years. Social factors also play a role. Boys with low heart rate were more likely to become violent adult offenders if they had poor relationships with their parents and if they came from a large family. Also, boys with low heart rate were more likely to be rated as aggressive by teachers if their mother was a teenager, if they came from a low socioeconomic background, or if they were separated from the parent by age 10 (Popma and Vermeiren 2008).

The psychophysiological response patterns among aggressive girls with conduct problems are dissimilar from those of aggressive boys with conduct problems. Conduct disorder behaviors in females may be driven by stronger socioenvironmental influences (Beauchaine et al. 2008).

Lack of empathy response to the suffering of others (callous-unemotional) is related to antisocial behavior. This deficit appears to reflect structural and functional deficits in neural circuits, such as the amygdala and the anterior insular cortex, that are involved in the recognition of emotional distress in other people. A structural study in adolescents showed a significant reduction in gray matter in bilateral anterior insular cortex and left amygdala in subjects with conduct disorder (Popma and Vermeiren 2008). Amygdalar dysfunction may be a key neurodevelopmental etiological factor in understanding callous-unemotional traits, and callous-unemotional symptom severity may reflect reduced connectivity between the amygdala and the ventromedial prefrontal cortex (Dolan 2008).

Blazei et al. (2008) reported strong evidence for the transmission of antisocial behavior from father to child. In both preadolescence and late adolescence, a father's antisociality significantly predicted all measures of a child's externalizing behaviors. The presence of an antisocial father in the child-rearing environment had a particularly detrimental role on a child's antisociality in late adolescence, whereas the correlation was weak during preadolescence. When the father was not present for most of the child's life, no association was found between his antisociality and the child's antisocial behavior. When the father was present for most of the child's life, a strong positive association was found between father's and the child's antisociality, suggesting that the transmission of antisocial behavior from father to son is not entirely genetic. The study only explained 11% of the variance at age 11 and 21% of the variance at age 17, leaving 79%–89% of the variance unexplained (Blazei et al. 2008).

Adolescents with callus-unemotional (CU) traits—those lacking empathy, guilt, and being unmoved by the suffering of others—show particular neuropsychiatric features. They engage in proactive, instrumental aggression, seeming to be impervious to sanctions (they are unable to learn from reinforcing information), and do not seem to share the affiliate need and goal of typical children (Viding and McCrory 2015). Recent functional MRI (fMRI) findings show low amygdalar reactivity to fearful faces in children with CU traits. This finding extends to more complex forms of social judgement with regards to other's distress, such as categorization of legal and illegal behaviors in a moral judgement task. Two recent studies reported atypical neural activity to other people's pain in children with CU traits. There in a reduced activity in a brain network areas associated with empathy for other's people pain: anterior insula, anterior cingulate cortex, and amygdala (Viding and McCrory 2015, pp. 972–973).

Impulse-Control Difficulties

Many children with neuropsychological deficits demonstrate impulsive behaviors and a low tolerance for frustration. They become readily aggressive when things do not go their way; they demand immediate gratification and are intolerant of postponement of any of their wants. When their wants are not gratified, they throw tantrums (or lose control; they become threatening or become destructive of the surrounding environment) or use intimidation to impose their wills. In these situations parents feel helpless and feel unable to assert themselves. Many parents feel that the only option left is to seek the help and protection of the police. Because of their aggressive behavior and lack of other social-interpersonal skills (e.g., sharing, empathy, reciprocity), these children have problems making and maintaining long-term friendships.

Impulsive behaviors reflect deficits in executive functions, and they may be a consequence of disinhibition secondary to brain impairment. These children show no sense of propriety or judgment regarding sexual, aggressive, or appropriate social behaviors. Impulsive behavior is common in children who have ADHD, conduct disorder, or psychotic disorders. Impulsiveness is also a prominent feature of bipolar disorders, particularly mania.

Mood and Affect Dysregulation

Impairments in the expression, stability, and appropriateness of affect are common disturbances in neuropsychiatric patients. Moria (i.e., an abnormal tendency to joke), apathy, and brain-stem emotional lability are several examples of well-known adult emotional disturbances that are associated with specific neurophysiological or neuroanatomical impairments.

Depression and mania can be secondary to brain disorders (see Note 12 at the end of this chapter). Explosive or blind rage in great disproportion to the eliciting situation is a common after lesions of the frontal or temporal lobes. Damage to the medial aspects of the frontal lobes renders the person incapable of initiating even primitive behaviors, such as getting out of bed or eating; the person also becomes devoid of affect or emotional responsivity (apathy). Even mild damage to this region produces a loss of spontaneity and creativity, accompanied by flattening of affect; these symptoms may be misinterpreted as depression by well-meaning but uninformed psychotherapists.

According to Dickstein (2015), Leibenluft defined irritability in 2003, in neuroscience terminology, as a markedly increased reactivity to negative emotional stimuli that is manifested verbally or behaviorally; this definition facilitated research distinctions between children with chronic irritability and hyperarousal ("severe Mood Dysregulation") with those with clear episodes of euphoria ("narrow phenotype bipolar disorder). This resulted in the inclusion of the diagnosis of disruptive mood disregulation disorder (DMDD) in DSM-5 (American Psychiatric Association 2013, pp. 603–604), to be discussed in the next paragraph.

In part, to counter the overextension of the bipolar disorder diagnosis, which spurted the use of polypharmacy in children so diagnosed, DSM-5 introduced the diagnosis of disruptive mood disregulation disorder. The diagnostic criteria for this disorder could be applied to many of children and adolescents who had previously been diagnosed with bipolar disorder. The criteria for DMDD include the following (American Psychiatric Association 2013, p. 156):

A. Severe recurrent temper outbursts manifested verbally (e.g., verbal rages) and/or behaviorally (e.g., physical aggression toward people or property) that are grossly out of proportion in intensity or duration to the situation or provocation.
B. The temper outbursts are inconsistent with developmental level.
C. The temper outbursts occur, on average, three or more times per week.
D. The mood between temper outbursts is persistently irritable or angry most of the day, nearly every day, and is observable by others (e.g., parents, teachers, peers).

E. Criteria A–D have been present for 12 or more months. Throughout that time, the individual has not had a period lasting 3 or more consecutive months without all of the symptoms in Criteria A–D.

F. Criteria A and D are present in at least two of three settings (i.e., at home, at school, with peers) and are severe in at least one of these.

G. The diagnosis should not be made for the first time before age 6 years or after age 18 years.

H. By history or observation, the age at onset of Criteria A–E is before 10 years.

I. There has never been a distinct period lasting more than 1 day during which the full symptom criteria, except duration, for a manic or hypomanic episode have been met.

J. The behaviors do not occur exclusively during an episode of major depressive disorder and are not better explained by another mental disorder (e.g., autism spectrum disorder, posttraumatic stress disorder, separation anxiety disorder, persistent depressive disorder [dysthymia]).

K. The symptoms are not attributable to the physiological effects of a substance or another medical or neurological condition.

This diagnosis excludes ODD, intermittent explosive disorder, and bipolar disorder but can coexist with major depressive disorder, ADHD, conduct disorder, and substance use disorders.

Bipolar Disorder

Axelson et al. (2015) reported, in a longitudinal study, that bipolar spectrum disorders (bipolar I, bipolar II, and bipolar not otherwise specified) were significantly more prevalent in high-risk offspring as compared with community controls even before the offspring had reached young adulthood. The high-risk offspring had higher rates of depressive episodes, and nearly all nonmood Axis I disorders were more prevalent in the high-risk cohort. Mania and hypomania in high-risk offspring were almost always preceded by identifiable mood episodes and non–mood disorders. Distinct subthreshold episodes of mania or hypomania were highly specific to the high-risk offspring cohort and were the strongest predictors of progression to full threshold mania and hypomania. Identifiable depressive episodes preceded the onset of mania/hypomania above and beyond subthreshold of mania/hypomania in about two-thirds of the cases, but only major depressive episode specifically predicted the onset of mania/hypomania above and beyond sub-threshold of mania or hypomania and the presence of a disruptive behavior disorder (Axelson et al. 2015, p. 644). The prognostic significance of subthreshold mania or hypomania may not be limited to youth, as subthreshold symptoms of mania and hypomania have been found to be predictive of future conversion to bipolar disorder in adults diagnosed with unipolar depression. Given the clear prognostic significance of subthreshold mania or hypomania in youth at familial risk for disorder, more research is necessary given that both major depressive disorder and disruptive behavior disorders also indicate risk for future bipolarity (Axelson et al. 2015, p. 645).

Children with bipolar disorder show significant neurocognitive impairment in areas of attention, working memory, verbal memory, and executive function (Pavuluri and Bogarapu 2008; see Note 12 at the end of this chapter). The neurocognitive deficits are present during the acute state and remain during remission. Cognitive flexibility is greatly impaired in children with narrow-phenotype bipolar disorder. Children with bipolar disorder also display social cognitive deficits in facial emotion recognition and emotional processing difficulties. Youths with bipolar disorder were particularly prone to misread peers' but not adults' expressions of happiness, sadness, or fearfulness as being angry (Pavuluri and Bogarapu 2008). This finding was corroborated by Perlman et al. (2013, pp. 1314–1325), who reported emotional face processing impairments in pediatric bipolar disorder, reflecting a functional impairment in the fusiform gyrus. Brotman et al. (2008) concluded that deficits in facial emotion labeling may be a risk marker for bipolar disorder.

Irritability is a very prominent symptom in pediatric psychiatry. It is a significant component of a number of DSM-5 pediatric disorders: bipolar disorder, anxiety disorders, PTSD, major depressive episode, and oppositional defiant disorder. Chronic irritability is the hallmark of DMDD. Youths with bipolar disorders and DMDD have similar levels of parent-reported irritability and did not differ in their behavioral accuracy in identifying emotional faces. They did differ in the relationship between irritability and neural activity. Neural activity in the amygdala was found to correlate with irritability across all intensities of all emotions in DMDD subjects, whereas in bipolar subjects, irritability correlated with amygdalar activity only in fearful faces (Dickstein 2016, pp. 653–654).

Children of mothers with bipolar disorder, when compared with children of mothers with major depressive disorder and psychiatrically healthy control subjects, demonstrated impairment in executive function and selective deficits in spatial memory and attention (Klimes-Dougan et al. 2006). Children of mothers with bipolar disorder differed from psychiatrically healthy control subjects in that the former had a greater number of ADHD symptoms and depression, as well as lower IQ scores. Deficits are unrelated to the presence of manic or depressive symptomatology. Neuropsychological deficits may be a trait factor (Klimes-Dougan et al. 2006). It is generally accepted that bipolar disorders with mixed states carry a poor prognosis and a high burden of associated comorbidities, including anxiety, substance abuse, and suicidality (Castle 2014, p. 39). Bipolar disorders with mixed features are particularly susceptible to worsening of manic-like symptoms upon exposure to antidepressants (Castle 2014, p. 40).

The strongest predictors of developing bipolar disorder were baseline depression/anxiety, baseline and proximal affective lability, and proximal subsyndromal manic symptoms. Having all these risk factors conferred a 49% predictive chance of developing bipolar spectrum symptoms compared with a 2% risk for those without these risk factors (Dickstein 2016, p. 654).

Depression

Of high relevance in the expression of depression are a number of psychosocial factors. The inner and outer stability of the child's role model is influenced by that person's chronic history of medical or psychiatric illnesses, including substance abuse or history of alcohol abuse, anxiety disorders, psychosis, and personality disorders. In addition, intrafamilial interactions and communication are important in the development of affective disorders. Emotional and physical deprivation, physical and sexual abuse, parental divorce, disharmonic communication in the family, sibling density, and family stresses such as change of employment, migration, and poverty increase the risk of depression. Personality factors such as emotional instability, interpersonal dependency, and aggressiveness indicate a high risk for depression (Bark and Resch 2008). All of these negative factors increase the allostatic load (Kapczinski et al. 2008). A traumatic experience in early childhood produces an increased risk of a depressive syndrome and an increased risk of suicide at a later stage of development (Bark and Resch 2008). The highest rate of depression occurs in traumatized children without social support and with a short allele (S polymorphism) rather than in children with an LL genotype (Bark and Resch 2008). An association exists between the short allele and the hyperactivity of the amygdala, as well as between the hippocampus and anxiety. Children are at high risk of developing a major depressive episode if they have poor or unreliable psychosocial support, in addition to a high number of mistreatments. The risk is higher if the amygdala is hyperreactive in response to adverse stimuli and a high release of adrenocorticotropic hormone occurs as a reaction to experiences of separation (Bark and Resch 2008) (see Note 13 at the end of this chapter).

Dysthymia is not a circumscribed condition and seemingly captures persistent depression and anxiety as well as a personality contribution (Rhebergen and Graham 2014). It is imperative to differentiate unipolar from bipolar depression. The old term, *melancholia*, is still relevant in psychiatric practice. DSM-5 (American Psychiatric Association 2013, p. 185) describes melancholia with a specifier—with melancholic features—as follows:

1. One of the following is present during the most severe period of the current episode:

    a. Loss of pleasure in all, or almost all, activities.

    b. Lack of reactivity to usually pleasurable stimuli (does not feel much better, even temporarily, when something good happens).

2. Three (or more) of the following:

    a. A distinct quality of depressed mood characterized by profound despondency, despair, and/or moroseness or by so-called empty mood.

    b. Depression that is regularly worse in the morning.

    c. Early-morning awakening (i.e., at least 2 hours before usual awakening).

    d. Marked psychomotor agitation or retardation.

    e. Significant anorexia or weight loss.

    f. Excessive or inappropriate guilt.

Melancholia has biologic markers: 1) a hyperactive hypothalamic-pituitary-adrenal (HPA) axis, producing high cortisol levels, and 2) reduced change in cortisol levels throughout the day. A positive dexamethasone suppression test was the first biomarker investigated in melancholia, but this finding is inconsistent. Research has also demonstrated increased plasma arginine vasopressin levels, corticotropin-releasing hormone (CRH) dysfunction, and basal hypothalamic-pituitary-thyroid ultrasensitivity (Parker and Paterson 2014, p. 3). Also elevated in melancholia are tumor necrosis factor–α (TNFα) and 5-hydroxytryptamine antibodies, indicating a relationship with the immune inflammation system. These findings are also inconsistent. Some investigators have found decreased white matter in the DLPFC and in regions associated with the limbic system, thalamic projection fibers, and the corpus callosum (Parker and Paterson 2014, p. 3).

Regarding mood disorders in adults, depression is most common in disorders that produce dysfunction of the left frontal lobe, the temporal lobes, and the left caudate nucleus (Cummings 1995a). Most of the focal lesions that produce mania involve the right hemisphere: the inferior frontal lobe, the temporobasal region, or the thalamic-perithalamic areas. Degenerative and infectious illnesses that affect the frontal lobes or frontal-subcortical systems are also associated with mania (Cummings 1995a). Analogous lesions and symptom expression in children await substantiation.

Depressive symptoms are frequent precursors of or a common trait at the beginning of adolescent schizophrenia. About 20% of adolescent schizophrenia cases are preceded by a depressive episode (Remschmidt 2008).

There is an increasing recognition of the role of inflammation in a number of psychiatric disorders. Soczynska et al. (2012) ask, "Are psychiatric disorders inflammatory-based conditions?" A preliminary pro-inflammatory gene expression signature has been reported in the offspring of individuals with bipolar disorder, and elevated mRNA levels, as well as protein expression levels of interleukin 1B, interleukin 6, and TNFα, have been reported in the prefrontal cortex of adolescent suicide victims (see Soczynska et al. 2012).

Anxiety

Early manifestations of anxiety are conceptualized through the presence of a temperamental trait called *behavioral inhibition.* Behavioral inhibition refers to the inherent tendency in young toddlers and children to display withdrawal and autonomic arousal in the face of novel situations and unfamiliar persons. Behavioral inhibition is a well-known precursor of later anxiety and is a rather specific antecedent of social phobia. When toddlers with behavioral inhibition are followed over time, they develop separation anxiety and performance anxiety and also show an increase of social anxiety by adolescence. In studies of children at high risk for anxiety disorders, agoraphobia and panic in the parents were associated with the same disorders in children, and major depression in parents increased the risk for social phobia in children. Parents' panic and depression were also associated with increased risk for separation anxiety disorder and anxiety disorders in children. An important realization is that a substantial number of at-risk children will not develop anxiety disorders in adulthood, whereas another group will develop mood disorders in adulthood. Threats of smothering and smothering sensations are associated with panic disorder in adults and anxiety in children. This physiological reflex is more common in separation anxiety disorder than in social phobia. A study of high-risk children demonstrated that early separation anxiety disorder led to specific phobias, agoraphobia, panic disorder, and major depression, whereas early agoraphobia led to generalized anxiety disorder (GAD) (Grados 2008).

Fear conditioning is a basic underlying mechanism in pathological anxiety. A conditional fear response may develop to a neutral conditioned stimulus. The basolateral complex and the central nucleus of the amygdala play a role in the generation and perpetuation of conditioned fear responses. The orbitofrontal cortex is likely to be a part of the neural circuitry that underlies the manifestations of anxiety in children and adolescents. The insula plays an important role in the process of body orientation and subjective emotional experience and may play a role in processing visceral states important for feelings and emotions. Hippocampal structures appear to play a central role in the contextual modulation of the acquisition of conditioned fear and of its renewal or reinstatement following extinction (Grados 2008).

Three processes are considered to encompass the range of anxiety reactions in children: attentional systems, threat appraisal, and learning. For the pathological anxiety response sequence to become established, an initial vigilant-monitoring tendency (automatic reactivity) needs to occur, determining a lower threshold for the appraisal of the threat. These findings support the notion that a stable general hypersensitivity to environmental stimuli in children with behavioral inhibition exists in the form of an enhanced reactivity of the fear circuitry of the brain to novel stimuli (Grados 2008). Elevated levels of CRH in early age may be involved in the reduction of hippocampal volume found in early trauma-related posttraumatic stress disorder (PTSD). This is not a consistent finding; other studies have demonstrated that patients with PTSD show small intracranial volumes, cerebral structures, and corpus callosum, but no differences in the hippocampus or the amygdala (Monk and Pine 2009). Neurocognitive impairments, mostly in learning and memory impairments, have been identified in subjects with PTSD.

Alterations in the circuit involving the amygdala, stria terminalis, and the HPA axis are implicated in the fear response and in the elicitation of anxiety symptoms. On the other hand, anxiety is related to difficulties of disengaging attention from threatening stimuli; thus, children's amygdala activation does not appear to discriminate between fearful and neutral facial expressions. Patients with GAD display enhanced activation in the ventrolateral prefrontal cortex, and adolescents with GAD and social phobia show enhanced engagement of the amygdala when viewing negative-valence face emotion photographs and rating experienced levels of fear. This enhancement is also observed in the medial and ventral areas of the prefrontal cortex when attention is directed toward experienced levels of fear (Monk and Pine 2009).

Latas and Milovanovic (2014, p. 58) report that 85% individuals with borderline personality disorder have a co-occurring lifetime anxiety disorder, and that there is a high proportion of personality disorders in all types of anxiety disorders: 35% in PTSD; 41% in panic disorder without agoraphobia; 47% in panic disorder with agoraphobia; 48% in separation anxiety disorder; 52% in obsessive-compulsive disorder (OCD) (now classified on DSM-5 as an obsessive-compulsive and related disorder); and 47% in GAD. The prevalence of personality disorder is: Cluster C: 39%; Cluster B: 19%, and Cluster A: 13%.

Aggressive Behavior

Aggressive behavior may have a neurological cause when 1) the patient shows personality change and dyscontrol not shown prior to the event; 2) the individual's aggressive behavior is extreme in intensity and frequency; or 3) the patient's rage, violence, or destructive behaviors are unprovoked. Sometimes, aggressive patients have a history of or indication of brain injury (e.g., children who have been physically abused may have sustained a brain injury). About 3,000 children sustain hemispheric damage every year as a result of physical abuse. If the patient is remorseful and expresses disbelief about the loss of control, a neurological cause needs to be considered and an appropriate referral should be made. Although complex partial seizures are frequently implicated in intermittent aggressive dyscontrol, limited evidence is available to support this claim.

PTSD, childhood bipolar disorder, DMDD, borderline personality disorder, and intermittent explosive disorder are associated with an increased risk for reactive aggression; disorders associated with reactive aggression are also associated with a dysfunction of the frontal systems involved with affect regulation. There are four systems that allow the control of emotional responding and, consequently, reactive aggression: 1) frontal cortex, via excitatory projections on inhibitory interneurons within the amygdala; 2) attentional manipulation of emotional responses; 3) detection of reinforcement of contingency changes mediated by the ventromedial prefrontal cortex; and 4) social response reversal mediated by the ventrolateral and other regions of the prefrontal cortices (Blair 2009).

Social and Interpersonal Difficulties

Some children have selective deficits in social behavior secondary to an inability to process and understand affective cues or nonverbal behavior. These deficits produce the so-called social and emotional learning disabilities. Children with receptive aprosody cannot read affect or other nonverbal cues in social contexts and thus do not respond appropriately in social situations. Children with expressive aprosody are unable to display or express emotion concordant with the meaning they want to convey or the affective norms of the social circumstances in which they find themselves. These children also have difficulties understanding jokes and metaphorical language.

DSM-5 (American Psychiatric Association 2013) recognizes social (pragmatic) communication disorder with the following criteria:

A. Persistent difficulties in the social use of verbal and nonverbal communication as manifested by all of the following:

1. Deficits in using communication for social purposes, such as greeting and sharing information, in a manner that is appropriate for the social context.
2. Impairment of the ability to change communication to match context or the needs of the listener, such as speaking differently in a classroom than on a playground, talking differently to a child than to an adult, and avoiding use of overly formal language.

3. Difficulties following rules for conversation and storytelling, such as taking turns in conversation, rephrasing when misunderstood, and knowing how to use verbal and nonverbal signals to regulate interaction.
4. Difficulties understanding what is not explicitly stated (e.g., making inferences) and nonliteral or ambiguous meanings of language (e.g., idioms, humor, metaphors, multiple meanings that depend on the context for interpretation).

B. The deficits result in functional limitations in effective communication, social participation, social relationships, academic achievement, or occupational performance, individually or in combination.

C. The onset of the symptoms is in the early developmental period (but deficits may not become fully manifest until social communication demands exceed limited capacities).

D. The symptoms are not attributable to another medical or neurological condition or to low abilities in the domains of word structure and grammar, and are not better explained by autism spectrum disorder, intellectual disability (intellectual developmental disorder), global developmental delay, or another mental disorder.

Children with affective aprosody may have problems with the motor programming of affective gesturing and, as a result, exhibit an emotional flatness, robotic speech, and an array of atypical social behaviors. They may be inappropriately affectionate and "sticky." Their lack of normal affective expression, their gaze disturbances, their tendency to violate social space, and their "stickiness" all contribute to the oddness of their speech and behavior. It is likely that these children do not understand the perspective of others and are apt to make disastrous social faux pas (Voeller 1997). In adults, these deficits frequently represent nondominant hemispheric dysfunction. The situation in the developing brain may not be as straightforward. These deficits may be dissociated from other academic and neuropsychological deficits associated with right-hemisphere impairments.

Psychosis

Psychotic symptoms are commonly observed in child and adolescent psychiatric practice. The significance of psychosis is not clear. In some cases it is a severity marker. Psychosis is more common in mania than in depression, but bipolar depression with psychosis is not rare, and psychotic depression in adolescence may be the harbinger of a future bipolar course (Carlson 2013, p. 570). In young people, a first episode of psychotic depression may portend a bipolar course; psychotic symptoms in a nonbipolar depression may portend a schizophrenic course (Carlson 2013, p. 571).

A variety of hallucinatory and delusional symptoms are caused by demonstrable neurological dysfunctions. Temporal lobe epilepsy (complex partial symptomatology), although elusive in its detection, must be considered in the differential diagnosis of psychotic disorders. As far back as 1987, Taylor et al. stressed this issue in adult psychiatry: "Even in the absence of a classic epileptic picture and course, temporal lobe disease should be considered in the differential diagnosis of psychosis" (p. 10). This is equally true in the differential diagnosis of psychosis in children and adolescents (see the case examples on Ralph [Case Example 8] in Chapter 8, "Documenting the Examination"; Myra [Case Example 10] in Chapter 9, "Evaluation of Internalizing Symptoms"; and Ricardo [Case Example 2] earlier in this chapter). Rick's and Troy's case examples [Case Examples 8 and 9, respectively, also in Chapter 9, involve a variety of neuropsychological deficits. See also Abe's case (Case Example 4), earlier in this chapter, for a connection between temporal lobe injury and psychosis.

When performing the perception portion of the mental status examination (see Chapter 8), the examiner should go beyond the customary questions regarding the presence of auditory and visual hallucinations and inquire about the presence of olfactory, gustatory, haptic, sensory, somatic, and other perceptual disturbances (e.g., out-of-body experiences, derealization, premonitions, déjà vu, jamais vu) and delusional symptoms.

For a comprehensive differential diagnostic list of medical, genetic, and neurological conditions in childhood, see the article by Benjamin et al. (2013) on congenital and acquired disorders presenting as psychosis in children and young adults.

Remschmidt (2008) recommended use of multiple sources to validate the diagnosis of schizophrenia; he recommends the use of the mnemonic PLASTIC: for **P**rospective, **L**ongitudinal, **A**ll source, **T**reatment, **I**mpairment, and **C**linical presentation. When the clinician is considering the clinical presentation of very-early-onset schizophrenia or early-onset schizophrenia, Remschmidt recommended a dimensional approach that attends to the following areas:

- *Cognitive symptoms:* distortions of thinking, delusions, hallucinations, and thought distortions (thought insertion, breaks and interpolation in the train of thought, thought echo, incoherent or vague thinking).
- *Delusions:* ideas of reference, persecutory beliefs, bodily changes, delusions of control, and others. Systematized delusions are uncommon in childhood but become more frequent in adolescence.
- *Hallucinations:* threatening voices, command hallucinations, and hallucinations without a verbal structure (humming, laughing, or whistling). Auditory hallucinations are by far the most frequent. Visual hallucinations

are more common before age 13. They are also common in intoxications and delirium.

- *Emotional issues and changes in social functioning:* blunted affect, mood disturbances (irritability, fearfulness, and suspicion), negative symptoms (apathy, paucity of speech), and incongruity of emotional responses resulting in social withdrawal and lowering of social performance. Positive and negative symptoms may be present years before overt manifestations of the disorder.
- *Disturbances of speech and language:* paucity of speech or logorrhea, perseverations, speech stereotypes, echolalia and phonographism, and neologisms.
- *Motor disturbances:* clumsiness, motor disharmony, strange postures (rocking), stupor or catatonia, bizarre movements or motor stereotypies (finger stereotypies), and compulsive acts or rituals.

According to Remschmidt (2008), various disorders should be considered in the differential diagnosis: autism (autism spectrum disorder), multiple complex developmental disorder, multiple developmental impairment, affective psychosis (psychotic depression, bipolar disorder), drug-induced psychosis, and organic brain disorders (in addition to DMDD). Remschmidt's constructs of multiple complex developmental disorder and multiple developmental impairment appear to be similar to the concepts of pervasive developmental disorder and schizophrenia, respectively. About 20% of patients with multiple complex developmental disorder develop schizophrenia later in life (Remschmidt 2008).

For a summary of the structural abnormalities in childhood and adolescent schizophrenia as described by Remschmidt (2008), see Table 12–8.

Recent studies suggest that microglia activation with ensuing neuroinflammation is a key mechanism dominantly affecting neuronal networks, brain morphology (e.g., oligodendrocyte alterations), white matter damage, and so on, as well as impairments in learning, memory, and behavior in schizophrenia (Debnath and Venkatasubramanian 2013, p. 433). A range of characteristics of schizophrenia, such as progressive structural brain changes, cognitive and functional decline, poorer treatment response, and increased vulnerability to relapse, now seem to be under the control of immune determinants (Debnath and Venkatasubramanian 2013, p. 434)

Zhang et al. (2015) studied a cohort of 25 unmedicated persons with chronic schizophrenia to ascertain the degree of neurodegeneration and to determine if the lack of antipsychotic treatment changed the findings of previous observations. In comparison to control patients, patients with schizophrenia showed less cortical thickness in the ventromedial prefrontal cortices bilaterally extending laterally to the orbitofrontal areas, in the left superior

Table 12–8.   Structural brain abnormalities in very-early-onset schizophrenia (childhood-onset schizophrenia) and early-onset schizophrenia

Reduction in total brain volume. The left hemisphere is smaller in males. Reduction of the left hemisphere in males and a decrease in rightward hemisphere asymmetry in females correlates with decreased IQ.

Decreased total cerebral volume in siblings with childhood-onset schizophrenia (COS); decreased frontal and parietal gray matter volumes.

Minor physical anomalies associated with ventricular enlargement, indicating an early prenatal developmental disturbance.

In COS, a progressive loss of cerebellar volume during adolescence.

Specific abnormalities in COS subjects: small brains, smaller amygdala and thalamus, and a large caudate.

Progressive brain volume loss, correlating with premorbid impairment and baseline symptom severity.

Gyrification abnormalities in COS (common).

Source.   Adapted from Remschmidt 2008. Modified from Cepeda 2010, p. 364.

temporal gyrus extending to the occipital lobe area, and in the right pars triangularis. There were faster age-related cortical decrements in the right ventromedial prefrontal cortex, left superior temporal gyrus, and right pars triangularis. These findings have also been observed in childhood-onset schizophrenia, in which the cortical decrements occur at a faster pace (Zhang et al. 2015).

Meier et al. (2014, pp. 98–99) demonstrated a substantial neuropsychological decline in schizophrenia from premorbid to the post-onset period. The extent of the developmental progression of decline varies across mental functions. These authors' findings suggest that different pathophysiological mechanisms may underlie deficits in different mental functions.

Genome-wide association studies show the strongest signal for schizophrenia on chromosome 6p22.1 in a region related to the major histocompatibility complex (MHC) and other immune functions such as the human leukocyte antigen (HLA) alleles (Sperner-Unterweger and Fuchs 2015, p. 201) (see Note 14 at the end of this chapter).

Is schizophrenia an autoimmune disorder? A recent publication by Sekar et al. (2016) links a number of genes in the major histocompatibility complex (MHC), on chromosome 6, with an increase in the risk for developing schizophrenia. The association arises in part from many structurally diverse alleles of the complement component 4 (C4) genes, mostly *CSMD1*, which encodes for a regulator of C4. The alleles generate diverse expression in the brain, C4A and C4B, secreted by neurons. The association of common C4 allele with schizophrenia is proportional to its tendency to generate greater C4A expression. Human C4 proteins localized to neuronal synapses, dendrites, axons, and cell bodies. In mice, C4 mediates synapse elimination during postnatal development. These results implicate excessive complemental activity in the development of schizophrenia and may help to explain the reduced numbers of synapses in the brains of individuals with schizophrenia. This risk is linked to the natural process of synaptic pruning, by which weak or redundant connections are discarded as the brain matures (Carey 2016). Genes located in the MHC get activated during adolescence and early adulthood to carry out synaptic pruning primarily in the prefrontal cortex (PFC). Persons who carry the genes that accelerate or intensify the pruning are at a higher risk of developing schizophrenia. These persons have diminished connections in the PFC in comparison with non-affected persons. It has been proposed (Carey 2016) that in persons with schizophrenia there is a group of genes that causes an aggressive "tagging" of connections and other neuronal structures for pruning, effectively accelerating the process, thus, suggesting that schizophrenia is an autoimmune disorder. Persons with schizophrenia have higher levels of the variant C4A protein than do control subjects. Sekar et al. suggest that too much C4A protein leads to inappropriate pruning during this critical phase of development (Carey 2016).

Cornblatt et al. (2015) proposed a predictive profile for the accurate identification of young people at risk for the development of schizophrenia and related illnesses. This profile consists of four variables: disorganized communications, suspiciousness, verbal memory impairment, and declining social functioning. The authors claimed that their profile increased the risk of positive prediction from 30% with the high-risk criteria alone to 81.8% with the predictive profile. The authors stated that contrary to expectations, depression, anxiety, role functioning, duration of symptoms, substance abuse, medications, or very young age (12–14 years) had a limited predictive value. Adolescents with a low risk index score would be considered to be at a low level of risk, whereas adolescents with a high risk index score would be considered to be at the high end of risk.

Autistic Behavior

Autism (now classified as autism spectrum disorder [formerly autistic disorder]), is one of the most severe psychiatric disturbances and is a particularly dehumanizing neuropsychiatric condition. Autism is characterized by 1) a lack of communication language, 2) a lack of interpersonal relatedness, 3) an unusual preoccupation with inanimate objects, and 4) a need for sameness. DSM-5 conceptualizes autism spectrum disorder as a broader diagnosis. The traditional triad of impairment domains—social interaction, communicative behavior, and repetitive and restrictive behaviors (RRBs)—was collapsed into two domains. RRBs remain separate and intact, with the addition of atypical sensory experiences. The social and communicative domains have been merged. Diagnostic specifiers include 1) known etiological factors (medical, genetic, environmental); 2) severity and level of support needed; 3) intellectual impairments; 4) language impairments; and 5) presence of catatonia (Foss-Feig and MacPartland 2016, p. 41). We should add the presence of a neurological condition (seizures or other).

The abnormal development of social reciprocity is one of the most striking features of autism and that the social, communicative, imaginative, and cognitive elements of the disorder are inextricably linked. The discovery by Bauman and Kemper in 1985 of a reduction in the number of Purkinje and granular cells in the cerebellum was a "clap of thunder." This unexpected finding, amplified in 2003, opened the gates to a flood of morphometric studies of the cerebellum and to a reconsideration of its role not only in autism but also in other complex human behaviors like language, attention, and affect. Overconnectivity of some cortical circuitry, and underconnectivity in others involved in subcortical relays, such as the basal ganglia, amygdala, and other limbic areas, and in the cerebellum, are at the forefront of current research (Rapin 2011, p. 7).

Autism is usually accompanied by a variety of profound neurodevelopmental problems. Brain anomalies and brain dysfunction(s) are considered the main cause of this perplexing syndrome. Kinsbourne and Wood (2006) stated that autism spectrum disorder represents a behaviorally defined set of developmental disorders that result from diverse biological, genetic, and ecogenetic factors. Research in autism spectrum disorder is complicated by the broad heterogeneity in clinical and biological characteristics. Intellectual disabilities are present in about 80% of patients with autism, and neurological findings are present in about 60%–70% of autistic children. By adolescence, up to 30% of children with autism have developed a seizure disorder. Autism is associated with conditions such as phenylketonuria, fragile X syndrome, varicella infection in utero, toxoplasmosis, cytomegalovirus infection, and many other identifiable illnesses.

The discovery of the mirror neurons (localized in the inferior parietal lobe and inferior frontal lobe—areas related to speech, theory of mind, and imitation) has placed autism's characteristic deficits of empathy and social reciprocity on a new neurobiological and evolutionary foundation. Mirror neurons are a group of cortical neurons that discharge when one executes a movement, as well as when one observes another individual's actions. The engagement of these cells is thought to reflect an understanding of others' intentions. Abnormalities in the development of mirror neurons have been proposed as the cause of autism (Moura et al. 2008). Hickok (2014), in his book *The Myth of Mirror Neurons: The Real Neuroscience of Communication and Cognition,* argues against the impairment of the mirror cells as a central tenet of the cause of autism.

Evolutionary theory posits the development of empathy as one of the most important abilities developed by human beings; empathic relationships strengthen interpersonal connections and permit more complex social organizations (Moura et al. 2008). The social brain is formed primarily by the amygdala, which contributes to the expression of normal socioemotional behaviors; other areas in the temporal lobes also contribute to the socioemotional behaviors. Autism, therefore, is a disorder of the social brain. Consistent with this theory, as well as the observation of an increase of brain mass in individuals with autism, is the finding of increased neuronal packing density in the hippocampus, subiculum, entorhinal cortex, medial septal nuclei, and several amygdalar nuclei. Cerebellar abnormalities are also involved in children with autism (Moura et al. 2008).

Contrary to prevailing misinformation, vaccinations are not associated with the etiology of autism. On the other hand, if one identical twin is autistic, the risk for the other twin to develop autism is between 36% and 95%. If there is damage to the cerebellum at birth, the risk is 37%. If a fraternal twin is autistic, the risk for the other twin is 31%. Other factors, such as prematurity, paternal age (>60 years), and maternal age (>35 years), have a low risk, 3% (Wang 2014).

Obsessive-Compulsive Disorder

DSM-5 includes, in the category of obsessive-compulsive and related disorders, the classic obsessive-compulsive disorder, body dysmorphic disorder (BDD), hoarding disorder, trichotillomania (hair-pulling disorder), excoriation (skin-picking) disorder, substance/medication-induced OCD and related disorder, OCD and related disorder due to another medical condition, other specified OCD and related disorder, and unspecified OCD and related disorder (American Psychiatric Association 2013, pp. 235–264).

OCD is not a unitary disorder; a number of studies have indicated that OCD is a heterogeneous disorder with many possible subgroups. Epidemiological studies reveal that OCD has two peaks of incidence: one peak in childhood with male predominance and a second peak in early adulthood with female predominance. The course of OCD is also heterogeneous. Onset may be insidious with a chronic waxing and waning course, and although symptoms may change with time, they keep an enduring thematic consistency (Rosário et al. 2008).

OCD in childhood is possibly more biologically driven or more genetic than its adult-onset form (see Note 15 at the end of this chapter). Hoarding is correlated with OCD measures of slowness, responsibility, and indecisiveness; doubt and higher depression severity are more common in girls (Grados and Riddle 2008; see Note 16 at the end of this chapter). We need to consider a fifth factor, to incorporate somatic concerns (BDD) and skin picking (excoriation disorder), both not uncommon in childhood.

Developmentally, most children and adolescents engage in a significant number of ritualistic, repetitive, and compulsive-like activities. For example, young children need to repeat certain behaviors until the behaviors feels "just right." Children often feel uncomfortable when these behaviors are not performed the same way every time. During their school years, children commonly collect items (e.g., coins, stamps, pens, CDs). For many adolescents, grooming rituals take a long time. It is not clear how these normal obsessive-compulsive behaviors relate to OCD. Research indicates that the earlier the onset of obsessive-compulsive symptoms in children, the higher the morbid risk for first-degree family members to develop obsessive-compulsive symptoms, OCD, tics, or Tourette's disorder. Family aggregation of OCD was largely concentrated among families of probands with early-onset OCD who had a very high comorbid risk (Rosário et al. 2008).

Clinically, children and adolescents show higher rates of aggressive and harm obsessions than adults, but they have a lower frequency of sexual obsessions. Religious obsessions are more frequent in adolescents than in children and younger adults. Hoarding compulsions were the only symptoms that were more frequent in children and adolescents. Also common in children and adolescents were the fear of losing one's parents and the need to perform rituals, such as reassurance seeking and asking the same questions repeatedly. Younger children are more likely to suffer from compulsions than from obsessions and to display higher frequencies of repetition, hoarding, tic-like compulsions, and sensory phenomena. The compulsions commonly precede the obsessions by about 2 years. In patients with late-onset OCD, obsessions and compulsions start at the same time (Rosário et al. 2008).

In the evaluation of sudden-onset OCD symptoms and tics, special attention should be paid to history of infectious illnesses and chronology of symptoms.

PANDAS (pediatric autoimmune neuropsychiatric disorders associated with streptococcal infections) is associated with the sudden, prepubertal onset of OCD or a tic disorder that is characterized with the acute or episodic appearance of symptoms that temporally coincide with Group A streptococcal infections. Questions regarding sore throats or recent strep throat infections (especially with regards to completion of the antibiotic course) should be examined. In addition, the examiner should pay close attention to the history of symptom worsening and abatement in regards to the development of infectious illnesses.

The broader PANS definition (pediatric acute-onset neuropsychiatric syndromes) helps to account for those cases that do not have an initially identifiable origin (Swedo et al. 2012). For the diagnosis of PANS, the acute onset of OCD or severe restriction of food intake is accompanied by two or more neuropsychiatric symptoms: anxiety, emotional lability/dysphoria, behavioral/developmental regression, deterioration in school performance, sensory or motor abnormalities, and regression in sleep and urinary continence. For example, sudden-onset separation anxiety without any identifiable trauma or change in environment may be observed. The handwriting of children with previously legible and age-appropriate script may deteriorate to scribbles or disorganized drawings. Previously "good sleepers" may begin to display sleep terrors or severe nightmares, difficulties with sleep onset, or frequent awakenings. Children who had been previously potty-trained may begin to display episodes of enuresis.

Sensory phenomena are defined as uncomfortable, disturbing sensations, perceptions, feelings, or urges that precede or accompany repetitive behaviors (compulsions or tics). Patients with OCD feel driven to repeat the compulsions until they experience a sense of relief from the uncomfortable sensations. The sensory phenomena could be physical or mental (e.g., sensations in the skin, the "just-right" perception, feelings of incompleteness). Evaluation of the sensory phenomena is relevant because some studies report that patients with early-onset and tic-related OCD have a higher frequency of sensory phenomena and that these symptoms might cause more distress than do compulsions for these patients (Rosário et al. 2008).

The following case example illustrates the development of OCD in a child.

Case Example 6

Donald, a 12-year-old Caucasian preadolescent male, was evaluated for possible ADHD and for behaviors that included stealing, lying, and cross-dressing. He had also voiced suicidal thoughts but had made no suicide attempts. Learning disorders and expressive language difficulties were identified. Donald was an adopted child. He lived with his mother and his brother, 4 years older, who was his parents' natural child. Donald's parents had been divorced for 7 years prior to the evaluation, and they maintained a hostile relationship. Each parent spoke badly about the other in front of the children. Donald's mother had been sexually abused as a child and had a mood disorder. She was in poor health and at the time of the evaluation was receiving medical, psychiatric, and psychotherapeutic treatment. She was frustrated with the uncertainties of Donald's diagnosis.

Donald had been mainstreamed at school. Teachers had made no serious complaints about his behavior in the classroom. At home, however, Donald created a great deal of distress: he procrastinated about his homework and chores, irritated his brother by getting into his "things," and frustrated his mother by his persistent argumentative, oppositional, and defiant behavior. Donald also had a history of fascination with fires.

The mental status examination revealed a small, meek, nonspontaneous male. He had an air of immaturity. He displayed frequent tics in the upper left side of his face. His speech was marked by significant hesitation and a considerable degree of stuttering. The examiner observed occasional grunting and throat clearing. Donald's mood appeared mildly depressed. His affect was appropriate but constricted. There was no evidence of thought disorder or of any perceptual disorder. Donald denied suicidal or homicidal ideation. He indicated no concerns about his cross-dressing. His sensorium was intact, and he seemed to be of an average intelligence. He displayed no insight into his problems and demonstrated marked passivity about what was going on with him and around him.

One year after the initial evaluation, Donald's mother reported that he was becoming progressively more preoccupied with sex. She suspected that he masturbated frequently using stuffed animals. There were indications that he used the dolls for his sexual practices because his mother frequently found the dolls with openings that corresponded to the genital areas. On more than one occasion, Donald's brother and mother had seen him wearing feminine undergarments. Donald's mother often could not find some of her pantyhose, panties, brassieres, or shoes. Furthermore, when trying on her shoes, mother would sometimes notice that they were stretched out. She suspected that Donald had worn them.

When Donald's mother received her latest telephone and credit card bills, she became aware that Donald had charged thousands of dollars in calls to various sex lines. Donald was obsessed with sex. Donald was experiencing powerful sexual compulsions. He started taking fluoxetine with very positive response; his sexual preoccupation lessened, and his compulsion to call the sex lines decreased.

In general, OCD accrues significant comorbidity both in breadth and in severity. Common associated conditions include mood disorders, anxiety disorders, oppositional defiant disorder, intermittent explosive disorder, ADHD, and psychotic disorders. Up to 60%–80% of children and adolescents with OCD have a comorbid disorder: 51% have ADHD, 47% have ODD, and 5% have pervasive developmental disorder (currently, autism spectrum disorder). ADHD is more common in boys (53%) than in girls (24%). Comorbid anxiety disorders not related to the OCD are common in all age groups but occur more frequently in children (56%) and adolescents (35%) than in adults (17%). However, major depressive rates are higher in adults (78%) than in adolescents (62%) and children (39%). Rates of tics in children range from 20% to 60%, compared with 9% in adolescents and 6% in adults; 48% of subjects with early-onset OCD present with tics or Tourette's syndrome, compared with 10% of subjects with late-onset OCD. A tic-related OCD subgroup has been identified, with a higher risk of transmission of OCD, subclinical OCD, and tics among first-degree relatives of OCD probands; higher male frequency; early onset of the disorder; and a different treatment response compared with other OCD patients (Rosário et al. 2008).

OCD occurs in conjunction with diseases of the basal ganglia. The caudate nucleus or the globus pallidus may be involved. In adults, most disorders that produce OCD symptoms affect the basal ganglia bilaterally (Cummings 1995a). Tourette's disorder is associated with OCD in 20%–30% of cases. An infection associated with the group A beta-hemolytic streptococcus (GABHS), or other infectious processes, including Lyme disease and Mycoplasma pneumoniae, are implicated. Family studies show that first-degree relatives of children with PANDAS have higher rates of Tourette's disorder and OCD, as well as an expanded expression of a trait marker for susceptibility to rheumatic fever, the monoclonal antibody D8/17. Having multiple infections with GABHS during 1 year was associated with an increase of Tourette's disorder, but the data concerning antibiotic prophylaxis have not been compelling (Roessner and Rothenberger 2008). Two longitudinal studies failed to show an association between GABHS infections and exacerbations of tics or OCD. The presence of antistreptococcal and antineuronal antibodies is inconsistent. However, immunological mechanisms seem to be involved: levels of proinflammatory cytokines (TNF and interleukin-12) are elevated, and regulatory T cells are decreased at baseline and during exacerbations (Roessner and Rothenberger 2008) (see Note 17 later in this chapter).

In a large sample of children and adults with Tourette's disorder, ferritin and serum iron levels were significantly lower but still within the normal range. Ferritin correlated positively with volumes of the sensorimotor, midtemporal, and subgenual cortices (Roessner and Rothenberger 2008, pp. 107–108). Lower iron stores appear to contribute to the hypoplasia of the caudate and putamen, increasing the vulnerability to developing or having more severe tics. Lower iron may also contribute to smaller cortical volumes, decreasing control of the tics. "In a group of treatment-naïve boys with Tourette's Disorder (TS), volumetric MRI revealed significantly larger left thalamus in TS whereas no group difference was observed for the right thalamus. The boys with TS also showed a significant reduction in rightward asymmetry in thalamic volume compared with healthy subjects" (Roessner and Rothenberger 2008, p. 107). There is an increase in the volume of the dorsal prefrontal, parieto-occipital, and inferior occipital cortices and a decrease in the volume of the premotor, orbitofrontal, and subgenual cortices in children with TS (Roessner and Rothenberger 2008).

OCD in childhood is a severe condition that rarely responds to single treatments. OCD response to psychotropic medications is modest. Multidimensional treatments are mandatory.

Obsessive-compulsive personality disorder (OCPD) and traits of OCPD were found to be relatively common among individuals with eating disorders, including those with anorexia nervosa, bulimia nervosa, and binge-eating disorder. Moreover, perfectionism was specially associated with eating disorders and, perfectionism, and rigidity, as OCPD traits in childhood were identified as important risk factors for the development of eating disorders, particularly anorexia nervosa (Starcevic and Brakoulias 2014).

Given the evidence that the glutaminergic system is involved in OCD, it seems reasonable to target this system in pharmacotherapy (Kariuki-Nyuthe et al. 2014) (see Note 18 later in this chapter).

Paraphilia and Hypersexuality

Regarding abnormal sexual behavior in adults, paraphilias have been associated with frontal lobe disorders (e.g., frontal degeneration, multiple sclerosis), basal ganglia diseases (e.g., Huntington's disease, Tourette's disorder, Parkinson's disease following treatment with dopaminergic agents), and epilepsy. Hypersexuality may be attributed to secondary mania, Klüver-Bucy syndrome, or septal lesions (Cummings 1995a). Similar neuroanatomical correlations in children need substantiation. In a number of cases described in this chapter, like those of Ruben (see Case Example 5) and Donald (see Case Example 6), there is a history of hypersexual and paraphilic behaviors.

Key Points

- The field of pediatric neuropsychiatry deals with the assessment and treatment of congenital or acquired neurodevelopmental disorders.
- The elucidation of the biological basis of behavior and emotions is being carried out at an accelerated pace in the field of child and adolescent psychiatry. Significant progress is being made in establishing the genetic, biochemical, neurophysiological, and neuroanatomical bases of psychopathology.
- In contemporary psychiatric thinking, the neurobiological basis of behavior is taking an increasing preeminence. Clinicians/examiners, no matter what their field of expertise, need to be familiar with basic neurobiological and neuropsychological concepts.
- The neuropsychiatric examination includes the assessment of attention, language, cognition, memory, visuospatial skills, motor function, sensory functioning, and executive functions.

- Clinicians need to be informed of the basic tenets of the most common neuropsychiatric conditions and be able to detect signs and symptoms indicative of neuropsychological or neuropsychiatric impairments.
- Clinicians also need to be knowledgeable about the indications and interpretations of neuropsychological testing.
- There is convincing evidence that socioeconomic disadvantage causes detrimental effects on the structure and function of the brain.

Notes

1. According to Holz et al. (2015, p. 366), the new field of *environmental imaging* is concerned with the impact of socioeconomic disadvantage (SED) on the structure and functioning of the brain. Poverty is the strongest predictor of SED. It has been known that SED increases the risk of psychopathology related to social defeat, the sense of being excluded, characterized by being in a subordinate position characterized by increased stress and isolation. Altered social stress processing may be the mediator. Decreased volume of the dorsolateral prefrontal cortex, and a male-specific reduction in the perigenual anterior cingulate cortex (ACC), could result in dopaminergic hyperactivity, a consequence of altered stress regulation that also links with increased risk for psychosis. Poverty is a major public health risk (physical and mental), particularly with disorders such as autism spectrum disorder and conduct disorder. Poverty entails exposure to a number of covariant risks: life stress, substance abuse, poor social support, and lack of access to resources such as nutrition, education, and medical services. In the past the concept of sociogenetic brain syndrome was aptly applied. Individuals exposed in early life to poverty exhibit a decrease in the orbitofrontal cortex (OFC), a key structure involved in emotional and reward processing. The association between poverty and conduct disorder is mediated by OFC volume. This finding cannot be explained by sex, obstetric adversity, lifetime substance abuse, or genetic risk. Children in SED have an overall reduction in gray matter (particularly in frontal and parietal areas) and in amygdalar and hippocampal volumes (mediated by support and stressful life events). Young adults followed since birth show reduced activation in the basal ganglia, including ventral striatum, during reward anticipation as a function of early adversity. This hyposensitivity was accompanied by hypersensitivity in the basal ganglia during reward delivery. The latter finding is linked to ADHD, explaining a connection of increased risk of externalizing behaviors following exposure to

early adversity. When the impact of early life stress, including adoption, orphanage upbringing, physical abuse, and low SES background, on limbic volume was compared, hippocampal volume was reduced only following physical abuse and with low SES. Higher levels of behavioral problems were mediated by decreased hippocampal volume but not amygdalar volume. Right amygdala is increased in volume after verbal/emotional abuse and physical mistreatment. Amygdalar volume is particularly susceptible to stress during ages 10–11 years. Maltreated children exhibit reduced cortical thickness in the ACC and OFC, and this is accompanied by a reduced surface in the temporal and lingual gyrus and by less gyrification in the lingual gyrus and the insula (Holz et al. 2015, pp. 366–370).

2. Impressive gains in the understanding of a number of neuropsychiatric conditions and technological advances in diagnostic testing have made possible what in previous years would have been considered fantasy or science fiction. Gothelf (2007) described the following scenario:

> A 15-year-old male is referred for a neuropsychiatric evaluation because of academic and behavioral problems at school. Psychiatric evaluation reveals that the adolescent presents with psychotic features and an indiscriminate, over-friendly approach to strangers. Upon neuropsychological evaluation, he exhibits deficits in working memory and in object recognition processes. Functional MRI evaluation reveals increased activation in the cingulate gyrus and dorsolateral prefrontal cortex during performance of a Go/NoGo task. There is also decreased activation in the region of the intra-parietal sulcus when performing a two-dimensional puzzle task. Based in the multimodal assessment, the child psychiatrist suspects that variants of several genes including COMPT, PRODH, elastin, LIM domain kinase 1 (LIMK1) are mediating the patient's neuropsychiatric and neurocognitive deficits. Consequently, a blood sample is drawn and a molecular work-up reveals that the patient's profile is consistent with the suspected high-risk genetic variants. Variations in the COMPT and PRODH genes explain the prefrontal cognitive deficits and psychotic symptoms, whereas variations in the LIMK1 explain the dorsal visual processing stream deficits and the over-friendly approach of the patient. The child psychiatrist presents the results of the clinical evaluation and laboratory tests to the patient and his family, and suggests medications that will regulate the activity of the COMPT enzyme and that will normalize the expression of the LIMK1 gene (p. xvii).

3. Shenton and Turetsky (2011, p. xiii) attribute most of the progress in the understanding of the neuropsychiatric disorders to the dramatic improvements in image resolution and the development of novel imaging techniques: computed tomography, positron emission tomography, single photon emission computed tomography, MRI and functional MRI,

diffusion tensor imaging, magnetic resonance spectroscopy, ultrasound, and magnetoencephalography.

4. Denckla (1997) has reservations about the diagnostic validity of graphesthesia in children. She thinks that this may not be an efficient test because little is known about the firmness of the association between mental image or visual memory of a letter, the name of the letter, and the dynamic-tactile experience of graphesthesia. The implication is that for these tests to be valid, a certain cognitive developmental level is required. Tactile sensory loss is common in children with cerebral palsy. Astereognosis and dysgraphesthesia are specific agnosia deficits observed in children with cerebral palsy. Denckla's reservations about the validity of graphesthesia in children may also be applicable to related tests.

5. According to Harris (1995a), "Neuro-imaging technology attempts to correlate specific aspects of information processing with specific brain regions. Structural imaging methods are used to link damage in particular brain regions with behavioral deficits; functional brain imaging investigates physiological changes associated with brain activity. Links to brain structure or physiology may validate neuropsychological assumptions for the developmental disorders" (p. 24).

6. There are numerous misconceptions about neuropsychological testing (Sbordone 1997), including that

- A detailed history and interviews of collateral sources are not necessary because such information may bias test interpretation. *This is not correct.* The neuropsychologist can simply rely on the patient's medical records to arrive at an understanding of the type of brain injury the patient sustained. *This is not correct.*

- Defective performances on neuropsychological testing indicate cognitive dysfunction and/or brain damage, and defective performances on particular tests indicate dysfunction or damage to specific areas of the brain. The neuropsychologist does not need to test or interview a particular patient if he or she has access to the patient's raw test data. *This is not correct.*

- Collecting reliable test data is the neuropsychologist's primary goal. *This is not correct.* Careful interpretation of test data, using appropriate norms, is essential in arriving at accurate opinions about the patient's cognitive impairments or the localization of brain dysfunctions. *This is not entirely correct.*

- Changes in cognitive functioning are best determined by careful examination of serial neuropsychological test data. It is unwise to continue testing a brain-injured patient if the patient becomes fatigued because the test data will become unreliable. *This is not correct. Brain-*

damaged patients should be tested in relatively quiet settings that are free from distractions or extraneous stimuli.

- The neuropsychologist's primary responsibility is to record the patient's specific responses to specific test stimuli during testing. It is not necessary to record the amount and type of practice, cues, prompts, or various strategies given to or used by the patient during testing, because the raw test data are sufficient to determine the patient's cognitive impairments. *This is not correct.*
- Test data can be interpreted accurately in the absence of information from other sources (e.g., historical information, medical records, academic records). Interpretations based on test data alone can predict the patient's ability to function at work, school, home, or in other real-world settings. *This is not correct.*
- It is not essential to observe the patient functioning outside the testing (laboratory) environment because careful interpretation of the test data will provide a sufficient basis for predicting how the patient is likely to respond in real-world settings. *This is not correct.*
- Patients who sustain traumatic brain damage will make most of their recovery during the first 6 months and continue to recover for up to 2 years after the injury. *This is not correct.* Intact performance on a standardized neuropsychological battery (e.g., Wechsler Intelligence for Children—4th Edition, Halstead-Reitan Neuropsychological Battery, Luria-Nebraska Neuropsychological Battery) rules out the likelihood that the patient has cognitive deficits or has sustained a brain insult. *This is not correct.*
- Neuropsychological test reports need to contain only a brief description of the reasons for referral, identifying information about the patient, the names of the tests administered, the raw test data, and interpretation of the test data. *This is not correct.*
- The neuropsychological test can reliably identify brain damage if it is present. Intact performance in a variety of neuropsychological tests (e.g., Category Test, Wisconsin Card Sorting, Trail Making Test) known to be sensitive to frontal lobe damage rules out the likelihood of frontal lobe pathology. *This is not correct.*
- The results of neuropsychological testing should be consistent with the patient's complaints. *This is not correct.*

7. Other findings in Frances's case.

Cognitive testing. Verbal test scores were below average; the highest score was 8. Performance scores were higher than the verbal scores; one subtest score was 9, whereas another was 13 (object assembly). These scores indicated that Frances's abilities based on visual perception and some forms of motor response were substantially better than her language-based abilities. Because of the large discrepancy between Frances's Verbal and Performance IQ scores, the Full Scale IQ was not considered a meaningful descriptor of her cognitive abilities. She had below-average (borderline) scores on tasks requiring verbal comprehension, reasoning, and expression.

Sensory-perceptual functions. Mild difficulty in maintaining fixation during visual-field tests was revealed.

Motor functions. Moderate to severe bilateral impairments were noted.

8. According to Barkley (2015, pp. 358–359), ADHD is highly hereditary: genetic factors account for more than 70%–80% of its expression. Family studies show a marked elevated risk of ADHD among relatives of children with ADHD (10%–35%), rising to as much as 55% risk if at least one parent was affected or if there are two or more affected children. Parents with ADHD convey as much as 57% risk to the offspring. The contribution of shared environment is negligible (0–13%) and not statistically significant. ADHD is polygenic. Genes that have reliably been identified include the serotonin and dopamine transporter genes *5HTT* and *DAT1*, respectively; the dopamine receptor genes *DRD4* and *DRD5*; the serotonin type 1B receptor gene *HTR1B*; and *SNAP25*, a synaptic regulating protein gene. There are many other genes under investigation that are suspected of having an influence in the expression of ADHD (p. 360). Children and adults suffering injuries to the prefrontal regions have long been known to demonstrate deficits in sustained attention, inhibition, regulation of emotion, motivation, and the capacity to organize behavior across time (dysexecutive syndrome, or "frontal lobe disorders") with symptoms that overlap with those of ADHD (p. 362). Some studies suggest that some cases of ADHD may arise or may be exacerbated by streptococcal infections, perhaps via the damaging effects on the basal ganglia (p. 373). Smoking during pregnancy is more frequent in mothers from low SES; smoking increases the risk for the externalizing disorders ADHD and conduct disorder in the offspring. Nicotine exposure may cause damage to the brain at critical developmental periods and may chronically affect the cholinergic and dopaminergic neurotransmissions. Subjects exposed to smoking during pregnancy had a reduction in the inferior frontal gyrus (IFG). Activity in the IFG was inversely related to lifetime ADHD symptoms, thereby closing the gap between environmental adversity, neurobiological correlates, and psychopathology. Cortical thinning in the dorsolateral prefrontal cortex has also been demonstrated in subjects exposed to cocaine in utero. Findings are more pronounced in the left hemisphere (Holz et al. 2015, p. 368).

9. According to Patankar et al. (2012), soft neurologic signs (SNS) are present in 84% of children with ADHD; of the timed motor movements, speed of movement and dysrhythmias are the most reliable findings. Synkinesias (movement overflow), which are present in 40% of cases, and mirror movements, which are present in 30%, are indicators of a developmental delay of motor inhibition. Dysrhythmias and slow speed are an indication of functional deficits of the cerebellum and the basal ganglia. The severity of symptoms decreases with increasing age. By age 7 many of the skills assessed by the Physical and Neurological Examination for Soft Signs (PANESS) have matured—that is, reached "adult" level of proficiency. Children with the predominantly inattentive type of ADHD have significant poorer fine motor skills, while children with the combined type have greater problems with gross motor skills. Children with impulsivity have more dysrhythmias indicative of cerebellar pathology.

10. The topic of concussion was the subject of a series of articles in *The New York Times* on September 29 and 30, 2015. Belson (2015) noted that because of concerns with brain injury, and "[d]espite the popularity of college and professional football, the number of male high school football players has fallen to about 1.08 million this year [2015], a 2.4% decline from five years ago" (B11, B15). Some schools have shut down the football programs all together. In a front page article, "Concussions in a Required Class: Boxing at Military Academics," Phillips (2015) brought the issue of concussion in military academies to the forefront. Ninety seven concussions were reported at West Point, where boxing is a required training, during the last three academic years for which data were available (2012–13, 2013–14, 2014–15. The Air Force Academy reported 72 and the Naval Academy 29 during that same period. Some medical experts say that the risks of the boxing requirement outweigh the rewards, and that even when there is no diagnosable concussion there can still be lasting brain damage. The Department of Defense attempted to block or delay this reporting.

11. Other findings in Ruben:

Physical examination. He had multiple self-inflicted bruises on the right arm and right foot, plus an old irregular scar in the lateral aspect of the right arm, corresponding to a self-inflicted burn.

Neurological screening. Ruben was left handed; he exhibited marked right-left disorientation and dysnomia (e.g., he called a cross "two lines," called a triangle "a rectangle," and did not know the name of the diamond.) This naming difficulty also reflected problems with abstract perception and thinking.

Psychological testing. Verbal tests scores were very poor; all were below 4 (10 is average). Performance test scores were below average, except object assembly, which was 11. Academic test scores were below third-grade level in reading, spelling, and arithmetic. Ruben's reading performance met the criteria for a diagnosis of a learning disability. His performance in spelling and arithmetic was substantially below expectations based on age and grade placement.

Projective testing. Ruben's performance was consistent with an affective psychosis with depressive features; significant organic impairment was present. He exhibited no psychosis at the time of testing, but his reality testing showed a propensity to deteriorate under minor stresses. Schizotypal personality features were suggested.

Neuropsychological testing. Ruben wore glasses throughout the testing. His fingernails showed signs of severe nail biting; otherwise, he was well groomed and appropriately dressed. When approached initially, Ruben was concerned he would receive an injection and said, "He is gonna kill me," but he didn't appear nervous or frightened. He willingly accompanied the examiner and was polite and cooperative throughout the test session. Ruben related to the examiner in a friendly and outgoing manner. Ruben's sentence organization was somewhat poor, although he managed to communicate his meaning. For example, he defined a thief by saying, "A thief is he's stealing stuff." Word usage problems contributed to his difficulty organizing his verbalizations. For instance, when attempting to communicate that a boy in the story wanted to be a violinist, Ruben said, "He just wants to be a violin. He wants to be a musical instrument thing. He wants to learn, I guess." Through such attempts to restate his thoughts, Ruben demonstrated awareness that his verbal communications were ineffective. The neuropsychologist elicited a history of head trauma at age 6 years, when Ruben fell from the monkey bars at school; Ruben did not lose consciousness. Ruben's speech and language were remarkable for problems of syntax, grammar, word usage, and content organization. He used the word "thing" when he did not know the correct name for something or substituted a less accurate term (e.g., he called lightbulb filaments "needles"). Ruben's expressive language suggested occasional loosening of the thought processes secondary to tangential thinking. His receptive language also appeared impaired. Ruben frequently did not understand instructions and questions. For example, when asked how many things make a dozen, he replied "Eggs." Ruben appeared to have difficulty remembering previously attempted combinations when using a trial-and-error approach. He lost points on timed tasks because of task behavior due to stopping to rub his forehead, and because he was overly concerned with noncritical aspects of his performance (perfectly lining up cards on a timed sequencing task). Although Ruben fidgeted and occasionally got out of his seat, he was able to sit and attend for long periods of time. His mood was cheerful and his affect congruent. Ruben's approach to the testing was varied but generally systematic and efficient. He appeared to use analysis when solving visuoperceptual problems and worked systematically back and forth across rows when doing a target detection task.

Visuospatial skills. Evaluation of visuospatial skills revealed impairment of orientation judgment, spatial target detection, and visuomotor integration. Speed and accuracy for detecting spatial targets were below normal limits for all symbols except complex embedded figure. Performance on constructional tasks using paper and pencil revealed very poor preservation of the spatial elements of the designs; Ruben's approach to this task was hurried and notably impulsive. Construction using puzzles and patterned blocks was within average range.

12. Pavuluri and Bogarapu (2008) described three pathways associated with bipolar disorder: two anterior—the frontostriatal cognitive circuitry and the frontolimbic affective circuitry—and one posterior—the face response visual circuitry. The anterior circuits modulate affect and cognition, whereas the posterior regulates the emotional facet. The frontostriatal circuit proceeds from the dorsolateral prefrontal cortex and projects majorly into the anterior cingulate cortex with further relays into the basal ganglia, and vice versa. The frontolimbic circuit comprises projections from the ventrolateral prefrontal cortex into the limbic areas of the amygdala, hippocampus, and cingulate and insular cortices. A significant amount of information from the anterior pathways is relayed into the thalamus (the so-called relay station). The deployment of the affective circuitry shuts down the cognitive circuitry. The posterior pathway has its origins in the primary visual area and in the visual association areas. Different emotional and expressive submodalities are relayed by feed-forward projections through different lobes en route to the prefrontal cortex, with particular projections to the amygdala and the superior temporal sulcus. Deranged development and/or deviant inputs and outputs from these circuits, present in some patients with bipolar disorder, could be considered as the neuroanatomical and neurophysiological basis for the dysfunctional disturbances in the affective, cognitive, and emotional areas common in this illness (Pavuluri and Bogarapu 2008).

13. Patients with major depression and psychosis show greater hippocampal and amygdalar volume reduction than do patients with major depression without psychosis (Keller et al. 2008). Smaller amygdalar volume may be a risk factor for future psychotic depression, and smaller hippocampal volumes seem to indicate a risk factor for stress-related psychopathology and therefore a greater likelihood of posttraumatic stress disorder (Keller et al. 2008).

14. Recently published genome-wide association studies indicate that MHC molecule–mediated glutamatergic receptor function may be related to cognitive impairments in schizophrenia. There is a converging evidence that interleukin-6 (IL-6), a predominantly pro-inflammatory cytokine related to the type-2 T helper (Th2) immune response, might be involved in the pathogenesis of schizophrenia. The relationship between functional IL-6 gene polymorphism and reduced hippocampal volume, recently observed in naive patient with schizophrenia, supports this evidence (Sperner-Unterweger and Fuchs 2015, p. 202). There is a correlation between IL-6 and tryptophan/kynurenine and kynurenic acid (KYNA) ratio, indicating that IL-6 interferes with the kynurenine pathway; earlier studies indicated that a shift in the kynurenine pathway toward enhanced KYNA formation might be involved in the pathophysiology of schizophrenia. Findings of low quinolinic acid/kynurenic acid ratio (QUIN/KYNA) in cerebrospinal fluid of patients with schizophrenia support that hypothesis. Thus, it seems that a shift from QUIN toward KYNA may represent a consequence of the shift toward Th2-type immunity away from type-1 T helper (Th1)–type immunity (Sperner-Unterweger and Fuchs 2015, p. 204).

15. Structural and functional neuroimaging studies in both pediatric and adult OCD subjects suggest a dysregulation of the fronto-cortical-striatal-thalamic circuitry. Morphometric studies in children and adolescents with OCD show reduced striatal volumes. Volumetric abnormalities in the frontal and anterior cingulate cortices appear to be specific to the gray matter in pediatric patients with OCD, whereas both gray matter and white matter are affected in adult subjects with OCD. The anatomical findings are consistent with anterior cingulate hypermetabolism, demonstrated in neuroimaging studies. Functional neuroimaging studies suggest that the metabolism of the orbitofrontal cortex, anterior cingulate, and caudate nucleus is abnormal in both pediatric and adult patients. Growing evidence indicates that the dopamine system may be involved in the pathogenesis of OCD. OCD frequently occurs as a comorbid condition with Tourette's disorder, Parkinson's disease, and Huntington's chorea, diseases in which dopaminergic neurons play an important role. Oxytocin might play an important role in late-onset OCD; neuro-

peptides may play a role as well. Extensive interactions have been identified in the brain between neuropeptidergic and monoaminergic systems (Rosário et al. 2008).

16. Recent factor-analytic studies have reduced obsessive-compulsive symptoms to four fairly consistent and clinically meaningful symptom dimensions: contamination/cleaning, obsessions/checking, symmetry/ordering, and hoarding. Studies demonstrate that these dimensions are temporarily stable and correlate meaningfully with genetic, neuroimaging, and treatment response variables (Rosário et al. 2008).

17. Knowledge of the etiology and immunology of Sydenham chorea spawned the concept of PANDAS. There is considerable debate among experts about the pathophysiological mechanism of PANDAS and the possible relationship to other movement disorder, including tics (Jankovic and Fahn 2010).

18. Potential glutamatergic agents include riluzole, memantine, and other N-methyl-D-aspartate antagonists (e.g., amantadine, ketamine) and other anticonvulsants with glutamatergic properties, such as topiramate, lamotrigine, N-acetylcysteine, and D-cycloserine (Kariuki-Nyuthe et al. 2014, p. 35).

CHAPTER 13

Comprehensive Psychiatric Formulation

The comprehensive psychiatric formulation is a conceptual, multidimensional etiological understanding of a clinical case. In this chapter, we discuss the different factors that are considered relevant in determining a clinical presentation. The psychiatric formulation helps the examiner reach diagnostic conclusions and understanding of the nature of psychosocial and cultural stressors. The comprehensive psychiatric formulation is an indispensable skill in clinical practice. The examiner should understand the concept of formulation and recognize common problems that are encountered in the formulating process.

The ultimate objectives of the diagnostic interview are the development of a psychiatric formulation and the creation of a comprehensive treatment plan. These goals involve determining a DSM-5 (American Psychiatric Association 2013) or an ICD-10 categorical diagnosis and developing an understanding of the nature of psychosocial and cultural stressors that influence psychopathology. The formulation process is an indispensable and overarching conceptual exercise of the child and family's functional level to generate a treatment plan. Skills in comprehensive psychiatric formulation are fundamental in clinical practice. In this chapter we focus on the psychosocial and cultural aspects of the psychiatric assessment.

In DSM-5, in the section "Use of the Manual," the following assertions about the approach to case formulation are made:

The symptoms in our diagnostic criteria are part of the relatively limited repertoire of human emotional responses to internal and external stresses that are
generally maintained in a homeostatic balance without a disruption in normal
functioning. It requires clinical training to recognize when the combination of
predisposing, precipitating, perpetuating, and protective factors has resulted
in a psychopathological condition in which physical signs and symptoms exceed normal ranges. The ultimate goal of a clinical case formulation is to use
the available contextual and diagnostic information in developing a comprehensive treatment plan that is informed by the individual [and family's] cultural
and social context. (p. 19)

DSM-5 makes reference to the concept and importance of the comprehensive formulation multiple times throughout the text. Furthermore, the manual includes a new emphasis on the cultural aspects of norms and psychopathology. This emphasis is necessary in a multicultural milieu like the United
States, and in the context of the massive current waves of migration across
the world.

In the DSM-5 section on cultural formulation, we read:

Understanding the cultural context of illness experience is essential for the
effective diagnostic assessment and clinical management. *Culture* refers to
systems of knowledge, concepts, rules, and practices that are learned and transmitted across generations. Culture includes language, religion and spiritual-
ity, family structures, life-cycle stages, ceremonial rituals, and customs, as well
as moral and legal systems. (p. 749)

The formulation process is a deliberate conceptual organization of the interview data with the purpose of understanding and explaining the different
perspectives of the child as a biological system, as a developing individual,
as a person, as a member of a family, as a school member, and as a member
of larger social systems (e.g., cultural and religious organizations). Formulations have an implicit philosophical grounding and are biased toward preferred
points of view and therapeutic practices; because of these varying viewpoints
and the lack of a unifying language, formulations are constructed with conceptual preferences and according to academic traditions. Against these draw-
backs practitioners need to follow evidence-based practices and concepts
that have peer review consensus (see Note 1 later in this chapter).

Background of the Formulation Process

Child psychiatry is by definition a contextual enterprise. By necessity, the field
is attentive to developmental issues and incorporates explanatory concepts
related to psychological and interpersonal evolutions (its origins, vicissitudes, and conflicts) and the ecology in which these functions operate.

Achenbach (2008) clearly explained that the diagnostic formulation involves the putting together of various kinds of information about a case to form

a comprehensive picture of the case. For children and adolescents, the information may include developmental history, family dynamics, physical liabilities, stressors, formal diagnosis, and prospects for change. In clinical practice, the diagnostic formulation may say more about the child's needs and the indications for particular treatments than formal diagnosis does.

The formulation process is a baffling exercise for beginners in the field of child and adolescent psychiatry. This is due in part to a progressively widening schism between 1) the expectation—as espoused by a sound ethical practice—that clinicians should have a comprehensive understanding of the child and his or her family; 2) the pragmatics of contemporary practice, based primarily on the descriptive psychiatric pathology, as espoused by DSM-5 and ICD-10, and the emphasis on psychopharmacological interventions that have relegated psychosocial interventions to other mental health professionals; and 3) an unfortunate deemphasizing of the formulation and the formulation process in many training and academic centers.

Even though the child psychiatrist may not be involved directly in providing individual or family therapies or other psychosocial interventions, he or she should have an overarching understanding of the patient's case and should be able to offer appropriate input or guidance when is indicated by the illness clinical course.

Some biologically oriented child psychiatrists pay lip service to individual dynamic and systemic issues involved in child psychopathology. In this regard, Muller (2008) argued that the concept of mind has been diluted in the DSM classification system and that, at the most extreme pole of reductionism, all psychopathology is explained as a result of a dysfunction or disease of the brain. Many psychodynamically oriented child psychiatrists disregard hereditary, constitutional, and organic factors that contribute to the child's dysfunction.

A conceptual polarity also exists between individual- and family-oriented theorists. The former emphasize individual psychopathology with some disregard for family and other systemic factors; the latter overlook individual characteristics (i.e., temperamental, hereditary, constitutional, and developmental factors) and focus exclusively on family systems points of view. Fortunately, the family field has begun to incorporate developmental thinking in its theoretical concepts.

In the cognitive-behavioral therapy field, Tarrier and Johnson (2016, p. 2) suggest that the clinician should collect and organize information from a number of areas: analysis of the problem situation, motivational analysis (reinforcers), developmental analysis (including "biological equipment" and sociocultural experiences), analysis of self-control, analysis of social relationships, and analysis of the sociocultural-physical environment. They recommend an action-oriented approach to formulation.

Advances in developmental psychopathology will force an integration among these conceptual approaches and will bridge these schisms. Research indicates, for instance, that children of depressed mothers are more likely to develop psychiatric illnesses, including depression, anxiety disorders, and externalizing disorders (Gunlicks and Weissman 2008), and that improvements in parental depression from either medications or various forms of psychosocial therapies are positively correlated with child gains (i.e., reductions in psychopathology and improvements in the level of functioning); (see also Hinshaw 2008).

In this chapter, we introduce guidelines that attempt to bridge the gap between descriptive psychiatry and the practice of psychosocial interventions. More specifically, we consider developmental, psychodynamic, and systemic conceptualizations to be important components of overall diagnostic assessment and treatment planning.

Psychiatric Formulation in the Child and Adolescent Psychiatric Literature

The child and adolescent psychiatric literature contains limited references to the topic of formulation. Anna Freud contributed greatly to the process of child and adolescent assessment. On the basis of her father's psychoanalytic concepts, she developed the *metapsychological profile*, an exhaustive inventory of mind functioning from drive, structural, and ego perspectives. The recommendations based on such an evaluation focus specifically on psychoanalytic psychotherapy. Of particular importance in the area of developmental assessment is Anna Freud's (1977, 1980) concept of *developmental lines*. We will discuss the relevance of these concepts later in this chapter (see also Rick's case [Case Example 8] in Chapter 9, "Evaluation of Internalizing Symptoms").

Cohen (1979) stated that "[i]n order to formulate and to make recommendations, obviously, one does not need to know everything. Indeed, a good part of the information collected may not necessarily be relevant to decision making and recommendation" (p. 634). Cox (1994) defended the need for the formulation process and described its conceptual and therapeutic roles as follows:

> A further process of diagnostic formulation is required to bring the qualities which are different and distinctive about the individual child and family. The formulation puts forward ideas and suggestions about which psychological mechanism might be operating, about underlying causes and precipitants of the disorder of this child, about factors leading to a continuation of the disorder and the potential strengths and ameliorating factors that could be used in formulating a treatment plan. (p. 26)

Cox stressed what the formulation should or should not be: "It's quite inadequate merely to collect a lot of facts in the hope that some sense will come of them when they're put together. Rather the clinician must be formulating hypotheses to be tested from the very first moment he meets the family. These hypotheses may concern family interactions or the nature of the child's problems" (p. 26).

Henderson and Martin's (2007) conceptualization complements Anna Freud's concept of developmental lines. They discuss the four P's of causality:

- **P**redisposing factors render the child vulnerable to the presenting symptoms.
- **P**recipitating factors relate to eliciting or inciting factors of the presenting symptoms
- **P**erpetuating factors favor endurance of the symptoms or condition.
- **P**rotective factors address strengths, resilience, and supports.

The simplicity of this model's mnemonic betrays its heuristic value, because this model, more than any other, addresses head-on the issues of the origin of pathology and symptom maintenance.

It is also recommended that the interview and observations be specifically tailored to the relevant issues in each child's problems. It is further advised that the interview systematically cover a range of situations and difficulties.

Shapiro's (1989) contribution to the conceptual aspects of the formulation is valuable because he attempts to integrate developmental psychoanalytic thinking with descriptive psychiatry. He reviews the misconceptions applied to adult and child formulations and disagrees with reservations about formulation, including the idea that the clinician will become too invested in the formulation to permit change. Shapiro also counters the misconception that "a formulation is only useful for those who are planning to do a dynamic therapy with a child"; in Shapiro's view, "dynamic understanding may guide the clinician towards other therapies as well" (p. 675). In creating a formulation, Shapiro stresses the importance of psychoanalytic developmental psychology, particularly the three subsystems of ego psychology, developmental lines, and separation-individuation theories. These points of view are of immense value in the developmental assessment component of a comprehensive formulation.

Relevant to the child psychiatry field is Henderson and Martin's (2007) discussion of the biopsychosocial model. This model is the best known and most accepted comprehensive conceptual explanatory model and the one that has gained application in a variety of medical fields: "Regardless of anatomical lesions, or clear psychological or social etiologies, this model insists that all three [realms] be accounted for, and in doing so has been a powerful and successful model for physicians in all fields of medicine" (p. 378). However, the model does not guide the clinician in determining how to weigh or measure the relative contributions of each realm in any given patient.

Pruett (2007) issued a warning about conceptual dissections: "It is extremely shortsighted to dissect out the child—even intellectually—from the family for diagnostic studies, economics of time, convenience of intervention or cost containment" (p. 2). Unfortunately, the DSM-5 taxonomy does that to a very large extent. The same reservations could be expressed about dissecting out the family from the social milieu and from its cultural environment.

Theory of the Comprehensive Psychiatric Formulation Process

The comprehensive psychiatric formulation serves as the integrative part of the child or adolescent psychiatric evaluation. The goal is to synthesize the collected information (e.g., referral information, patient and family interviews, testing) to reach an integrated understanding of the data. The formulation creates hypotheses that need to be tested in clinical practice.

The formulation considers endogenous factors (hereditary, constitutional, biological, developmental, intrapsychic) and exogenous factors (familial, interpersonal, social, cultural, and others) related to the chief complaint of the disorder under discussion. Consideration and assessment of each factor are essential in the diagnostic formulation and are relevant for the delineation of a rational and comprehensive treatment program. Rarely is an illness or disorder produced by one factor alone. Maladaptation and illness are frequently the result of an interaction of forces.

Explanatory models are being extended beyond a sole emphasis on the medical basis of individual pathology to acknowledge the importance of cultural identity and other exogenous factors in a comprehensive assessment. Lewis-Fernández et al. (2016, p. 13) state that many aspects of experience shape a person's identity and that the assessment of cultural identity should be comprehensive. This assessment should document ethnicity, race, geographical origin, language, acculturation, gender, age, sexual orientation, religious and spiritual beliefs, socioeconomic class, and education. The authors stress that personal identity may shift across time, context, and expectations and that identity is always framed in relation to the person's past history, current concerns, and future prospects. Furthermore, the way people talk about and describe their identity depends on the setting and the interlocutor. According to Kratochwill et al. (2008), the medical model is a disease-based model, the pathology is assumed to be within the individual, although the cause may be environmental. Some theorists consider biological deviations to be necessary and sufficient factors in the development of pathology; others claim that chemical or neurological anomalies are necessary but not sufficient for pathogenesis. Here environmental conditions may or may not catalyze a constitutional predisposition to pathology. (p. 14)

Applications of the medical model influence assessment and treatment in various ways. Organic factors may not always be the cause of an observed medical or physical problem. There is growing recognition that psychological factors may affect a physical condition and that physical symptoms may have no known organic or physiological basis (Kratochwill et al. 2008).

In contrast to the medical model, the comprehensive formulation attempts to explain the problems or issues of the child as an individual and as a member of a family and other systems. A complex dynamic interaction occurs among the factors that contribute to the expression of an illness. All factors need not be addressed in the formulation of every case; each factor plays a role to a greater or lesser degree. In a given patient, certain factors are more relevant than others, and factors combine in unique ways to express or maintain a disorder. Factors cannot be understood in isolation, and for most disorders, research does not yet support granting central etiological status to any single risk or causal factor (Mash and Dozois 1996).

A satisfactory formulation stresses both protective and risk factors. Protective factors are those that promote normative development and optimal adaptation; resilience allows a child to respond and to recover from stress without significant or enduring loss of developmental acquisitions or adaptive functioning. Risk factors create vulnerability to developmental psychopathology.

Tarrier and Johnson (2016, p. 4) assert that

case formulation is thus translation of theory into therapy, but it is the function of all theories to be disproved if possible. The clinician should create explanatory structures or heuristics for understanding the client's problems but proceed with caution not to muster evidence selectively only in their support but to examine critically why their heuristics and hypothesis may be incorrect and can be shown to be so.

The diagnostic formulation has two objectives: one is diagnostic and the other therapeutic. A comprehensive descriptive (syndromic) diagnosis is essential for a comprehensive psychiatric formulation and a valid treatment plan. We focused on DSM-5-guided diagnoses in Chapter 9, "Evaluation of Internalizing Symptoms"; Chapter 10, "Evaluation of Externalizing Symp-

Table 13–1. Objectives of the comprehensive diagnostic formulation

I. Descriptive (syndromic) DSM-5-based diagnosis

II. Assessment of intrinsic (endogenous) and extrinsic (exogenous) factors (psychosocial assessment)

   A. Intrinsic factors

      1. Developmental factors

      2. Psychodynamic factors

      3. Other intrinsic factors

   B. Extrinsic factors

      1. Parental and family dynamics

      2. Developmental interferences

      3. Other extrinsic factors

Source. Adapted from Cepeda 2010, p. 390.

toms"; and Chapter 11, "Evaluation of Abuse and Other Symptoms." The evaluator should consider how the identified syndromes (e.g., mood disturbances, anxiety, psychosis) organize and distort the patient's perceptions about his or her internal and external worlds. Table 13–1 summarizes the objectives of the diagnostic formulation.

Finally, the formulation should be written in a flexible format and as a working hypothesis; by no means should the formulation represent a fixed conceptualization or a negative prognostication. There is no such a thing as a hopeless case, because the psychiatrist could contribute to improving the quality of life and the level of functioning of any given patient. The psychiatrist will make every effort possible "to help families grow with their vulnerable [impaired] children" (Pruett 2007, p. 2).

Assessment of Intrinsic (Internal) Factors

Developmental Factors

Psychoanalytic developmental psychology concepts are relevant in the assessment of developmental factors. This assessment addresses the degree to which the child is mastering the developmental tasks associated with his or her developmental phase. For instance, in assessing a preadolescent, the examiner notes the child's adaptation to the extra-familial environment (e.g., school, neighborhood), the child's progressive immersion in same-sex peership, the child's involvement in fantasy-oriented play, and the child's progressive internalization of rules, among other tasks. When evaluating an adolescent, the examiner explores how the adolescent is coping with adolescent developmental tasks, such as separation-individuation, sexual exploration, identity consolidation, career orientation, formation of supportive groups in the extra-familial social milieu, and so on.

The concept of developmental phases is broad and nonspecific; more relevant, specific and clinically useful is the concept of developmental lines, which addresses the developmental vicissitudes of important ego-psychological and object relations functions. The assessment of developmental lines provides clinical focus and assists in the identification of areas of disturbance. Anna Freud added to Sigmund Freud's implicit developmental lines (i.e., psychosexual development, maturation and development of ego defense mechanisms, and anxiety transformation) the following: from individual dependency to self-reliance, from egocentricity to peer relationships, from inability to manage the body and its functions to the child's control of them, and from play to work. She also suggested a developmental line from anaclitic (i.e., need-satisfying) relationships to object constancy. The number of developmental lines is not complete, and the lines are not independent of one another. Future progress in developmental psychology and child psychoanalysis may bring forward new developmental lines and conceptual refinement of the ones already described.

Anna Freud (1965/1977, 1979/1980) suggested that the examiner should pay attention to the harmony or disharmony of the progression of the developmental lines. The following case example illustrates disharmony in the developmental lines.

Case Example 1

Steve, a 14-year-old Caucasian male, who weighed 250 lbs. and was over 6 feet tall, was being evaluated for suicidal behavior. He was in conflict with both of his divorced parents but had received a great deal of nurturing from his maternal grandfather, who died less than 1 month before the psychiatric examination. Steve felt that there was no point in living after his grandfather passed away. Steve appeared older than his stated age; he was intelligent and a very good student and was also successful on his school's football team. Steve's mother had limited emotional sources of support and attempted to lean on him for emotional support.

Steve's advanced physical development contributed to a major disharmony in the developmental lines: because he looked older than his chronological age, his mother and other people had expectations of him that were not congruent with his emotional or psychological development. This misperception promoted pseudo-maturity and precocious ego development. Steve had strong, ungratified dependency needs. He had ongoing power-control fights with his mother; he opposed her rules, saying that he was too big to depend on her. Because both parents were insensitive to his dependency needs, Steve found a group of troubled adolescents to gratify his unmet narcissistic needs and to provide him with modeling, guidance, protection, support, and a sense of belonging that, he so much longed for. Behind Steve's robust adolescent body was a big "needy baby." His body size made him feel that experiencing dependency needs was proper only of a smaller or younger child. In contrast, because of his large size, his parents overlooked that he was still in need of tender and loving care.

Circumstances in which developmental disharmony is present (e.g., in precocious puberty, delayed sexual development, precocious cognitive development, chronic medical illness) bring about psychopathological risks (see Rick's case [Case Example 8] in Chapter 9, "Evaluation of Internalizing Symptoms"). If the child is at variance with developmental expectations, this variance and its implications need to be explained. The developmental assessment will determine areas of developmental progression, regression, or arrest.

The diagnostic formulation distinguishes between normative developmental conflicts of a transitory nature (i.e., those commonly found at a given developmental stage, such as enuresis after a prolonged separation, or limited regressions, such as clinginess or attention seeking, after the arrival of a newborn) and internalized conflicts or character (personality) traits of an enduring nature. The latter indicate problems in the mastery of previous developmental tasks.

Pertinent questions in assessing internal factors or developmental areas include the following: Is the child mastering the tasks appropriate to his or her developmental state? Is the child progressing in the different developmental lines? Does the child show evidence of internalized conflicts? Does the child demonstrate lags in development from previous phases?

An important evolving point of view is emerging from the field of developmental psychopathology. Longitudinal research has consistently demonstrated that most of the adult disorders have childhood roots and that most childhood disorders have sequelae that persist into adult life (Maughan and Collishaw 2015, p. 5).

Psychodynamic Factors

In the assessment of psychodynamic factors, the examiner evaluates the child's internal mental operations and corresponding dysfunctions. He also evaluates the psychological forces that motivate the child's behavior. This assessment aids in the understanding of the quality and strength of the child's personality traits.

In the following sections, we discuss the dominant psychodynamic points of view: ego psychology, object relations theory, separation-individuation theory, self psychology, attachment theory, and interpersonal theory.

Ego Psychology

As its name implies, ego psychology emphasizes the ego. According to Sigmund Freud's (1923/1962) tripartite conception of the mind, commonly known as *structural theory*, the ego perceives the physical and psychic needs of the self and the qualities and attitudes of the environment (including objects), and it evaluates, coordinates, and integrates these perceptions so that internal demands can be adjusted to external requirements. The ego accomplishes these goals by utilizing the so-called conflict-free ego functions of perception, motor capacity, intention, anticipation, purpose, planning, intelligence, thinking, speech, and language, among others. The ego also deploys defensive mechanisms to protect the individual against the conscious awareness of the conflictive demands of the id (e.g., primitive urges, impulses, biological needs) and the superego, insofar as these may arouse intolerable anxiety (Moore and Fine 1990).

Examiners who use ego psychology as the basis for the dynamic formulation should pay attention to the following ego functions:

- Ego boundaries
- Reality testing and preponderant ego defenses
- Impulse control and superego functioning
- Capacity for sublimation, insight, and verbalization
- Intelligence and other adaptive ego strengths
- Motivation and long-term planning
- Capacity to develop a therapeutic alliance

Object Relations Theory

Object relations theory bases its psychological explanations on the premise that the mind is concerned with elements (issues) taken from the outside, primarily aspects of the functioning of other persons (objects). The processes of internalization are emphasized. This mind model explains mental functions in terms of relations between the various internalized elements (Moore and Fine 1990).

Examiners who use object relations theory as the basis for the dynamic formulation should pay attention to the following functions:

- Quality of object relations
- Integration and stability of self and object representations
- Degree of guilt, envy, and reparation
- Degree of projective identification and splitting in psychological functioning

Separation-Individuation Theory

Separation-individuation concepts apply to a developmental theory, to a process, and to a complex stage of development. In the development of the individual, Mahler et al. (1974) proposed normal, autistic, and symbiotic phases and the separation-individuation process, which comprises differentiation, practicing, rapprochement, and object constancy subphases (Moore and Fine 1990). Mahler's autistic phase has been severely criticized because evidence demonstrates that infants start relating to their primary objects beginning at birth and probably before:

> Contemporary developmental scientists are, by contrast, amazed by how early and successfully the young child begins to grasp the mental states of other people, even when those emotions, beliefs, and desires are different from the child's own, even infants begin to comprehend that subjective mental states are the key to understanding people's behavior. (Thompson et al. 2006, p. 4)

Examiners who use separation-individuation theory as the basis for the dynamic formulation should pay attention to the following functions:

- Evidence of progression throughout the separation-individuation process
- Evidence of a rapprochement crisis
- Evidence of object constancy

Self Psychology

Self psychology emphasizes the vicissitudes of the structure of the self and the associated subjective, conscious, preconscious, and unconscious experiences of selfhood. This point of view recognizes as the most fundamental essence of human psychology the individual's needs to organize his or her psyche into a cohesive configuration, the self, and to establish self-sustaining relationships between the self and its surroundings; these relationships evoke, maintain, and strengthen the coherence, energy, vigor, and harmony among the constituents of the self (Moore and Fine 1990).

Examiners who use self psychology as the basis for the dynamic formulation should pay attention to the following functions:

- Self concept and self-esteem regulation
- Self-esteem stability
- Self cohesion versus self fragmentation
- Role of affirmation and twinship
- Nature of narcissistic injuries
- Nature of grandiose and exhibitionistic needs

Attachment Theory

Attachment theory has gained a great deal of interest because it has a strong empirical foundation and its principles can be subjected to research—characteristics that set this model apart from its counterparts. John Bowlby (1969) proposed that children have an innate (evolutionary) predisposition to become attached to a primary figure, usually the biological mother. The concept of attachment describes both the underlying psychological constructs and the selective patterns of proximity seeking that a young child strives to maintain at times of stress. Although the process of attachment is clearly reciprocal, the term *attachment* usually refers to the behavior of the child in relation to the primary figure. Although patterns of selective attachment develop during the first year of life, the notion of attachment is applicable throughout the life cycle (Volkmar 1995). In the research arena, the development of valid and reliable instruments for assessing attachment patterns and psychological constructs such as alexithymia (failure of symbolization and mentalization) has led to many empirical investigations that have confirmed that interpersonal relationships can influence illness behavior and physical health (Taylor 2008).

Examiners who use attachment theory as the basis for the psychodynamic formulation should pay attention to the following functions (Bacciagaluppi 1994; Belsky and Cassidy 1994):

- Quality of the attachment experience provided to the infant
- Attachment-exploration balance
- Hierarchy of attachment to major caregivers
- Presence of a secure base
- Nature of internal working models
- Presence of a secure or insecure attachment

Please refer to sections on attachment and bonding and on maternal pathology and attachment subtypes in Chapter 7, "Psychiatric Evaluation of Preschoolers and Very Young Children."

Interpersonal Theory

Interpersonal theory, originated by Herbert ("Harry") Stack Sullivan, postulates that a person's impulses, strivings, and personality patterns need to be understood in the context of interpersonal relationships. Interpersonal relationships are a human concern from the very beginning of existence. The primary striving of the mind is the satisfaction of physical and emotional needs, especially the need for human contact and the achievement of a sense of security. Anxiety is aroused when these needs are threatened. Anxiety is an interpersonal experience and the primary motivator of human behavior (Weiner and Moll 1995). Specific therapeutic interventions based on Sullivan's concepts have been effective in the treatment of depression (Mohl 1995) and other disorders.

Examiners who use interpersonal theory as the basis for the dynamic formulation should pay attention to the following functions:

- Sense of security or evidence of anxiety and loneliness
- Predominance of modes of experience
- Nature of the security operations
- Presence of consensual validation

Other Points of View

Alternatively, other conceptual frames, such as family therapy, cognitive-behavioral therapy (CBT), and other behavioral or ecological models, may be used as the basis for the conceptualization of the formulation.

Other Intrinsic (Internal) Factors

The examiner must consider 1) other factors that influence the way the personality becomes organized and 2) the manner in which the primary caregivers respond to the developing child (e.g., temperamental traits, other individual qualities) (see Note 2 at the end of this chapter). The psychiatrist also must explore other developmental acquisitions (e.g., psychosexual development, social and interpersonal functioning) and, when pertinent, other levels of functioning (e.g., physical functioning, motor coordination, cognitive and moral development). Other skills and abilities that affect the child's sense of competence, adaptive capacity, and self concept should also be surveyed.

Competence in developing peer relations requires special attention. This capacity is a good measure of a number of intrapersonal and interpersonal skills such as self concept, level of self-esteem, problem-solving skills, and capacity for reciprocity and empathy. Children's peer relations serve vital functions, have important short-term and long-term consequences, are linked to children's competence in coping with major social tasks, and can be facilitated by systemic interventions aimed at increasing social competence (Asher et al. 1994). Poor peer relations predict school dropout, whereas aggressive behavior predicts criminality (Asher et al. 1994).

When intellectual impairment, learning disabilities, or other handicaps are present, the examiner must evaluate how these impairments affect the child's self concept and self-esteem regulation. For example, how do the child and the family cope with these limitations, and what adaptive compensatory mechanisms are called into play? Denial of a handicap is a common phenomenon; often, the denial in the parent is far greater than that in the child.

Adolescents with behavioral and academic difficulties require careful assessment. A number of psychiatric syndromes, including developmental language and learning disorders and other neuropsychological deficits, need to be identified. Frequently, emotional and behavioral difficulties at school are merely surface behaviors caused by those unidentified problems. Adolescents with academic and learning disorders have low self-esteem and a deficient sense of competence, among other problems. These children may require speech and language assessment, psychological or neuropsychological testing, a pediatric evaluation, and other pertinent testing.

Assessment of Extrinsic (External) Factors

Parental and Family Dynamics

Assessment of parental and family dynamics relates to the degree to which the parents or family as a whole promotes normative child development (through, e.g., provision of basic care, nurturing, love, consistent limit setting, gratification of healthy narcissistic needs, support for autonomy, identity formation) and the degree to which the parents or family provides a warm and supportive environment with reliable and consistent boundaries. Issues related to social learning, modeling, conditioning, and other behavioral aspects within the family are relevant in this area (Mash 1989) (see Note 3 at the end of this chapter).

When the examiner is assessing difficulties in the area of family dynamics, the following issues could be addressed: Where is the preponderance of the dysfunction—in the parenting function, in the marital subsystem, or in the family system as a whole? Are the parents allied in the provision of discipline? How cohesive are the marital system and the sibling subsystems? Do any of the parental figures have identifiable problems? Do any of the parents exhibit overt psychiatric pathology? Is alcohol or drug abuse a problem in the family? What are the family's strengths? Is abusive behavior going on in the environment?

Psychopathology in the parents (i.e., mood disorders, substance abuse) is recognized as having a deleterious effect on the development of the child. Because important gains in the child's symptomatology and level of functioning have been demonstrated when the parent improves, it behooves the psychiatrist to identify parental psychopathology and to implement a prompt intervention.

Developmental Interferences

The concept of *developmental interference* relates to factors within the rearing, school, or social environment that are outside the child's control and that have a negative influence on the child's psychosocial development. In addition to marital or family dysfunction, such interference commonly includes other adverse events, such as illness, trauma, or loss, as well as persistent stresses in the physical, psychological, educational, or cultural environment. Bullying at school is a common developmental interference (see Chapter 11, "Evaluation of Abuse and Other Symptoms"). If the adversity is too intense or prolonged (see related concept of allostatic load in Chapter 14, "Symptom Formation and Comorbidity"), it may be internalized and transformed into an internalized conflict—a destabilizing developmental factor that then becomes part of the child's psychopathological organization (Nagera 1966). A developmental interference occurs when the child does not receive the care needed at a given developmental phase or when the gratification goes beyond what a particular phase requires. Each developmental stage, or each developmental line, may be interfered with as a result of deprivation or overgratification.

Research suggests a strong link between early trauma, loss, and family disturbance and later interpersonal dysfunction. Parents create developmental interference by omission or by commission. Interference due to omission is associated with situations of neglect, abandonment, or undue permissiveness, at one extreme, or with the inability to set consistent limits (i.e., to enforce rules and monitor boundaries through appropriate discipline and consistent limit setting) at the other extreme. Interference due to commission is secondary to physical, emotional or sexual abuse, to reversals of the child and parent roles, or to overindulgence (now called "affluenza"). Physical and sexual abuse, overindulgence, and lack of appropriate and consistent discipline are common developmental interferences.

Other Extrinsic (External) Factors

Chronic illness in children has a major negative effect on the boundaries between children and their parents, and it interferes profoundly with the process of separation-individuation. Compensatory overdependency may develop because of frequent separations (due to hospitalizations) or fear of death (see Rick's case [Case Example 8] in Chapter 9, "Evaluation of Internalizing Symptoms," and Cory's case [Case Example 2] later in this chapter). Parents may overindulge or overprotect the child, thus impinging on the child's autonomy, self concept, and moral codes. This behavior has a negative effect on the child's sense of competence and on other adaptive functions. Parents of handicapped children often feel guilty and responsible for their children's limitations. These parents have problems with self-blame and letting go and with setting consistent limits.

School refusal problems have multiple causes, including separation anxiety. Many children are afraid to attend school because they fear intimidation by older children (see Chapter 11, "Evaluation of Abuse and Other Symptoms"), pressure to join gangs or use drugs, or other factors. For example, an intelligent 12-year-old boy began to skip school. After an intense exploration of the reasons for his behavior, he confided that he had been beaten up regularly by a group of children belonging to a gang.

Pertinent questions in assessing external factors include the following: Is the school milieu favorable to learning and positive development? Is the school system meeting the child's psychoeducational and psychosocial needs? What kind of influence does the peer group have on the child's behavior? Is the neighborhood safe, or is it infested with insecurity, drugs, and crime? Are the child's and the family's behaviors culturally syntonic?

When a psychiatric syndrome is present, the formulation should postulate what developmental factors and environmental circumstances are facilitating the expression of the disorder in question. Precipitating and perpetuating factors are important concerns.

No assessment of external factors is complete without an examination of the child's and family's areas of strength. The assessment should include observations on the regulatory functions within the child and within the family. Answers to questions such as these are important: When the child or family members are involved in a crisis, how do they attempt to solve it? What do they do? Whom do they call for help? Is there any organized way of solving the problem? What soothing mechanisms help the child or family to get back on track? What mechanisms does the child activate to stop escalation of the problem and to initiate its resolution? Is there any cognitive dissonance in the parents' approach to problem solving? Do the family beliefs in empirical medicine get mixed with beliefs in spiritual medicine, supernatural or paranormal healing?

Pragmatics of a Comprehensive Psychiatric Formulation

There is no standardized way to complete a comprehensive psychiatric formulation. Adherence to a particular explanatory model will influence the way the formulation is conceptualized. The model used (e.g., biopsychosocial, psychodynamic, cognitive, behavioral, family-based) will influence the emphasis of the formulation and generally reflects the conceptual preferences and practice modality of the formulator. The details and emphasis of some aspects of the formulation vary, depending on the circumstances at the time the formulation is done.

Coherence and comprehensiveness are two important elements in the formulation. The formulation needs to be relevant to the presenting problem(s) and to the most important developmental aspects of the case.

In this section, we suggest a format for a comprehensive psychiatric formulation, comprising six components, or sections; each section is illustrated with case examples of three children of different ages.

1. A succinct explanatory statement that indicates the major psychopathological issues. This statement answers the question "What is this case about?"

   John is an 8-year-old Caucasian male with a history of suicidal behavior, aggressiveness, and disorganized thinking.

   Andrew is a 13-year-old African American male with a long history of impulse-control difficulties and a recent history of violence, depressive affect, and suicidal behavior.

   Maria is a 17-year-old Mexican American female with a long history of major depressive disorder and borderline personality traits.

2. A succinct explanatory statement that indicates the perceived main problem (i.e., core issue or conflict). This statement answers the question "What are the main issues of the case?"

   John's main conflicts seem to be related to his perception of rejection and the threat of abandonment by his very ill adoptive mother. He perceives this threat as a psychological death because, in his own words, "There is no reason for me to live anymore."

   Andrew's main conflict is confusion over his primary maternal object.

   Maria struggles with developmental issues of autonomy and individuation in a very pathological, nonsupportive environment: her father was psychotic, and her mother (who also had psychiatric problems) was controlling and lacked empathy for Maria.

3. A succinct explanatory statement indicating the hereditary, constitutional, or organic factors related to the main problem. Any medical or neurological difficulties may be included here. This statement answers the question "What are the contributory biological factors of the case?"

   John's natural mother was a drug abuser. John was exposed to drugs in utero. Previous psychological assessments had shown a disparity between his verbal and performance abilities. He also exhibited language deficits and electroencephalographic abnormalities and possibly had poor nutrition. John had asthma and inconsistent bladder control.

Andrew's mother had a background of alcohol and polysubstance abuse, and she probably abused drugs during pregnancy. Genetic factors were probably involved, because Andrew's mother had a chronic psychiatric disorder and his maternal grandmother had an affective disorder.

Maria had a severe depressive disorder and strong anxiety disorder features. Management of the depressive syndrome with antidepressants was difficult because of cardiovascular complications.

4. A succinct explanatory statement of the dominant intrinsic factors that contribute to the problem(s). This statement answers the question "What are the predominant developmental and psychodynamic factors of the case?"

For John, the threat of parental loss had precipitated significant regression, including impairment of thought organization and reality testing. He also displayed prominent somatization, which represented an affective regression and identification with his very sick adoptive mother (she had severe diabetes with multi-organ complications). Recurrent somatic symptoms ensured gratification of John's unmet narcissistic needs and likely represented an identification with his sick mother. John sometimes expressed intense ambivalence toward his mother and family as a whole. His self concept was very negative. He felt hopeless and showed marked desperation and torment. He attempted to take responsibility for the perceived rejection by psychotic guilt, the latter secondary to his intense aggression. Anger against his rejecting objects taxed his ego capacities and stimulated regression and serious compromise of his adaptive capacity. John's capacity to bond emotionally to other people was also a concern.

Andrew's loyalty conflicts were strong. His mother and grandmother competed for his love and affection. Andrew displayed impairment in the development of object constancy and lacked stable object and self-representations. Competition for Andrew's love had blocked the resolution of infantile omnipotence and facilitated the creation of manipulative interpersonal traits. Lack of object constancy rendered him vulnerable to separations and impaired the separation-individuation process; these difficulties also contributed to an unstable self concept and to a faulty superego development. Parent-child role reversal was a prominent feature in Andrew's development; he worried continuously about his mother.

Maria struggled with identity consolidation issues; she had a rigid system of defenses and had very high expectations for herself. Her strong defenses against sexuality appeared to be eroding. Control was a major coping defense for Maria. Anger and hostility were pervasive maladaptive features and highly valued coping mechanisms.

5. A succinct explanatory statement of the relevant extrinsic factors (e.g., developmental interferences and other risk factors). This statement answers the question "What are the detrimental factors (developmental interferences) in the child or in the rearing environment that have a bearing on the case?"

> John had a history of multiple placements and ongoing rejection by his adoptive mother (she had made explicit threats to reverse the adoption). Questions regarding abuse and neglect were ongoing. His adoptive mother was very sick, and his adoptive father had been given the diagnosis of organic affective disorder, secondary to a stroke. Other siblings also had emotional problems: a younger sister had a history of psychiatric problems and had been hospitalized previously.
>
> Andrew's family situation was extremely chaotic and confusing. His mother was dysfunctional and had alcohol and drug abuse problems. He had never had a male parental figure as a source of masculine identification and as an appropriate model for aggressive expression.
>
> Maria's family was highly dysfunctional: violence, scapegoating, and rejection were common. Parents and siblings had severe psychopathology.

6. A succinct explanatory statement of the protective factors—in the child, within the family, or in the rearing environment—that promote normative development and adaptive resolution of the problem(s) or conflict(s). Issues related to resilience and self-regulatory functions for the child or the family may be mentioned here. This statement answers the question "What are the strengths of the child or the family?"

> John was likable and engaging; he was verbal and intelligent. He did well in supportive and structured environments. He was attached, though ambivalently, to his adoptive sister. Finally, John had a strong bond with his natural sister, who had been adopted along with him.
>
> Andrew was handsome and very intelligent and had some degree of insight. His grandmother was genuinely involved with him. Appropriate placement of Andrew and stabilization of his rearing environment were considered essential to regulate his inner world and to ameliorate his pervasive psychological turmoil.
>
> Maria was a likable, honest individual who displayed integrity. She was tenacious and determined. She was intelligent, insightful, and very committed to helping herself and her family. Although her father was

prone to intermittent psychotic functioning, he was the main source of affection for the children.

While advancing in the formulation process from sections 1 through 6, the clinician should gain a progressive understanding of the child or adolescent's circumstances. Note that sections 2–6 address areas or factors that could become the target of specific therapeutic interventions. These sections could be considered to represent circumscribed or specific formulations themselves.

After the examiner has identified the factors that contribute to the creation and maintenance of symptoms, he or she should go one step further in the formulation by making conceptual or explanatory bridges among the different factors. As the examiner advances through the six sections, he or she should attempt to make relevant connections among the components of the formulation. According to the clinical evidence and the examiner's theoretical bias, any of these sections could receive particular emphasis or amplification; this format is flexible.

Brevity in the presentation of the formulation is stressed. A very long and elaborate write-up renders this exercise impractical and clinically cumbersome. Because the formulation is offered as a conceptual guide to clinicians who have different levels of sophistication and expertise, it should be written without technical language.

The following case example demonstrates the six-section format for a comprehensive psychiatric formulation of an adolescent with a definitive neuropsychiatric disorder.

Case Example 2

1. Cory was a 15-year-old African American female who had significant difficulties with anger control (she pulled a knife on her brother twice and had done the same to her father 2 years earlier). She had poor interpersonal relationships and was oppositional and unruly toward her mother.
2. The main issues in Cory's case were 1) lack of stabilization of a partial seizure disorder secondary to poor compliance with anticonvulsant medications and 2) frequent power-control struggles with her mother.
3. Hereditary and constitutional factors were involved. Cory's mother had made a suicide attempt in her youth, and Cory's brothers had problems with aggression and impulsiveness. At birth, Cory almost died and underwent major abdominal surgery. More fundamental was the presence of complex seizure symptomatology (i.e., a positive electroencephalogram with right-temporal spiking). Furthermore, features of a receptive aphasia were present. Other symptoms, such as paranoia and perceptual distortions, were compatible with complex partial symptomatology (psychomotor seizures). Cory would become disoriented in space; a number

of times, she lost her way home and would become helpless. She would wander around and start crying.

4.　Salient issues regarding Cory's internal developmental factors centered on massive denials and pervasive externalization of blame for her persistent and recurring problems. She did not take any responsibility for her aggressive and impulsive behaviors and was prone to blame others when she lost control. Cory defended against strong dependency needs toward her mother with hostility and was very ambivalent about her. Her feelings toward her mother vacillated from open rebellion to regressive behavior characterized by baby talk and the need for frequent body contact with her. Somewhat aware of her perceptual inaccuracies, Cory relied on her mother a great deal for consensual validation. Seizure phenomena and twilight states contributed to her idiosyncratic experiences and her conviction that what she felt and experienced was real. Cory felt that everyone misunderstood her, and she was very suspicious of most people. Her lack of insight was remarkable (anosognosia).

5.　Cory's mother had been overprotective and lenient with Cory because she feared for Cory's life. Her mother was also inconsistent with discipline. Cory's mother was a single parent with a limited support network. Because of strong denial, Cory did not comply with her medications, which were essential to control her seizure disorder, the main cause of a great deal of her psychopathological functioning. Cory needed her mother's supervision and needed tighter controls because she was very impulsive, misjudged situations, and was prone to distort interpersonal events. She regularly broke her mother's rules and failed to meet her mother's expectations. Cory was sexually active and had sneaked some partners into her bedroom. She believed that people were out to get her.

6.　Cory was a tall, attractive, and intelligent adolescent. In spite of her neuropsychological problems, which affected her learning, she liked school and was motivated to do schoolwork. Cory's developmental features and her conflicts with her mother were major factors in her dysfunction. No progress was possible with Cory until the therapist understood and validated Cory's idiosyncratic experiences.

The case examples provided in this section could have been written with a different emphasis or from other theoretical perspectives, or with a different systemic or ecological focus. The proposed model allows alternative conceptualizations. No single theory supports the psychodynamic aspects of the formulation. Each theory has an explanatory richness that needs to be exhausted before using alternative theories to fill the conceptual gaps. Knowing one theory in depth is preferable to knowing a variety of theories superficially. The clinician needs to know the explanatory power and the limits of a chosen theory, as well as the advantages of choosing one theory over the others. When the limits of a theory are reached, the clinician can appeal to other theories to satisfy explanatory gaps. For an example of a formulation based on self psychological concepts, see Note 4 at the end of this chapter.

Cognitive-Behavioral Therapy

CBT is now broadly used as a conceptual model and as an intervention modality. CBT evolved from behavior therapy with the addition of cognitive theory. CBT emphasizes the importance of social information processing (memory, attention, flexible thinking) and cognitive distortions in psychopathology. Thus, CBT brought "mind" back to psychology, positing that one's interpretation and processing of stimuli and events impacts behavior. Rigid and distorted beliefs about oneself, the world, or the future are targeted in CBT. Altering one's belief system can modify behavior (Kendall et al. 2015, p. 496).

The framework of CBT posits that patients with generalized anxiety disorder overestimate the level of danger in their environment, have difficulty with uncertainty, and underestimate their capacity to copy. CBT for generalized anxiety disorder involves cognitive restructuring to help patients understand that their worry and avoidance are counterproductive; promotes the practice of exposure therapy to enable patients learn that their worry and avoidance behavior are malleable, and stimulates the practice of relaxation training to counteract raising anxiety (Stein and Sareen 2015, p. 2065). The following is a vignette illustrating the psychiatric formulation for an anxious child as conceptualized in a CBT framework.

Case Example 3[*]

Philip, a 9-year-old male, was the youngest of three boys; his older brothers were 8 and 6 years older than Philip. Philip was quite ill at age 2 years, and as a result of meningitis, he required an extended stay in hospital. His mother never left his side during his stay. Philip was very close to his mother, while his brothers were closer to their father.

He was referred by his school counselor because of concerns about his constant worrying and anxiety. These problems were manifested most often in the classroom and when Philip was on the playground. Philip was academically bright and tried very hard in his class work. Philip became upset when he didn't complete assignments perfectly. He felt particularly anxious with his male math teacher, because the teacher often raised his voice in the class. Philip didn't want to complete math assignments fearing he would make mistakes, and he was concerned that his teacher would yell at him.

Philip did not have any close friends at school. He was often teased by the other boys, mostly name-calling; on one occasion, he received a physical threat by a same-age peer. What bothered Philip more was that his two older brothers were quite popular at the school when they had attended the same campus.

---

[*]We thank Mr. Rick Edwards, Clinical Director of Inpatient Services at Clarity Child Guidance Center at San Antonio, for this case illustration.

Incorporating CBT into the formulation, the therapist was able to outline background information and experiences that caused Philip to be so anxious. There was a gap in the ages of the boys, leaving Philip to feel like an only child. Coupled with the lengthy illness at age 2 and his mother being quite protective of Philip, he often saw the world as overwhelming, intimidating, and challenging beyond his ability to be successful. With the increasing school demands, both socially and academically, Philip developed a pattern of negative thoughts and often anticipated failure; furthermore, his harsh and negative view of himself interfered with his abilities to do well in school and being successful at making friends.

Because Philip automatically anticipated potentially threatening scenarios ("the math teacher was going to yell at me"; "none of the boys liked me"), he would do his math assignments over and over until he made sure they were error free; he also avoided being in the playground altogether during recess. Philip's mother reinforced his beliefs by rewarding his efforts at having no mistakes on his work and arranging access to solitary activities he enjoyed, such as reading and video games.

Initial treatment sessions focused on common cognitive distortions that Philip experienced. This was done in order to develop a better understanding for the child, parents, and therapist about Philip's causes of anxiety and worrying. Cognitive restructuring was used in sessions to change the cognitive distortions and work to build positive self-talk. Although, the negative thoughts did not occur in the actual therapy sessions, parents were present during some sessions so they could recognize when the cognitive distortions occurred and could offer a countering realistic thought to replace the negative thinking.

An anxiety ladder was used to formally outline the causes of Philip's anxiety and fears in an ascending order, starting with the least anxiety-producing situation on the bottom rung and working up to the most challenging, the most anxiety-producing situation, as the top rung of the ladder. From there the therapist and Philip began the process of systematic desensitization, whereby Philip could practice progressive exposures, with Philip and the therapist monitoring toleration of the anxiety-producing situation starting at the lowest level and building up to the most anxiogenic one. The therapist worked with Philip to visualize the first step, while discussing accompanying thoughts, and encouraged positive self-talk and self-soothing until Philip could visualize the step without anxiety. After these exercises or training, Philip was exposed to the real-life situation. The process continued up the ladder progressively to the most challenging situation. Visualization practice was used to provide relief from troubling thoughts or emotions. By imagining a safe, calm place, and using as much detail and sensory information as was possible, Philip could master any degree of emerging anxiety. "Finding a place" that was stress free, where Philip could go to whenever he needed was of utmost importance.

Phillip responded well to this therapeutic approach, and as a result his anxiety and enduring worrying improved.

Common Problems in the Elaboration of a Comprehensive Formulation

Common deficiencies may be encountered in reviewing formulations. Some formulations

1. Recite or agglomerate the data without integration.
2. Lack an orderly presentation of the explanations. They mix concepts and lack clarity or internal consistency.
3. Do not "grasp" or represent the core problem.
4. Overlook the patient's subjective issues (i.e., internal factors). They overemphasize external factors at the expense of developmental, intrapsychic, and interpersonal conflicts.
5. Are psychodynamically incoherent. Clinicians new to the formulation process frequently use a confusing mixture of concepts or explanatory models to explain internal factors.
6. Fail to explain the presenting problem.
7. Are not comprehensive.

Reformulation

The formulation is a dynamic process. The psychiatrist needs to change the formulation when new clinical data emerge, when a negative development occurs in the clinical course, or when no progress is made after the treatment plan has been implemented. Theresa A. Piggot's (personal communication, 1996) approach to refractory obsessive-compulsive disorder is relevant in cases that need reformulation as a result of lack of progress. When there is no progress, she advised the following:

1. Review the accuracy of the diagnosis.
2. Review the comorbid conditions.
3. Review the adequacy of the treatment trials.
4. Review the integration of the treatment modalities.
5. Review compliance.
6. Review whether expectations about the therapeutic objectives are realistic.

To the preceding list, we add several additional recommendations:

1. Review the status of the developmental interferences.
2. Review the status of the therapeutic alliance.
3. Consider the possibility of countertransference factors (see Chapter 16, "Countertransference").

At times, a re-interview may provide data or observations that have previously been missed and may allow a reconceptualization of the formulation.

Key Points

- The comprehensive formulation should be a component of every diagnostic interview.
- The comprehensive formulation assists the psychiatrist in the conceptualization of the presenting problem and in determining the areas that need focused therapeutic attention, both in the rearing environment and in the psychological realm.
- The examiner needs to be familiar with child developmental issues and with broad family concepts to determine the nature of the rearing environment.
- The examiner needs to explore for the presence of developmental interferences.

Notes

1. Kratochwill et al. (2008) explained the situation well:

   Tremendous amounts of data have been accumulated concerning the origins, development, influences, and variations of human behavior. Nevertheless, the wealth of information has clearly not resulted in an integrated view of human performance. Indeed, the current state of knowledge generated from the various conceptual models has not only resulted in the lack of an integrated view of human functioning, but has yielded various conceptual positions that are diametrically opposed and has spawned debate in the evidence-based practice movement....Because our understanding of human behavior is influenced by the basic assumptions concerning the "why" of behavior, assessment and treatment practices often become inextricably interwoven with the particular conceptual model of human functioning held by the psychologist [or psychiatrist]. (p. 13)

2. Cloninger et al. (1996) defined temperament as "the dynamic organization of the psychobiological systems that regulate automatic responses to emotional stimuli. Individual differences in temperament are known to be moderately heritable and stable throughout life regardless of culture or ethnicity" (p. 3). Cloninger (1987) proposed "three dimensions of personality that are genetically independent and that have predictable patterns of interaction in their adaptive responses to specific classes of environmental

stimuli. The three underlying genetic dimensions of personality are called novelty seeking, harm avoidance and reward dependence" (p. 574). Novelty seeking, which involves a dopaminergic pathway, is a behavioral activation system; harm avoidance is a serotonergic, behavioral inhibition system; and reward dependence is a norepinephrine-mediated behavioral maintenance system that facilitates the acquisition of conditioned signals of reward or relief from punishment. Each system has discrete neuroanatomical areas of influence. Cloninger developed a personality typology based on these dimensions. For instance, antisocial personalities are high in novelty seeking and low in harm avoidance and reward dependence, obsessive individuals are high in harm avoidance and low in novelty seeking and reward dependence, and so on. According to Cloninger, advances in gene mapping promise to elucidate the genetic architecture of a variety of temperamental traits.

3. Concepts such as "the average expectable environment" or "good enough mother" do not do justice to the role of the rearing environment. They imply that the developmental environment plays a passive, unimportant, and often detrimental role. Rarely is there an explicit articulation or recognition of the positive contributions of the environment in the developmental process; the whole issue of the nature of the developmental environment (the role of the mother or caregiver, in particular) seems to be taken for granted. Neuroscience and developmental research are seeking to elucidate the specificity of factors that promote optimal development. Schore (1994) presented the following summary of evolving views on this subject:

> We now know that the early environment is fundamentally a social environment, and that the primary social object who mediates the physical environment to the infant is the mother. Through her intermediary action environmental stimulation is modulated, and this transformed input impinges upon the infant in the context of socioaffective stimulation. The mother's modulatory function is essential not only to every aspect of the infant's current functioning, but also to the child's continuing development. She thus is the major source of the environmental stimulation that facilitates (or inhibits) the experience-dependent maturation of the child's developing biological (especially neurobiological) structures. Her essential role as the psychobiological regulator of the child's immature psychophysiological systems directly influences the child's biochemical growth processes which support the genesis of new structure. (p. 7)

4. Rudolf, a 19-year-old Asian American male, exhibited poor self concept and chronic self-esteem difficulties. His compulsive sexualization reflected evidence of an ongoing narcissistic disturbance and a lack of affirming and supportive self-objects. His compulsive anal masturbation reflected the transformation of body functions into soothing self-objects

when supportive self-objects were not available to him. This autoerotic involvement represented a substitutive restorative (reparative) self-object. His fantasies during masturbation expressed exhibitionistic gratification of his arrested primitive grandiose self. His feeling that people were looking at him during his compulsive activities was another manifestation of his projected grandiose self. Rudolf's need for a heating pack on his back at night represented a longing for a restorative self-object (it stood for the absent grandmother who used to warm his back as a child). A body sensation was transformed again into a soothing self-object. Suicidal ideation emerged when his sense of self was at risk of fragmentation. Because he had not internalized his supporting self-objects, he was hopelessly dependent on others for his self-esteem regulation. Rudolf's drug use was an additional method with which he attempted to avert fragmentation of his enfeebled self. This formulation alternative is interesting; there is a sense of coherence in the systematic application of self psychological concepts, even though other psychodynamic propositions could be equally useful.

CHAPTER 14

Symptom Formation and Comorbidity

Certain clinical syndromes are commonly associated with particular descriptive symptoms; they also have corresponding psychosocial contexts or psychodynamics. For example, patients who have panic attacks display traits of helplessness, dependency, passivity, and behavioral avoidance. Similarly, patients who are depressed feel unmotivated, devalued, and hopeless. When these syndromes are clinically active, certain psychological and psychodynamic traits are expected to be present. These traits are considered state dependent, meaning that the traits are present when the patient becomes panicky, depressed, or the like. Those personality traits become submerged or are less salient when the syndromes (e.g., depression, anxiety) are under control. The intimate relationship between certain syndromes and associated psychodynamics (personality traits) is such that clinicians are advised to defer making personality disorder diagnoses when dealing with active syndromes (formerly, Axis I disorders) (see Note 1 at the end of this chapter).

Do psychodynamic constellations unleash clinical syndromes? This does occur. The most common example is a person's response to a loss. People have different thresholds for and different ways of responding to loss. Many factors, including constitutional and temperamental factors, family dynamics, and other psychosocial variables, determine this variability. In the so-called psychosomatic disorders, an intimate connection is assumed between the somatic and mind realms. In these illnesses, people become ill in response to a variety of stresses. The mechanisms implicating stress as a major factor in the development of a number of diseases are yet to be determined.

The intricateness of the somatic and the psychiatric is described in the following observations.

Hajek et al. (2016) assert that type 2 diabetes mellitus (T2DM) or insulin resistance affects not only somatic outcomes but also psychiatric outcomes. Bipolar disorders complicated by T2DM are associated with greater morbidity, lower treatment response, and poorer outcome with greater chronicity and disability (p. 2). Similarly, patients with hypercalcemia and insulin resistance (even without diagnosed T2DM) are at greater risk for developing mild cognitive impairment or dementia (p. 3). The authors reported the effect of two proof-of-concept studies demonstrating that 8–12 weeks of treatment with pioglitazone in patients with unipolar or bipolar depression and metabolic syndrome reduced depressive symptoms across clinician- and patient-rated assessments. Furthermore, pioglitazone was associated with improvement in inflammation, fasting glucose level, triglyceride level, and total body insulin resistance. The authors also mentioned that two double-blind, placebo-controlled trials showed greater reductions of depressive symptoms when pioglitazone was added to citalopram in unipolar or to lithium in bipolar depression. An emerging body of evidence shows that treatment targeting glucose regulation, such as insulin, metformin, and glucagon-like peptide-1 agonists (i.e., liraglutide, exenatide), have positive effects on brain-related outcomes (Hajek et al. 2016, p. 4).

Stress could be defined as the imperative adjusting to change. The concept of allostatic load is germane to the present discussion. Allostatic (adaptive) systems enable individuals to respond to a variety of situations other than strictly physiological changes. *Allostasis* is defined as the capacity to achieve stability through multi-systemic changes. This concept is akin to the concept of resilience. A price is paid for the forced resetting of parameters as a result of stress adaptation, particularly if the process becomes extreme, persistent, or inefficient. The cost of these processes is called *allostatic load*. Allostatic load is related to the cumulative, multi-systemic impact (the physiological toll) that is required for adaptation. It is the "wear and tear" of the body and brain resulting from chronic overactivity or inactivity of physiological systems that are involved in adaptational change. (This is like an exhaustion of the adaptive capacity.) When a person experiences too many unpredictable events, the allostatic load can increase dramatically, causing an allostatic overload (i.e., a "breakdown") that is associated with pathological conditions (Kapczinski et al. 2008). In general, a breakdown is followed by regressive behavior. From this perspective, comorbidity could be considered as the exhaustion or spilling over of the adaptive organismic failures.

Apparently, psychiatrists are failing to diagnose comorbidity; this is important because patients often want help not for the primary condition but instead for the associated morbidities (Zimmerman et al. 2008). Detecting comorbidity is clinically important; a logical assumption is that this practice will increase diagnostic accuracy, and a better diagnostic practice may result in greater patient satisfaction, improved alliance with the treating clinician, and, consequently, improved treatment adherence and better outcomes (Zimmerman et al. 2008).

The vulnerability to stress probably depends on response thresholds and on individual organ stress targets. The coping dysfunction, or breakdown, may be in the "somatic" realm or in the "mental" realm; either diathesis may have an underlying genetic predisposition. When children break down, they do it in different ways: one child may become depressed, another may become psychotic, a third may activate a psychosomatic illness, and a fourth may evolve a mysterious inhibition of the release of growth hormone.

What happens when a chronic syndrome, such as anxiety or depression, improves or remits? Common clinical observations show that control of chronic mood disorders may produce only partial improvement in personality functioning. Although the depression or anxiety may be controlled, many areas of the patient's personality dysfunction may remain. In chronically anxious patients, patterns of avoidance or inhibition, pervasive doubting, and strong dependency traits may remain. In chronically depressed patients, patterns of passivity, inhibition, low self-esteem, and fear of failure outlast the improvement of the affective disorder symptoms. In either situation, patients have a greater vulnerability to stress. The lasting dysfunctional traits may become impervious to further psychopharmacological treatment. These observations have made it mandatory to use a combination of treatment modalities. On the other hand, the presence of major depressive disorder, a disruptive disorder, or a substance use disorder in childhood or adolescence increases the odds for personality disorder in adulthood (Schulenberg et al. 2008).

In persons with chronic conditions such as bipolar disorders, the concept of allostatic overload is useful for understanding apparently unrelated findings, such as vulnerability to stress, cognitive impairment, and high rates of physical morbidity and mortality (Kapczinski et al. 2008). The model of allostatic load predicts that increased vulnerability to environmental stress would bring about an increased allostatic reaction: hypothalamic-pituitary-adrenal axis and circadian rhythm disturbances, abnormalities in the immune-inflammatory systems, and structural and functional brain changes (Kapczinski et al. 2008). In the later regard, Mah et al. (2016, p. 58) pose the question of whether anxiety can damage the brain. The authors note that in a variety of anxiety disorders, the amygdala, which processes cues predicting a threatening or aversive stimulus during fear conditioning, is hyperactive, whereas the prefrontal cortex and the hippocampus, which play a key role in down-regulating the amygdala, are hypoactive. Chronic activation of the stress sensitive systems can lead to eventual "wear and tear" of the neuroendocrine system, and over time this effect impinges on the functioning of other interconnected physiological systems, including the immune, metabolic, and cardiovascular systems.

This breakdown (i.e., allostatic load) is associated with an increased risk of diseases, such as cardiovascular disease, diabetes, metabolic syndrome, and neuropsychiatric disorders. For a long time it has been appreciated that stress exacerbates mental illnesses, contributing to a risk of depression and anxiety; it may also trigger the onset of schizophrenia or bipolar disorders or the development of posttraumatic stress disorder. It has been recently reported that women who experience significant psychosocial stress in middle age are at increased risk of developing Alzheimer's disease. Chronic stress and excessive glucocorticoid exposure may compromise the integrity of the hippocampus. This is evidenced by hippocampus atrophy and the decrease of the hippocampus neurogenesis (Kapczinski et al. 2008).

In the etiology of mental disorders, the contribution of temperament is infrequently considered in spite of the fact that this factor has an enduring quality. To add to the complexity of the etiology of anorexia nervosa, as Rotella et al. (2016) note, there is a large body of research showing that childhood neurotic and anxious traits are frequently present in patients with anorexia nervosa. Furthermore, perfectionism, neuroticism, obsessive-compulsiveness, impulsivity, narcissism, and sensation-seeking have been demonstrated to be more common in patients with eating disorders compared with healthy individuals. The Cloninger model has been widely used in eating disorders, and, generally, high harm avoidance, low self-directiveness, and low cooperativeness are associated with all eating disorder diagnoses (pp. 77–78).

What is the relationship between dysfunctional personality traits and affective dysregulation? One could postulate that chronic mood disorders promote maladaptive patterns of coping that gain stability or even functional autonomy. One could also argue that affective dysregulation and associated personality traits have different but parallel origins. Alternatively, the affective disorder could interfere with adaptive processes of learning and skill development in interpersonal relationships and in other areas; the unresolved symptoms could represent lags in adaptational learning (see Note 2 at the end of this chapter).

The precise nature of the phenomenon of comorbidity is a challenge in the ongoing elucidation of the origin and expression of psychopathology (see Note 3 at the end of this chapter). Is comorbidity, the presence of multiple psychiatric disorders, a real phenomenon? Is it an artificial result of the DSM taxonomies, DSM-5 (American Psychiatric Association 2013) included? The concept has important implications for the understanding of the different facets of illness and symptom formation, and of course for treatment. Without a doubt, the concept of comorbidity is the major culprit for the polypharmacy epidemic that is ongoing in contemporary clinical psychiatric practice. There are many critics and detractors of this practice. According to Achenbach (2008), DSM-IV-TR (American Psychiatric Association 2000) did not have well-validated markers for distinguishing childhood disorders from one other, and apparent comorbidity may reflect a lack of clear boundaries between disorders (see Note 4 at the end of this chapter). We doubt DSM-5 is any better in this regard. In other words, the diagnostic criteria for different nosological categories may not accurately represent the true existence of different disorders. This controversy notwithstanding, the notion of comorbidity has become reified in clinical practice.

Several studies suggest that certain psychopathologies precede early drug experimentation (before age 13 years) or regular drug use. For example, oppositional defiant disorder in children is strongly associated with drug experimentation with psychoactive substances, and the presence of a mental disorder in childhood is associated with marijuana abuse in adolescence. Dependency on psychoactive substances is higher in children and adolescents with conduct disorder, oppositional defiant disorder, affective disorder, anxiety disorder, and bipolar disorder. Debate is ongoing about the role of attention-deficit/hyperactivity disorder in psychoactive substance abuse (Szobot and Bukstein 2008). A diagnosis of conduct disorder between ages 11 and 14 years was found to be a strong predictor of substance use disorders by age 18, and children and adolescents exposed to trauma (physical or sexual) were found to have a higher prevalence of substance use disorders (Szobot and Bukstein 2008).

Factors that stabilize a syndrome or that are important in symptom expression or maintenance may not have anything to do with the origin of the disorder. The complexity of interactions in the process of symptom formation and symptom maintenance can be observed in the following case example.

Case Example

Kirk, a 16-year-old Caucasian male, was being evaluated for depression and suicidal ideation. Kirk's mother had a history of chronic depression; she was chronically suicidal and episodically self-abusive. His father, a scientist, qualified for the diagnosis of obsessive-compulsive disorder (OCD). He would repeatedly check his laboratory door to ensure that it was locked, and in the parking lot, he would walk around his car several times, checking all the door locks. On occasion, he would return to the laboratory at night to ensure that his lab had been securely locked.

Kirk's parents were involved in an ongoing conflict over issues of power and control. Kirk's mother complained that her husband was tyrannical and very controlling. When tension in the marriage increased, Kirk's mother would become depressed, self-abusive, and suicidal. At these times, Kirk and his 13-year-old sister (who exhibited regression) would come to their mother's rescue and unite against their domineering father. Kirk's father found himself progressively isolated and felt rejected and undermined. At those times, the father's insomnia and OCD symptoms would worsen, and Kirk's acting-out behaviors would escalate.

Kirk's mother undermined his father's efforts to set limits on the children. Kirk, in spite of superior intelligence, was flunking most of his school classes. School authorities earmarked Kirk as a problem child. He was very unconventional in his manner of dressing and was associated with troubled peers; he used drugs, too.

The preceding case example illustrates the additive influences of negative factors. For Kirk, some psychiatric features (e.g., depression) had biological-hereditary contributory factors (probably coming from both parents). These factors, added to prolonged exposure to parental psychopathology and marital discord, created significant developmental interferences, promoting negative social learning, negative internalizations and ultimately, a defective self-concept formation (see Note 5 at the end of this chapter).

A caregiver's affective disorder may have multiple effects on his or her parental functioning. Maternal depression is a very important diagnostic clue. Keitner and Miller (1994) agreed with this conceptualization: "It is not certain whether problematic family relationships predispose to or facilitate the emergence of depressive illness or whether the depressive illness and its attendant impact on patients' interpersonal styles create family difficulties in coping. There is evidence to support both points of view. In addition, the combination of a number of different stressors can obviously have an additive effect in leading to family dysfunction" (p. 22).

Kirk's case example also demonstrates the formation and stabilization of psychopathology in a developing child through concomitant parallel systems. Although Kirk's affective disorder improved, the developmental, internalized conflicts and the negative learning persisted. A protracted course of family therapy was required to disentangle Kirk from maternal enmeshment and to facilitate a closer relationship between Kirk and his father. The improved relationship was necessary for the consolidation of Kirk's masculine identity. The case example also showed mutual balancing, or stabilization, of the parents' individual pathologies: the mother's chronic affective disorder with periodic acute reactivations and the father's OCD and unremitting insomnia.

We have followed a number of adolescent patients who exhibited chronic, stable, maladaptive regressions. Crucial in the stabilization of the psychopathology is the symbiotic link of these children to their mothers. Positive steps in the treatment have been achieved every time the symbiosis has been fractured. A positive sign in this respect is the development of depression in mothers when their children begin to separate from the enmeshed relationship.

Negative factors in the development of psychopathology, as in Kirk's case example, may act additively or may potentiate themselves by synergism. An example of the latter is that a criminal outcome at age of 18 years was found to be more likely when the following two conditions occurred together in a male infant: 1) complications at birth and 2) maternal rejection by age 1 year. Neither condition in isolation produced the adverse development (Raine et al. 1994). The aggregate of negative factors may unfortunately have combined results that are far more negative than the mere presence of the individual factors.

Contemporary conceptualization of the nature-nurture relationship establishes a mutual influence between the factors. As Pike and Plomin (1996) explained, environmental factors, both shared and nonshared, have been found to be important to varying degrees. Parents who are negative cast a shadow over their families and put all children in these families at risk for depression in adolescence. Nonetheless, nonshared family environment also appears to have some effect. Non-shared environment is a fresh way of thinking about the environment of the family. It suggests that important experiences lie within the families, not just between families. For example, adolescents who are the object of more maternal negativity than their siblings are more likely to be depressed, independent from the effects of genetics or shared family environment (Pike and Plomin 1996, p. 568) (see Note 6 at the end of this chapter).

Key Points

- Comorbidity is a very common finding during comprehensive diagnostic evaluations.
- Diagnosis of comorbid disorders is important because comorbid symptoms may be more influential in maladaptation than the explicit presenting symptoms that prompt the psychiatric evaluation.
- Comorbidity complicates the diagnosis and treatment of any given disorder.
- Diagnosis of comorbidity enriches the evaluation and has a positive influence on fostering engagement and therapeutic alliance.

Notes

1. Lampe (2016) describes the characteristics and underlying development and genetics of avoidant personality disorder (AVPD) and social anxiety disorder (SAD). AVPD has been considered a more severe case of SAD. Three groups have been studied: AVPD, AVPD associated with SAD, and SAD without AVPD. Only about 25% of AVPD subjects have comorbid SAD, but the two disorders share a genetic vulnerability: relatives of subjects with SAD were frequently diagnosed with AVPD, whereas relatives of AVPD subjects received the diagnosis of SAD more frequently. There is research supporting the distinction between SAD and AVPD conditions and the decision not to consider them as part of a spectrum. Individuals with AVPD have a background of attachment difficulties and have poor self-esteem and a negative self-identity. Commonly, AVDP subjects have less experience of physical or sexual abuse but were raised in homes who were exceedingly critical, neglectful, or emotionally cold. There was a trend for more severe abuse than for persons with SAD. Avoidant and anxious attachment styles were common in schizoid and AVPD; however, social anhedonia was predictive of schizoid personality, and internalized shame (shame-aversiveness), heightened personal sensitivity, and the need to belong were predictive of AVPD (Lampe 2016, pp. 65–66).

2. Kandel (1998) proposed that behaviors that characterize psychiatric disorders are disturbances of brain function, even in those cases in which the causes are clearly environmental in origin. Genes and their protein products are important determinants of the patterns of interconnection of the neurons and the details of their functioning. Learning, including learning that results in dysfunctional behavior, produces alteration in gene expression. Kandel discussed the gene's template and transcriptional (phenotype) functions. The template function can be altered only by mutation and is not regulated by social experience of any sort. The transcriptional function, in contrast, is highly regulated, and this regulation is responsive to environmental factors. This epigenetic regulation is influenced by internal and external factors, including brain development, hormones, stress, learning, and social interaction. The regulation of gene expression by social factors makes all bodily functions, including those of the brain, susceptible to social influences. In humans, the modifiability of gene expression through learning in a nontransmissible way is particularly effective and has led to a new kind of evolution: cultural evolution (Kandel 1998; see also Note 5).

3. In the 1970s, Puig-Antich and colleagues made interesting observations concerning the association of major depressive disorder with the concom-

itant manifestation of anxiety and conduct disorder (Puig-Antich and Gittelman 1982; Puig-Antich et al. 1978). For the latter association, they noted that in a group of depressed preadolescents, the conduct disorder features waxed and waned, according to the reactivation or improvement of the affective disorder. When the depression was active, the conduct disorder features were active, and when the depression was in remission, the conduct features were also in remission. In the same vein, a strong association exists between conduct disorder and bipolar disorder: the conduct disorder may precede, be concurrent with, or follow the onset of bipolar illness. According to Kovacs and Pollock (1995), conduct disorders are equally likely to antedate or postdate the onset of the first episode of bipolar disorder.

4. According to Achenbach (2008), "If formal diagnosis of behavioral, emotional, social, and thought problems validity discriminate between disorders that are as distinct as physical diseases such as cancer, measles and diphtheria, it would make sense to use multiple specific treatments for children who qualify for multiple diagnoses. However, because neither physical etiologies nor other physical abnormalities have been identified as underlying nosological categories for children's behavioral, emotional, social, or thought problems, treatments cannot be aimed at different physical abnormalities marked by different formal diagnoses. Instead, treatments are aimed at altering behaviors, feelings, and thoughts that may overlap among nosological categories. Consequently, research is needed not only in the effectiveness of specific treatments for specific diagnoses but also on the effectiveness of treatments for the many children who qualify for multiple diagnoses" (p. 443).

5. Epigenetic factors (physical abuse) influence the gene coding for neuropeptide S receptor (*NPSR1*). The more active T ("risk") allele has been linked to panic disorder in women, induces increased heart rate and severe behavioral avoidance in panic disorder, and is related to environmental risk factors: T/T homozygosity has been shown to interact with child maltreatment experiences and result in higher scores in the higher sensitivity index (i.e., Anxiety Sensitivity Index [ASI]) (Gottschalk and Domschke 2016, p. 33). This allele causes significant amygdalar activation and is correlated with harm avoidance and increased activation of the locus coeruleus; high ASI scores were negatively correlated with prefrontal activity, suggesting corticolimbic dysfunction of the inhibitory cortical control over subcortical circuits (Gottschalk and Domschke 2016, p. 34). In line with the hypothesis of a dysfunctional corticolimbic interaction, *NPSR1* T allele carriers display lower glutamate/glutamine-to-creatine ratios in the anterior cingulate cortex during a cholecystokinin tetrapep-

tide (CCK-4)–induced episode of panic. The oxytocin receptor gene (*OXTR*) has received increased attention in the study of anxiety. Homozygous A/A carriers predicted high scores of negative affectivity and neuroticism (Gottschalk and Domschke 2016).

6. Pike and Plomin (1996) summarized a number of concepts related to behavioral genetic research: *Quantitative genetic theory* postulates that variation observed among individuals in a population can be ascribed to genetic and environmental sources; this stems from individuals' genetic variability and the variability of the environments experienced by the individuals. Genetic effects can be either additive or non-additive. *Additive genetic influence* refers to genetic effects that add up linearly in their effect on the phenotypic variance. *Non-additive genetic influence* refers to effects caused by interactions among the genes. *Environmental influences* consist of two categories: those shared by siblings reared in the same family (i.e., shared environment) and those not shared by siblings in the same family (i.e., non-shared environment). *Environment* in behavioral genetics is defined more broadly than is typically the case. It includes all sources of variations not explained by heritable genetic effects. In addition to psychosocial experiences, the environment includes perinatal factors, accidents, illnesses, and even chromosomal events, such as chromosomal anomalies, that are not inherited.

CHAPTER 15

Diagnostic Obstacles (Resistances)

When an examiner encounters difficult or complex situations during a psychiatric examination, he or she might appeal to the concept of *resistance*. Only by making a dedicated effort to understand the patient's circumstances, no matter how complex, daunting, intractable, frightening, or hopeless they may appear, the examiner will aspire to deal with issues surrounding difficult and complex diagnostic presentations. If the examiner simply appeals to the concept of resistance every time difficulties are encountered during the psychiatric examination, he or she will lose many opportunities for both professional and personal growth. The statement "the child is resistant" could easily be transformed into "the examiner is unable to engage the child" (see Note 1 at the end of this chapter). In the same way that a good chess player knows different openings and knows how to respond to the opponent's moves, the psychiatrist should know different strategies for responding to diverse clinical presentations (see Chapter 3, "Special Interviewing Techniques"). The psychiatrist needs to have a variety of engagement skills and other rapport-enhancing strategies readily available to meet difficult clinical challenges during the diagnostic examination.

Katz (1990) suggested a number of skills or qualities the examiner needs to have at his or her disposal. These include knowledge, understanding, empathy, and a positive and warm approach toward patients. To these, we add equanimity and a solid awareness of the child's developmental level.

The psychiatrist should remember that challenging or difficult children (and their families) are not creating difficulties anew for the examiner; the pathology that children and their families display during the psychiatric examination represents enactments or scripts of long-standing patterns of maladaptive behaviors (e.g., internalized conflictive relationships). These patterns require elucidation and understanding.

Resistance is a paternalistic concept. It implies that the mental health professional is right about the theory of disease that afflicts the child or the family, or worse, that the expert knows best about what to do regarding the problems that have been identified. Both assumptions may be incorrect. The concept of resistance is easily applied when the child or the family did not follow the expert recommendation and particularly when there is a lack of medication compliance. Arthur Kleinman (2016, p. xvii) introduced the concept of *category fallacy*, which results from the application of professional biomedical categories in places where those categories had no local cultural significance but instead imposed an alien ideology on indigenous illness experiences and treatment practices, thereby distorting both.

Technically, the concept of resistance relates to intrinsic protective factors that block an individual (group, system) from self-awareness of patterns of behavior or internal conflicts and/or from a willingness to change. Because the concept of resistance puts the burden of the diagnostic difficulties on the patient (discounting the contextual factors or the examiner's shortcomings in the interview process), and because this concept somehow conveys that the patient is somehow opposing the psychiatrist's efforts, we prefer the terms *interviewing difficulties* or *interviewing obstacles*.

A child who is not verbally productive is not necessarily resistive. Conditions such as deafness, elective mutism, communication and language deficits, attachment disorders, and developmental learning disorders may interfere with optimal verbal communication. Language and communication disorders, intellectual limitations, or other neuropsychological deficits also impair receptive or expressive communication processes.

If a child indicates that he or she does not want to participate in an interview, the examiner should review with the child what the examiner knows about the reasons for the evaluation (i.e., the so-called contractual aspects of the examination) and should invite the child to explain what he or she thinks is the reason for the evaluation. Children are often cajoled or manipulated into a psychiatric evaluation by deceptive means. For example, parents may say to a child, "Let's go see a doctor" or "We'd like you to see a counselor." Correspondingly, the child may go to the evaluation intending to "get mom or dad (or both) off my back." In circumstances of passive compliance, the examiner is uncertain whether the child is aware of any emotional or behavioral problem or if the identified patient acknowledges any feeling of internal distress or that his or her behavior is maladaptive.

In each diagnostic interview, the examiner needs to ascertain how the child was prepared for the examination. If the examiner suspects deception, he or she should attempt to understand why the family needed to manipulate the child. If deception has been identified, the examiner should attempt to discover other patterns of manipulation or communication deviancy within the family; family deception may be secondary to the power and control the child has gained over the family.

The challenge with a defensive and uncooperative child is to transform the child's mistrust and defensiveness into a working alliance so the examiner can conduct a productive diagnostic interview.

If the examiner needs to release information to the authorities (e.g., police, school officials, abuse investigators) or other agencies, he or she needs to let the child and family know the need for such a disclosure. The examiner should also convey that he or she is working on the child and family's behalf and that no step in the evaluation process will be taken without their participation.

The examiner needs to continually safeguard the purpose of the interviewing process. If the patient is uncooperative or plainly antagonistic, the examiner may be greatly tempted to plead for cooperation. Pleading is not recommended; the patient will likely react by providing only partial or even deceptive information, which will leave the nature of the difficulty unclarified and unresolved, and the obstacles of the communication unexplored. A better approach is for the examiner to attempt to understand every obstacle presented. Clarifications and interpretations are the optimal means for dealing with any difficulties with communication or rapport, or any obstacles in building an alliance.

The following vignette illustrates a novice examiner's inadequate management of interviewing obstacles:

> A 14-year-old Caucasian female with a history of conduct problems, self-abuse, suicidal behavior, and polysubstance abuse entered the interviewing room and sat facing away from the examiner. The examiner asked the patient to "sit more appropriately"; she complied. The examiner then pleaded for cooperation and received passive compliance on a number of occasions. The quality of the ensuing interaction was bland and detached; no rapport was established.

In this vignette, the emotional tone of the evaluation could have been different if the examiner had addressed the resistance from the very beginning by saying, for example, "It seems you do not want to talk to me" or "It doesn't seem that you want to participate in the interview." This approach also addresses negative affect that motivate the patient's lack of cooperation. The same approach should be taken when a patient acts out during the interview. Novice examiners take what seems to be the easiest way out approach when they simply ask the child to stop misbehaving. The preferable approach is to say to the child, "Now I am beginning to understand why your parents are concerned about your behavior" or "Now you are showing me why your parents brought you to see a psychiatrist [or other mental health professional]."

Effective and therapeutic interventions connect the child's acting out with the presenting problem and appeal to the child's adaptive ego (the part of the ego struggling for optimal adaptation). These approaches help the child to improve his or her participation in the examination by increasing the patient's self-awareness of what he or she is doing and by stimulating the patient's internal self-controls. A better intervention than asking the child to stop misbehaving would be for the examiner to make the child aware of an overall pattern of maladaptation by saying, for example, "The way you are behaving during this examination makes me wonder if this is the way you behave in other situations. I am beginning to understand why people complain about you." Demanding passive acquiescence or taking over the patient's controls is an intervention of last resort. Occasionally, the interviewer has no alternative but to take over the control of the situation for the sake of the patient's or the examiner's safety.

Classification of Interviewing Obstacles

For clinical and practical purposes, interviewing obstacles may be classified as either *pseudo-resistances* or *true resistances*. The latter category may be subdivided further into categories of superficial, moderate (approachable), or severe (insurmountable) interviewing obstacles.

Pseudo-Resistances

Pseudo-resistances are obstacles to the interviewing objectives that are not created by the child's defensiveness or unwillingness to participate. Pseudo-resistances can be considered from both the examiner's and the child's perspectives. A failure in the interviewing process may occur secondary to the examiner's inability to engage the child, lack of skill, lack of sensitivity to the child's problems, or lack of attunement to the child's developmental level. For example, the examiner may not be attentive or sensitive to the presence of language disorders or neuropsychological deficits. In these cases, the obstacles are apparent only because the communication deficits interfere with the child's ability to participate in the diagnostic interview. An attentive examiner should notice the child's efforts or attempts to communicate. Other factors may obstruct the process of establishing an alliance and ensuring a productive interview. As Lewis-Fernández et al. (2016) note, "Despite clinicians' best efforts, the [initial] medical encounter may be influenced by stereotyping, discrimination, racism and subtle forms of bias" (p. 18). To this list we need to add the interviewer's countertransference.

When the child obviously does not understand what he or she hears or seems to have a hearing deficit, the examiner should attempt to ascertain the child's communication intent by paying special attention to the child's nonverbal behavior (e.g., pointing, signaling, gesturing) or to the child's use of elementary vocabulary. If the examiner concludes that the child has communication difficulties, he or she should try to maximize the use of nonverbal media (e.g., play observation, drawing) to attain access to the child's internal world. If the child is hearing impaired, the presence of a qualified sign language translator is mandatory.

Other pseudo-resistances may occur in psychiatric practice. Abused children often act "dumb" and learn not to say anything that might bring the family in contact with the law or other agencies. These children appear superficially to be resistant; they have learned that being silent prevents them from getting into further trouble. On the other hand, children who are very anxious frequently become inhibited and freeze in the presence of strangers. Elective mutism should also be considered in the category of pseudo-resistances (see Pedro's case [Case Example 10] in Chapter 3, "Special Interviewing Techniques").

The examiner needs to be sensitive to each child's inner sense of internal disorganization and chaos. A child who is on the verge of a psychotic breakdown displays strong denials and avoidance, with all the external appearances of resistance; this is the patient's attempt to cope with impending psychological fragmentation.

True Resistances

Superficial Interviewing Obstacles

Interviewing difficulties that are readily amenable to cognitive, educational, or reassuring interventions are classified as superficial. They may be approached in the following ways:

1. The examiner clarifies the reasons for the evaluation (i.e., the contractual elements, see above), if these reasons are unclear.
2. The examiner stresses the importance of the child's participation.
3. The examiner deals with deceptive issues and openly and honestly explains to the child what the evaluation entails, what may be gained by it, and how the examination may help the child.
4. The examiner expresses concern and empathy for the child's plight.

Children and adolescents who display superficial obstacles commonly use a number of avoidant strategies. For instance, they commonly or repeatedly say, "I don't know," "I don't remember," "I forgot," and so on. In general, these responses indicate a deliberate decision not to participate in the interview or not to tell the truth. The examiner should not take these statements at face value. Suggested responses to these evasive and avoidant statements are "Tell me what you know," "Tell me what you remember," or "Let's talk about what you've forgotten." Frequently, the child may give an opening after these simple interventions, and the interview may be elevated to a more productive level; the child may become more revealing or more straightforward, and the new material may improve the diagnostic alliance.

Children who respond to prompts or questions with repetitive and unproductive answers such as "I forgot" and "I don't remember" are frequently avoiding, lying, or hiding or distorting the truth. The examiner should attempt to transform lying into a problem for the child or into an issue that may cause problems for the child. For example, the examiner may state, "It seems to me that you do not want to participate in the interview" or "I have the feeling you don't want to tell the truth." The examiner could also ask the child, "What happens when you don't tell the truth?" or "What happens to you when you lie?" When children respond with meaningless shrugs or other nonverbal behaviors, the examiner can respond by saying, for example, "My ears cannot understand what your shoulders are trying to say" or "Can you tell me what your shoulders are trying to say?"

Sometimes children become evasive and selective about information shared because they do not want to say anything that may jeopardize their significant others. They do not want to get anybody into trouble. Some children have been ordered not to disclose what is going on in their homes or in their lives. Abused children may have been threatened by the perpetrators not to tell anybody about the abuse. The examiner needs to be aware of these possibilities.

Moderate Interviewing Obstacles

Moderate interviewing obstacles involve situations characterized by a great deal of externalization of blame and responsibility, overt oppositional stance, bullishness, scapegoating, and intimidating and aggressive behaviors. These obstacles may be approached as follows:

1. The examiner should follow steps 1–4, listed above in the subsection "Superficial Interviewing Obstacles."
2. The examiner attempts to help the child gain insight into her current behavior. In a calm, nondefensive manner, the examiner asks the child what happens at home, at school, or in other places when the child behaves as

she is behaving in the office. The examiner also asks how the child feels while behaving this way and how other people react. The child may gain some awareness of how much she enjoys upsetting people. The child may also state that she likes to be in control or that she protects herself against the anticipation of being controlled by others. These new observations may provide an understanding of the child's problems and may provide new opportunities to establish or further the diagnostic alliance.

3. If the previous approaches do not work, the examiner uses the oppositional behavior (e.g., bullishness) to make connections between the child's problems in the real world and the examiner's observations of the child's behavior during the interview. The examiner attempts to connect the provocative enactment in the interview with the presenting problem. For example, if a provocative and oppositional child becomes defiant or evasive and keeps externalizing blame and responsibility onto others, the examiner should make the child aware of the similarities between the presenting problem that others complain about and the provocative enactment during the interview.

As the oppositional patterns of behavior unfold or begin to be enacted during the interview, the examiner must attempt to deal with such behavior by pointing out, for instance, "I'm having a hard time trying to understand you" or "You are giving me a very hard time." Comments like these usually elicit some affective response—a smile, a gesture of satisfaction, a sense of control, or verbalizations indicating that the child likes to be provocative or give people a hard time. When this issue is brought into the open, the examiner interprets the child's characterological trait or enactment and then attempts to make the child aware of how acting out in that way can create problems for her. The examiner can also attempt to connect the enactment with the presenting problem, by saying, for example, "I imagine that when you act like this, you may bring problems upon yourself" or "What happens to you when you act like this?" The first statement is more empathic; the second is more confrontational. These reflective statements place the examiner in the child's realm, in the sphere of the child's subjective state.

A similar approach can be taken in dealing with openly aggressive, provocative, or seductive children. The examiner can say, for example, "I am beginning to see why you are here. If you behave like this at school (or at home), it's no wonder that your teachers (or parents) are getting so upset or so mad at you!" This approach is the most risky because it is the most confrontational; however, if done with compassion or tenderness, it may have a powerful effect.

The following case example illustrates a moderate but approachable interviewing obstacle.

Case Example 1

Carlos, a 14-year-old Hispanic male, had a history of severe neurodevelopmental problems, including Tourette's disorder and a developmental aphasia (with speech apraxia and fluency difficulties), when he was evaluated. Carlos also displayed psychotic features and had become aggressive at home. On several occasions, he had threatened to kill his mother and her boyfriend. Carlos was interviewed because of complaints that he had molested a 5-year-old boy and had attempted to bite the boy's penis. In the past, allegations had been made of homosexuality and inappropriate sexual behaviors.

During the interview, Carlos displayed a great deal of shame: he tried to cover his face with either his T-shirt or his hands. Carlos was extremely self-conscious of his expressive language problems but had been able to respond to most of the questions until the examiner chose to explore the molestation.

The examiner started by saying, "Let's discuss what you did to the boy." Carlos exhibited signs of shame or embarrassment. The examiner proceeded, saying, "I understand you bit his penis." Carlos took a defensive stance and said, "I don't remember what happened." The examiner quickly replied, "I don't see any reason why you can't remember. You don't want to discuss this… There is no reason why you can't remember what happened." The examiner asked again, "What happened?" Carlos began to report what happened with the boy. He said that he had tried to molest a number of children before, adding, "I was going to do to other kids what was done to me."

Carlos then reported that when he was 7 years old, five or six men had raped him on a number of occasions. He said that no one knew; he had not told his mother, fearing that the disclosure could send her to the hospital. He showed significant relief after revealing this victimization.

The examiner's confrontations and challenges to Carlos's defensive denials were effective and quite productive. Issues related to sexual abuse, posttraumatic stress disorder, and enactment of sexual abuse with other children had been previously missed.

The following case example illustrates the management of a moderate to severe interviewing obstacle through the use of confrontation, interpretation, and humor.

Case Example 2

Jackie, a 12-year-old Caucasian female with cerebral palsy, was evaluated for suicidal behavior. She was wheelchair-ridden. She had been living in a group home for a number of months prior to the assessment. During the 48 hours preceding the psychiatric evaluation, Jackie had put a knife, a screwdriver, and a fork to her neck. She had tried to kill herself many times before.

Jackie was not living at home because of her violent behavior toward her mother and younger sister. She also had attempted to fall from her wheelchair in an effort to harm herself. The staff at the group home felt they could no longer take care of Jackie because she was very disruptive to other children and to the program in general. Jackie claimed that she was hearing voices telling her to kill herself. She had been hospitalized a number of times previously for similar suicidal and aggressive behaviors. Jackie also had mild cognitive impairment and some degree of language disorder—in particular, expressive language difficulties related to cerebral palsy.

Jackie came to the evaluation accompanied by her mother and two female staff members from the group home. She had dictated a suicide note to one of the staff members the night before. When a child psychiatry resident-fellow entered the room, just before the attending examiner arrived, Jackie gave the suicide note to her. The fellow advised Jackie to give the note to the examiner, at which time Jackie crumpled up and destroyed the note.

As soon as the examiner entered the evaluation room, he became aware of a very small, spastic child in a big wheelchair. The examiner had many feelings and intuitions about Jackie's situation and about how much Jackie hated to be a person with disabilities.

After the examiner sat down and began the interview, Jackie kept making eye contact with one of the group home staff members, ignoring the examiner. When the examiner called her attention to this behavior, Jackie said that she was hearing voices and added that the voices were telling her not to listen to the examiner. She told one of the staff members that she could not understand the examiner because of his accent. To this, the examiner replied that he also had problems understanding Jackie (because of her expressive language difficulties), saying, "We are in the same boat." Jackie smiled and made direct eye contact with the examiner. The examiner realized that the child was very manipulative and that she could be deceptive and "tricky."

As the examiner began to explore Jackie's suicidal behavior, Jackie said again that the voices were telling her not to pay attention. The examiner countered, "The voices do not want you to get any help. I expect you to block the voices so we can go ahead with understanding what is the matter with you!" The "alleged voices" stopped interfering.

When the examiner asked Jackie why she was not living with her family, she ignored the examiner again. The examiner said to Jackie in a humorous manner, "You are full of tricks" and "You are a tricky girl." Jackie smiled and began to talk about her violent behavior, emphasizing with emotion that this was why she was not living with her mother.

When the examiner asked Jackie why she was mad at her mother, Jackie became evasive and turned her head away. The examiner proposed that Jackie was mad at her mother for a number of reasons. The examiner suggested that Jackie blamed her mother for her being in the wheelchair. Jackie smiled and renewed eye contact. By this time, she had begun to use the word "trick" and "tricky" in a playful and insightful manner. For example, she said, "My mind plays tricks on me," to which the examiner replied, "Like when your mind tells you that the reason you aren't living with your mom is because she doesn't love you?" Jackie said that she wanted to go home. The examiner asked Jackie what was expected of her before she could go home, and Jackie said she didn't know. The examiner then advised Jackie that she could ask her mother what she was supposed to do. Jackie's mother said that they had already discussed this issue and that she expected Jackie to control her temper before returning home.

The examiner then focused on why Jackie wanted to kill herself. The group home staff members indicated that they had the distinct impression that Jackie believed that if she were to be expelled from the group home, she would be returned home automatically. "That's not the right way to return home," the examiner told Jackie, adding, "You need to learn to control yourself first."

The examiner explored Jackie's problems with self-concept and her sense of hopelessness. He said, "You probably feel that you're worthless and not good for anything because you're in a wheelchair." He then asked Jackie, "What kinds of things are you good at?" Jackie immediately replied that she liked to take care of plants. The examiner praised her for that. The staff members added that Jackie liked listening to the radio and watching television, especially a couple of comedy programs. The examiner asserted that the reason Jackie felt worthless and suicidal was that she blocked the positive qualities she had and paid attention only to her limitations. The examiner added that in the same way that Jackie was able to block the voices, she would have to learn to block bad feelings about herself. The examiner continued, saying that instead of focusing mainly on her limitations and bad aspects of herself, Jackie needed to pay more attention to her positive qualities and the things she could do.

Humor was used a number of times during the interview, especially when the examiner discussed how "tricky" Jackie could be and when he discussed Jackie's current use of blocking and the other kinds of blocking she needed to do. Although this interview started out with a negative, resistive, and aversive tone, it changed into a very productive exchange. Major gains were made in the therapeutic alliance. The examiner's active stance against a variety of obstacles (e.g., avoidance, denial, opposition, manipulation, dissociation, and activation of "psychotic symptoms") was very productive.

After Jackie was admitted to an acute psychiatric program, her case was assigned to another psychiatrist. Jackie's mother complained about the change and asked that the attending examiner be in charge of the case. The examiner thought the mother was satisfied with the way he had conducted the evaluation, but he felt that Jackie should have a say in this matter. The examiner went to the unit to speak with Jackie and told her that her mother was upset because of the change of doctors. The examiner asked Jackie, "What do you have to say about this?" Jackie replied, "I kind of…want you to be my doctor." The examiner responded with humor, "But I gave you a hard time!" To this Jackie replied, "You helped me!" This response seemed to confirm that the interview had been effective and had promoted insight.

Clinicians are very apprehensive about using confrontational techniques (see Chapter 3, "Special Interviewing Techniques"). Clinical observations are reassuring in this regard. Older, experienced clinicians often found, as Anderson (1968; quoted in Hopkinson et al. 1981, p. 413) notes, that "[c]onfrontations given by warm, empathic interviewers increased self-exploration, whereas this was not the effect with the interviewers who lacked these qualities." Turner and Hersen (1994) agreed with the value of confrontation during the clinical interview: "Mild confrontation, when accomplished with skill and interviewer openness, will also prove to be beneficial in cutting through patient denial and defensiveness. However, the clinician will realize, with increasing experience, how far to push a given patient. Of course with aggressive patients, the issue may become one of safety, for the interviewer and those others in the surroundings" (p. 16).

Confrontational techniques are usually contraindicated in children with severe oppositional traits and in those with very strong passive-aggressive features. In these cases, there is a risk of a hostile withdrawal or, worse, an unleashing of overt aggressive behaviors. In either situation, the diagnostic alliance will be lost. Attempts to reengage these children after an episode of lack of control are very trying. Confrontation should not be used in working with children who have psychosis or prominent organicity.

Children with a long-standing history of encopresis use marked denial, splitting, omnipotent control, isolation of affect, and dissociative defenses to deal with this humiliating symptom. Confrontation should be avoided with these children, as the following case example illustrates.

Case Example 3

Billy, an intelligent 14-year-old Caucasian male, presented for a clinical consultation at the local state hospital. The consultation was requested because of Billy's lack of progress in the adolescent acute program and because of conflicts between the program staff and Billy's mother regarding discharge criteria. Billy had been admitted to the program because of suicidal behavior and serious conflict with his siblings. Encopresis had been a significant complaint, and both Billy's mother and his siblings were upset over the offensive smell and the associated behaviors. Billy had been in the hospital for almost 4 months, an unusually long stay for an acute admission. Two weeks before the consultation, Billy had been furloughed home; he was returned to the hospital 1 week later because of the encopresis. During the time that Billy stayed in the hospital, encopresis had not been active, and he had denied having such a problem.

The examiner had difficulty engaging Billy during the individual interview; Billy came across as passive and distant. He denied knowing why he had been in the hospital in the first place and denied knowing why he was back. The examiner's efforts to find out what was going on at home were unsuccessful. The only thing Billy was clear and explicit about was that he didn't like the hospital and wanted to go home. During the interview, Billy's only active behavior was frequent glancing at his watch. Sensing a major resistance, the examiner promised that Billy would be allowed to leave in about 15 minutes. Billy responded by turning around his chair to face away from the examiner. He slouched and stretched out in his chair, clearly conveying that he was going to sleep and that he did not want to be bothered. As Billy started to withdraw, he began to breathe deeply.

The examiner interpreted these behaviors as involving self-regulating mechanisms and acknowledged to Billy that he understood that he was trying to calm himself down. The examiner took advantage of Bill's behavior and reframed and redefined his behavior as an adaptive attempt, thus removing its provocative and confrontational connotations. The examiner began to direct Billy's breathing, asking him to breathe deeply in and out. The examiner also periodically informed Billy how soon he could leave. Billy remained calmed. When the time was over, he stood up and left right away. The examiner stayed calm throughout the session and did not respond to or confront Billy's passive-aggressive and provocative behaviors.

Adolescent patients with encopresis are very passive-aggressive and markedly oppositional. In discussing the case with the staff, the examiner agreed that the best way to deal with Billy's encopresis and denial was for Billy's mother to take him on leaves of absence, making it explicitly clear to Billy that he would be taken back to the hospital every time he became encopretic. It would thus be very hard for Billy to hold on to his tenacious denial and blame the hospital for his separation from his family.

Severe Interviewing Obstacles

Children and adolescents with major behavioral and emotional problems display severe resistances. These children externalize blame and responsibility for their actions and defend themselves with very strong denials and projections. They are also mistrustful, if not overtly paranoid. The following is an example of a patient with severe resistance.

Case Example 4

Johnny, a Caucasian adolescent male, was 14 years old at the time of his diagnostic psychiatric evaluation. He had been in an unending conflict with his parents during the previous year, and the situation had deteriorated during the previous 4 months. In spite of ongoing outpatient therapy for Johnny and his family, no significant progress had been achieved. Johnny had been in a child psychiatric hospital twice when he was 8 years old. He had received antidepressants in the past but had stopped taking medications 3 months earlier.

A couple of days before the evaluation, Johnny announced to his family that he was going to orchestrate his getting kicked out of school, and he accomplished this goal a day before the examination. Johnny had been extremely provocative at school; he had a history of multiple school suspensions for behavioral and aggressive problems. At home, he was unruly: during the previous week, he had come and gone as he pleased. He was defiant and had threatened to kill his mother and father many times. Two months earlier, he had taken his grandparents' van without permission and had stolen a gun from them.

During the previous 3 months, Johnny's parents had carried out the following routine before retiring at night: they unplugged the phones, collected their money and other valuables, and put a theft-deterrent device on the car to ensure that Johnny would not call gang members to steal it during the night. Johnny's parents suspected that he was associating with gang members. His mother had discovered aerosol cans in his room, and the day before the psychiatric examination, he was found with evidence of spray paint around his mouth and nostrils. When confronted, he cried and appeared remorseful, claiming that this had been the first time he had done something like this.

At age 10 years, Johnny had sustained a brain injury in a car accident. After the accident, Johnny forgot and had to relearn many things.

At the time of the evaluation, Johnny was very angry and contemptuous. He constantly externalized blame for his conspicuous acting out, not taking responsibility for his multiple transgressions. He pinned all the blame for his problems on his parents, accusing them of not loving him. He had felt unloved all his life and was quite jealous and hostile toward his younger sister; he was convinced that his parents favored her. His parents were at their wit's end and didn't know what to do about their son's behavior. They felt totally helpless in the face of Johnny's provocative and defiant behaviors. They also feared for their lives.

Johnny's father had been a peripheral figure in the family and in Johnny's life. He had delegated all forms of discipline to his wife, and to make matters worse, she had been incapacitated because of a fractured foot. Doctors were not optimistic about her prognosis for unassisted walking. Johnny believed that his father was his ally, and he boasted that he could manipulate his father. Johnny's father undermined his wife's efforts to provide consistent discipline. Partly because of this perception, Johnny's hostility, antagonism, and vicious verbal attacks and intimidations of his mother were limitless.

The family's financial situation had worsened since Johnny's mother had become ill. She had had a highly paid skilled job before becoming incapacitated. Johnny seemed oblivious to economic realities and continued making demands the family couldn't meet. Finally, Johnny's parents were concerned that he was turning into a delinquent and anticipated that he would end up in jail.

One might suspect that this child was anxious to leave home and that he would welcome any placement recommendations, but that was not the case. Johnny strongly rejected any suggestion of placement. Whenever placement was suggested, Johnny would blame his parents for wanting to get rid of him; obviously, this reaction baffled his parents. He threatened suicide when placement was discussed, because he wanted to continue living at home.

Johnny said that the examiner didn't like him either. From the start, he didn't believe that the examiner was on his side. He doubted the examiner could help him. The examiner sensed that Johnny wanted to get into a conflict with him from the very beginning.

Johnny seemed angry; he was also depressed, and his mood was labile. He denied suicidal ideation but acknowledged homicidal intentions against his parents. Johnny displayed a very rigid projective system, refused to acknowledge any responsibility for his behavior, and perseverated in blaming everything on his parents. The examiner was unable to engage Johnny and couldn't undermine his projective system.

This is a severe example of a child caught up in a very conflictive, deeply ambivalent relationship with his parents. Strong dependency and regressive tendencies opposed separation-individuation strivings. Jealousy of paranoid proportions was present. Furthermore, the previous brain trauma had left Johnny cognitively impaired, which was reflected in his rigid and narrow cognitive coping style and in his primitive defense mechanisms. Other factors such as discord within the family and stressors in the marriage, as well as the mother's recent incapacitation, contributed to Johnny's maladaptation. In spite of the examiner's efforts, the child rejected his suggestions of help.

The following example illustrates another adolescent's marked denial and severe "resistance."

Case Example 5

Robert, a 17-year-old Caucasian male, was evaluated after making a suicidal gesture. He had cut his right wrist, expressing a desire to kill himself. Six months before the evaluation, Robert had undergone an above-the-knee amputation of his left leg to prevent the spread of bone cancer (osteosarcoma). The cancer had been discovered when he was examined in an emergency room after his left foot was run over by an all-terrain vehicle. X rays taken at the time revealed the malignancy. Robert had received chemotherapy treatment, and he was using a prosthesis at the time of the psychiatric examination.

Robert had been very athletic and had participated in track and field events at school. He dropped out of school after the surgery. According to Robert, the school objected to his presence because a boy on crutches "could pose liability risks." Robert had always been in special education classes for learning disabilities. When Robert was 10 years old, Robert's brother (who was 5 years his senior) "accidentally" shot Robert in the abdomen with a gun. The circumstances surrounding the accident were unclear. One year before the evaluation, Robert's father had left home. Robert explained that his father was gay.

Robert limped into the interviewing room, sat quietly, and displayed a polite, pleasant demeanor. When Robert was asked to explain why he was in the hospital, he said that he had tried to cut his wrist "to stop his mother from threatening suicide." He displayed an anxious and peculiar smile that had an inappropriate quality; this smile resurfaced frequently throughout the evaluation. He denied any previous suicide attempts. He added that his mother was "crazy," reporting that she yelled at herself in the mirror and had threatened suicide many times before. He made all of these statements while exhibiting bland affect and his peculiar smile.

Because the loss of his leg seemed to be such an important issue, the examiner asked Robert to describe what it was like for him to hear about the cancer. He responded in a nonchalant manner, "It was okay." When the examiner encouraged him to discuss the loss of his leg or the changes that it brought to his life, he blandly answered, while smiling, that he could no longer run or do a number of things he used to do.

The examiner's multiple attempts to draw from Robert any emotional reaction regarding the loss of his leg and the impact that it had on his self-concept and self-image were met with strong denials. The examiner's use of countertransference (e.g., the sense of loss, of being handicapped, of being unattractive to the opposite sex) met with no success.

The examiner was not surprised, then, that his attempts to explore with Robert the accidental shooting by his brother, having a gay father, having a "crazy" mother, and other potentially emotion-laden experiences were met with the same blandness encountered when the examiner probed Robert's emotional response to the loss of his leg. Robert displayed massive denials, marked isolation of affect, affect reversal or reaction formation, and repression (of aggression). He was also a very immature adolescent. Factors that may have contributed to Robert's affective disturbance were severe learning disabilities, expressive affective aphasia, and cognitive impairments, plus major developmental problems associated with defective parenting (Robert's mother had alcoholism and had abused alcohol throughout her pregnancy with him). A fetal alcohol syndrome was considered.

Building a diagnostic and therapeutic alliance is impossible with patients who show intense mistrust (and are unable to believe in the goodness, or at least in the neutrality, of the examiner) as a result of strong psychopathology (e.g., severe trauma, fears of psychotic disintegration, or suspicious-paranoid behavior). When the examiner senses panic of fragmentation in prepsychotic children, he or she should respect the adaptive defenses and support reality testing and any efforts at self-control. Abused adolescents are very apprehensive about psychological evaluations, and this makes any trustful engagement difficult. The examiner should empathize with the adolescent's feelings about previous betrayals of trust and should encourage verbalizations regarding misuse (or abuse) of prior psychological or psychiatric evaluations.

If an adolescent persists in being resistive and remains uncooperative, the examiner should be wise to "lose a battle" rather than to "lose the war." When the accounts about the adolescent do not raise questions regarding safety to self or others, the examiner should concede that no understanding or conclusions can be reached without the adolescent's participation. The examiner should indicate to the adolescent that without his participation, there is no point in continuing the process. The examiner should tell the adolescent that as soon as he is willing, the examiner will be available for further contact and work. However, when the examiner is dealing with an uncooperative adolescent who is suicidal or homicidal or who has severe functional impairment secondary to mental illness, the examiner is obligated to pursue involuntary commitment.

If the examiner concludes there are not risks of safety, he might opt to tell the child that since the child does not see the need for any help right now, the examiner would like to check bases with the adolescent in an agreed period of time: a month? 2 months? and so forth.

On the other hand, the examiner needs to tell the family that safety is paramount: parents should not hesitate to call the police if they feel that their child may endanger them or if they feel that he may harm himself. In such a case the parents need to call an ambulance or the police to ensure a prompt admission to an emergency room or a child psychiatric unit. Furthermore, the interviewer may consider contacting Child Protective Services (CPS), to alert the agency that there is an impaired parent that may be at risk by her own son or daughter. CPS also needs to be informed when a child is suicidal or homicidal, or is making terroristic threats, and the parents are unwilling to take action.

Obstacles in Interviewing Families

Families and other complex systems also present obstacles to interviewing. The next case example illustrates the phenomenon of defensiveness within the family system.

Case Example 6

Marta, a 15-year-old Mexican American female, was referred to an acute psychiatric program after an almost successful suicide attempt. She had decided to hang herself with a dog chain after a fight with her boyfriend. She was unconscious for an undetermined amount of time before she was found. Marta had neither a history of suicide attempts nor a psychiatric history. She was admitted to a pediatric hospital for a complete neurological assessment. A computed tomographic scan of the brain was unremarkable, and a cervical spine series was normal. The extent of the neuronal damage caused by hypoxia was uncertain. A psychiatric consultation in the pediatric ward indicated severe thought disorganization and severe impairment of the sensorium, compatible with delirium.

After Marta was stabilized, she was referred to the acute psychiatric unit. The referring physicians met a significant obstacle when they requested family permission for the transfer. The family insisted that there was nothing wrong with Marta, that this was an accident, that she didn't mean to try to kill herself, and so on. Only by using strong persuasion were the physicians able to convince the family to agree to the transfer.

Marta spoke blandly about the events preceding the suicide attempt. She referred to the incident nondefensively and without any emotion. The most striking results of the mental status examination were abnormal findings in mood and affect: her affect was markedly blunted, and she was not dysphoric in any significant way. Her thought processes were unremarkable, but Marta was concrete. She denied suicidal ideation and denied that she would ever try to kill herself again. Marta did not endorse any feelings of sadness or any other depressive feelings. Her sensorium was intact at the time of the assessment.

When the family came to the acute unit, they demanded that Marta be released. They stressed once again that nothing was wrong with her. They said that if she were to need treatment, they would take her to the local mental health center. Any attempt to diminish the family's resistance was unsuccessful. Marta was discharged from the acute program against medical advice but the physician contacted CPS to let them know of the adolescent's ongoing risk, the adolescent's need of psychiatric care, and the parent's lack of response to the child's suicidal circumstances.

Cultural issues may have an important bearing in cases like Marta's. Shame about accessing psychiatric help is common in Mexican American families and families from nonmajority cultural and ethnic backgrounds. Some religious groups believe that God can take care of psychiatric problems, and others do not have any trust in Western medicine. The uninsured, out of desperation, may resort to indigenous and unreliable practices.

Marta's family is by no means an exception. In this case, denial within the family was as prevalent and as impervious as it was within the child. In severe family resistance, the identified or symptomatic child is likely a stabilizing figure in the dysfunctional family. In such cases, the family will interfere with any change in the child that may jeopardize the family's homeostasis. Gross denials are common in dysfunctional families in which the family's parental subsystem is impaired and the child is necessary to keep the family together. In severe cases of family "resistance" (see Johnny's and Robert's cases [Case Examples 4 and 5, respectively] earlier in this chapter), the examiner often encounters families that display multidimensional problems.

Key Points

- During psychiatric examinations, children (and families) are often defensive or wary about revealing personal information; commonly, these apprehensions are resolved when a positive engagement is achieved.

- During the diagnostic assessment, a number of obstacles imperil the objectives of the psychiatric examination. Denials, dissociation, projects, and paranoia are factors that commonly mediate obstacles during the psychiatric evaluation.

- Examples of good and inadequate management of the diagnostic interview can help the examiner learn how to approach difficult situations during the psychiatric examination.

Notes

1. Marianne Eckardt, the daughter of the famous and influential psychoanalyst Karen Horney, who, at over 100 years of age, is still a practicing analyst, contended in one presentation at the American Academy of Psychoanalysis and Dynamic Psychiatry annual meeting in 2014, in New York City, that the term "resistance" should be substituted for a "lack of therapeutic resources."

CHAPTER 16

Countertransference

The topic of countertransference is discussed last in this book because it is the most subjective and probably most complex area of the psychiatric examination. Although the ideas presented here are tentative, we hope they will stimulate examiners to think about these difficult, intriguing, and interesting (and sometimes mystifying) factors of the diagnostic interview. These suggestions may help evaluators to improve their own introspection and insight while conducting diagnostic interviews; this, undoubtedly, will result in improved interviewing skills and elaborating unfettered formulations.

The diagnostic interview is a transactional process between the child and family and the examiner. During the interview process, the examiner may be stimulated by a number of emotions or affective states. Sometimes, patients can "infect" examiners with positive or negative emotions. At other times, the examiner unexpectedly experiences unwelcome emotions or negative ideation during the diagnostic assessment. Countertransference difficulties are at the root of engagement failures and many diagnostic and therapeutic mistakes. The experienced interviewer uses the understanding and articulation of his or her own personal affective or cognitive responses during the interview to increase diagnostic information and to further the diagnostic and therapeutic alliance.

A professional attitude, the wish to help, compassion, sensitivity, and other empathic emotions are positive affective states that aid or assist the interview process. Technically, these positive emotions would not be termed *countertransference*. In this book, we define this term as *the emotions or affective states that interfere with the goals of gathering diagnostic information, establishing a diagnostic and treatment alliance, developing a treat-*

ment plan, or helping the patient and family. Any emotional state or thought process that diverts the examiner from helping the patient and family in the diagnostic process or formulating process will be designated as countertransference.

Countertransference occurs, for instance, when the examiner, out of frustration with the child or family, makes a hasty diagnostic closure or overlooks important diagnostic data. Countertransference is present when the examiner assigns a poor prognosis to a child because of an aggressive counterresponse to the child or family, or when the examiner interrupts the diagnostic process and dismisses the child and family. Prejudice related to socioeconomic status, race, gender, sexual orientation, religion, political orientation, or feelings about a child/family's country of origin, and others, could become the sources or negative countertransference.

For the purposes of this chapter, we will consider the concept of countertransference in a broader sense, paralleling Khan's definition of the term, as a nonpathological incapacity of the interviewer's affectivity, intelligence, and imagination to comprehend the total reality of the patient (and family). Khan's definition of the concept corresponds to a contemporary meaning of the term.

Weinshel and Renik's (1996) considerations regarding the analytic process are applicable to the psychiatric diagnostic examination. A broader definition of countertransference is considered advantageous. It is now assumed that the entire array of an examiner's emotional responses—those specifically induced by the child and the family and those brought by the examiner from his personal background—must be taken into account in studying the diagnostic and therapeutic process.

Children with aggressive, provocative, and negative defiant behaviors tend to elicit primary responses in examiners; the same is true of children who are callous, narcissistic, and manipulative. Parents who are physically or sexually abusive and those who are overtly neglectful also elicit strong negative affective responses in the examiners.

Parents who are provocative and challenge the psychiatrist's expertise and experience, questioning any advice or suggestions, elicit defensiveness and annoyance in the interviewer.

Simplistic notions of the psychopathological process increase the risk of countertransference. The examiner may attribute the child's problem to the parents, thinking, for example, that the parents are bad. Alternatively, the examiner might think that the child is constitutionally defective (i.e., "a bad seed"). However, psychopathology is complex and multidetermined. Another conception that promotes primary responses is the attribution of linear causality. In examinations of interpersonal psychopathology, circular causality has a better heuristic value.

The emotions that most frequently interfere with the diagnostic interview are anger, frustration, boredom, and dislike toward the patient or family. These emotions are not difficult to identify and could be transformed and worked through productively for the benefit of the patient and family; however, these same emotions may interfere with the thoroughness of the diagnostic process and may contribute to diagnostic and therapeutic mistakes.

Other emotions (e.g., sexual feelings, desires to obtain gratification from the patient) are more insidious and subtler to detect, and their negative influence may be more difficult to identify, understand, and transform. The examiner has more difficulties acknowledging and working through these emotions, which may be ego-syntonic (i.e., related to the psychological problems of the examiner).

Lewis (1996) discussed a number of issues that may elicit countertransference in clinicians working with children and adolescents; he also indicated common difficulties in these transactions. Aggressive children tend to mobilize strong defenses (or counterresponses) in clinicians. Children with intellectual disability (or other neurodevelopmental disabilities) are often overlooked and inadequately served, and children with physical deformities may repel some examiners. Lewis listed a number of diagnostic circumstances in which the examiner's countertransference may become problematic (Table 16–1). The list by no means exhausts the range of complexities or potential complications of countertransference responses.

The management of countertransference responses is complex. Good introspective capacity and self-awareness, equanimity, and extended supervision are fundamental requirements for mastering this problematic area. In this chapter, we sketch only a few practical ideas for dealing with negative countertransference responses that may occur during the interview process.

Beginning interviewers tend to avoid or put aside any feelings or emotional reactions that patients evoke in them. When emotional reactions are stimulated, these reactions are commonly disregarded because the interviewer finds these feelings unacceptable to her professional or moral standards. The feelings thus evoked are dissociated from the diagnostic process. In contrast, experienced interviewers pay close attention to their subjective responses and attempt to use them to gain further information about the patient's problems. In this manner, the experienced examiner deepens his or her emotional understanding of the patient or family and increases his or her knowledge of the patient's pathology.

To be able to accomplish this process in an effective and sensitive manner, the examiner needs to have a good level of self-awareness and satisfactory emotional self-knowledge. The examiner must be familiar with his or her usual affective range and emotional tone so that when this range or tone level

**Table 16–1.   Diagnostic circumstances in which
countertransference may be problematic**

Persistent difficulties in understanding the child's point of view

Failure to recognize the child's developmental level

Expectations that are not commensurate with the child's developmental
level

Regressive pull; identification with the child's acting out; wishes to encourage the
adolescent to act out against parents or other authority figures

Failure to understand the child's transference enactments (i.e., misperceiving the
child's relationship with the examiner or failure to detect the child's seductive
behavior toward the examiner)

Reactivation of previous conflictive areas in the examiner's life (i.e., problems with
aggression or sexuality or prior problems with parents)

Reactivation of affective states in the examiner (e.g., depression or activation of
affective states such as frustration, boredom, anger)

Projection of prior psychological or interpersonal problems onto the child or the
family

Need for approval from the child or the parents and repeated arguing or
competing with the child or parents

Negative response to children with certain personality traits (e.g., conduct
problems, drug abuse, promiscuous behavior)

Negative reaction toward children with deficits or handicaps

Lack of understanding or dislike for parents who are abusive or neglectful

Lack of sensitivity to gender, racial, cultural, or religious differences

Counterresponding to parents' devaluating attitude

Source.   Lewis 1996. Modified from Cepeda C: "Countertransference," in *Clinical Manual
for the Psychiatric Interview of Children and Adolescents.* Washington, DC, American Psychiatric Publishing, 2010, p. 446.

changes, the examiner will register the change and note that a particular emotional or affective state has been activated during the examination.

The examiner masters the countertransference through introspection.
When the examiner's emotional tone changes in quality or intensity, the examiner needs to wonder whether he or she is taking part in a patient's or
family's emotional enactment. The examiner may suspect, then, that the patient is dramatizing or enacting an emotional transaction with the examiner.
The patient may be unaware of this interpersonal influence on the examiner. In
other words, the patient may be completely unaware that he or she is reliving

an emotional script (a pattern of interaction) with the examiner. In these circumstances, the patient attempts to provoke particular emotional responses from the examiner. This occurs most frequently because the child or the family projects certain emotional states onto the examiner (i.e., projective identification).

The examiner could attempt to integrate the information gathered from his subjective response and introspective awareness with the data obtained throughout the interview process; this is accomplished by bringing the elicited emotions into a contextual understanding. When the examiner takes into account the context in which these emotions have been activated, he or she may gain an understanding of the patient's conflictive emotions and may gain further meaning from the intruding affective states.

Countertransference feelings are helpful in aiding the patient to verbalize and to understand certain emotional problems. Some patients are unable to verbalize their emotional problems for a variety of reasons; they act them out or dramatize them instead. Technically, they act out the emotional conflict with the examiner rather than expressing it verbally. By verbalizing the how the examiner feels when the patient talks about a given problem, the examiner helps the patient become aware of affects or emotional states that the patient may be unaware of or be disconnected (dissociated) from. The examiner may state openly that he or she feels a particular way when the patient talks about a given subject. The patient usually responds productively to this intervention, abreacting an emotion that had been difficult for the patient or family to put into words, making connections with other aspects of his or her life, bringing forward new material, or reaching a new level of understanding.

Whatever feeling is evoked during the interview (e.g., fear, anger, anxiety, sexual arousal), the examiner should attempt to make sense of it within the context of the interview. Frequently, the examiner is able to feel or experience affects that the patient has difficulties acknowledging and verbalizing.

Several situations present an opportune time for the examiner to use subjective responses to help patients find meanings or connections that have eluded them. These include instances when the examiner notices that the patient is struggling to find the words to verbalize a problem or to express what he or she feels, or when the patient does not make connections that are rather obvious to the examiner.

If the experienced interviewer becomes aware of a change in his or her normal affective tone, he or she may begin to ask a number of private questions: I am feeling overwhelmed, why is this happening right now? What is the reason I am feeling angry or anxious now? What is it about what the patient is saying or attempting to say that makes me feel fearful or bored? In trying to make sense of these questions, the examiner gains important information about the patient's inner conflicts.

How does the interviewer move from his or her subjective realm to the interaction and reality of the interview? When the examiner is contaminated or infected by the patient's prevailing affect, a simple sharing of the examiner's emotional state may be productive. Thus, if the examiner begins to experience depression or hopelessness, he or she may disclose these feelings to the patient and may wonder aloud what they have to do with the patient's circumstances, with what the patient is talking about, and with the way the patient is feeling or with what the patient or family has difficulties talking about. The patient's response may help illuminate his or her conflicts or the source of the patient's emotional problems. If the examiner feels drawn to the patient's emotional state, senses compassion for the patient's situation, or experiences a need to save or to rescue the patient, the examiner may wonder about the patient's sense of helplessness and a dire need for help. If this protective feeling is activated by preschoolers or by children who have difficulties verbalizing their needs, the examiner needs to consider deprivation, neglect, or abuse in the rearing environment.

At times, the understanding and handling of the countertransference responses is more complex, requiring careful introspection, discrimination of the examiner's affective state(s), assessment of the context of the examiner's responses, and the choice of an appropriate language to stimulate the patient's own introspective abilities.

If, for example, an interviewer begins to feel scared, and this feeling represents a change from his normal affective tone, he can take one of the following approaches to dealing with this emotional response. In the first, an indirect, approach, the interviewer reflects on his fear, becoming aware that the patient has limited control over her aggressive impulses. The examiner proceeds with the interview, inquiring whether the patient feels any sense of control when she becomes angry, how close she feels to losing control when he gets upset, what things would help her to stay in control, and so on.

In the second approach, which is a direct approach, the interviewer becomes aware of his fear and tells the patient the feeling he is experiencing by saying, for example, "As you talk about this, I am feeling scared" or "You are making me feel scared." Depending on the patient's response, the examiner may connect his response with the presenting problem or with responses that people have when they feel scared or intimidated by the patient. For example, the examiner could say, "I wonder if this is the way some people feel about you," or, better, "I wonder if that is the way you make people feel." These first two approaches are helpful when the patient is provocative or is acting out during the interview.

An even better direct approach, which is applicable when the patient has difficulties connecting her feelings with her thoughts, is for the examiner to pay close attention to his own emotional reactions and attempt to link those responses to the patient's narrative. For example, if the patient begins to talk about problems with her father and the examiner senses fear, he may approach the awareness of his emotional response in the following manner: "As you begin to talk about the problems you have with your father, I began to feel fearful. Is that the way you feel about him?" Or the examiner might say, "I am feeling fearful. Is that the way your father makes you feel?" Notice that both responses are very empathic; they connect with the patient's emotional responses. Interventions like these improve the patient's trust and engagement with the examiner and build the therapeutic alliance. This tentative exploration could be continued in many alternative ways.

When the intervention is correct and timely, the patient's response or the information that follows may validate the interviewer's assumptions through the emergence of new data. Such data may provide new diagnostic evidence, which, of course, enriches or broadens the interview process.

Sometimes, the examiner is overcome by subjective responses with meanings that may be somewhat familiar. The following is an example of an examiner's drowsiness response to an overwhelming, probably hopeless, clinical situation.

Case Example 1

Martin, a 14-year-old Hispanic male, was brought for a psychiatric evaluation because of progressively worsening difficulties at school, including academic and behavioral problems. According to Martin's mother, school officials were fed up with Martin's lack of response to progressively harsher disciplinary measures. Martin was now scheduled to attend an alternative middle school, the most restrictive and structured form of special education programming. According to his mother, this was the last step the school would impose on him prior to expulsion. Martin's mother believed that her son was no longer welcome at school because he had been relentlessly provocative and didn't seem to care about the consequences of his behavior. He had earned such a poor reputation that whenever something bad happened at school, his name was at the top of the list of suspects. Martin also had a problem with stealing, and the school had pressed theft charges against him; because of the latter, he was on probation. In one of the walls of her home, Martin's mother had found a hiding place where Martin kept money he had taken from her. To complicate matters, Martin was experimenting with drugs, and his mother was unaware of the extent of his experimentation. He also was running around with troublesome peers and was failing most of his classes.

Martin continually argued with his mother about her rules. He told the examiner, "I would be better off if my mother stopped bothering me." His mother was concerned that he had become more isolated, that he stayed in his room a great deal, and that he appeared withdrawn and sad. He cried when he talked about his father's death. His father had died in a plane crash 3 years prior to the examination. Apparently, his father was an experienced pilot and was giving flying instructions at the time of his death. The circumstances of the crash were unclear and were the subject of ongoing litigation. Martin had been a marginal student before his father's death, and he and his father reportedly had a close relationship. After his father's tragic death, Martin's life began a progressive decline: he was asked to leave a private school because of poor academic achievement, and he was placed in a public school with the expectation that more psychoeducational resources would help him with his learning difficulties. Instead, his behavioral problems worsen.

Understandably, Martin's father's death had been a shocking experience for the whole family. Martin's parents had marital difficulties and had been separated prior to the accident. Martin's mother had been devastated by the accident; she struggled with the loss and had attempted to reorganize her life by going to college. She also had started working on a law degree. Martin's only sibling was his 21-year-old sister, who was married and doing well.

Martin had a limited grief reaction after his father died. His mother had complained that Martin had not cried during the funeral and that he was averse to talking about his father's death.

The examiner had evaluated Martin 6 months earlier for oppositional behaviors and limited interest in schoolwork. At that time, his symptoms were not as severe as they appeared during the new evaluation.

Martin's mother was very confused and was feeling overwhelmed by her son's problems and by his lack of response to the school's and the family's efforts. She had some unrealistic academic expectations for him and was hoping that putting Martin back in a structured private school would get him on the right path. Martin had told his mother that he wanted to quit school. At some point during the interview, Martin's mother started crying; she confessed that she feared Martin could end up in jail.

At the time of this examination, Martin and his mother displayed behaviors that had been observed during the previous assessment: Martin sat impassively and quietly, offering no comments about any of his mother's concerns. His mother cried frequently, conveying a sense of helplessness and confusion. She was puzzled over Martin's lack of any interest to change. This small adolescent's passivity, his silent opposition, and his lack of introspective capacity had struck the examiner before. After hearing about the worsening of the overall symptomatology, the examiner asked Martin's mother to leave. The examiner then made an effort to engage Martin.

Soon after beginning the individual interview, the examiner began to feel so drowsy that he had difficulty staying awake. He was aware that he was prone to experience drowsiness when 1) the clinical situation was overwhelming (hopeless) or 2) the patient was actively opposing or resisting his efforts (see Note 1 at the end of this chapter). After the examiner recognized his drowsiness, he attempted to understand and to mobilize the drowsiness to continue with the clinical reexamination. The examiner said to Martin, "You don't want to be here." Martin responded, "I'd rather be at home playing." The examiner asked, "What is your view? What is going on?" Martin said, "If only my mother were to leave me alone, everything would be okay." The examiner asked, "How come you are getting into so much trouble?" Martin said that he didn't know. There was a pause, after which Martin displayed a brief smile. The examiner wondered what had made him smile, what had gone through his mind. He said, "It was funny the way you are looking at me." Martin responded, "Maybe I am running around in circles, maybe I'm confused." The examiner praised Martin for saying this. He told Martin, "This is the most honest and positive thing you have said today."

When the examiner recognized the emerging drowsiness and began to connect it to Martin's passive-resistive behavior, his drowsiness started to clear. He began to refocus his cognitive, diagnostic, and therapeutic functions on the case. In this manner, by dealing with the overt obstacle to the examination (i.e., Martin's resistance), he was able to resolve his drowsiness and regain his optimum level of awareness. The examiner was able to proceed with this difficult examination.

Patients with obsessional personalities have difficulties communicating emotions and often display marked isolation of affect during the psychiatric examination. They evoke a variety of countertransference responses from the examiner, as illustrated in the following case example.

Case Example 2

Amy, a 15-year-old Caucasian female, was evaluated for aggressive and destructive flare-ups. She had a history of suicidal behavior at age 11 years, and before the evaluation she had overdosed on fluoxetine. Amy was intelligent and had been in the gifted and talented program at school; however, her academic performance had deteriorated during the preceding year. When Amy was 3 years old, her 8-month-old brother survived a near-drowning experience; he was comatose for 18 months and sustained severe and permanent brain damage; he continued to require intensive daily care. She was 8 years old when her parents divorced. She believed her father divorced her mother because he couldn't stand to see his "brain-damaged child." Apparently, Amy's father complained that after the accident, his wife focused so exclusively on the injured child that he and their other children were neglected. Amy had displayed some antisocial acting out during the previous year.

Amy was an attractive and articulate adolescent. She elaborated her thoughts with extreme ease, used sophisticated language, and described events with great detail. After interacting with her for a while, the examiner began to feel bored and became aware that he was not listening. The examiner realized that the patient was not expressing any emotions (the examiner considered that his boredom was a sign that the patient was not communicating affectively). Her productions were filled with rationalizations, marked isolation of affect, displacements, intellectualizations, and strong denials, common defense mechanisms in patients with strong obsessional features.

When the examiner became aware of his boredom, he began to pay closer attention to the process of Amy's communications and commented on it. He told Amy that she had problems expressing emotions. Amy responded positively to this simple intervention: the emotional tone of the interview changed. She began to place less emphasis on factual issues and began to verbalize more affect-laden communication. Her stiff posture, rapid speech, and dry tone changed; her demeanor softened; and she became more at ease and more animated. Also, the quality of her speech improved, becoming more melodious and lively.

Thereafter, the examiner emphasized questions with affective content, and Amy rose to the task; however, she sometimes reverted to affectless communication and to her circumstantial verbalizations. Amy displayed no emotion when narrating her brother's accident, her parents' divorce, or her problematic behavior. She displayed more affect when asked what kind of help she needed. She said, with lots of emotion, that she needed individual therapy and therapy with her mother. She explained that she and her mother depended too much on each other. Amy struggled with her mother around issues of control and Amy's increased need for autonomy.

The preceding case example demonstrates the constructive use of countertransference. The case also exemplifies the importance of providing feedback about the patient's communication style or communication process (see the subsection "Process Interviewing" in Chapter 2, "General Principles of Interviewing"). This approach of indicating to the patient that she had problems expressing and verbalizing emotions helped to make the interview more productive.

In the next case example, the examiner experiences anger and transforms this dystonic feeling into a therapeutic understanding.

Case Example 3

Britt, a 13-year-old Asian American female, was experiencing hallucinations and was talking about killing herself. Her school counselor called the examiner to request an emergency evaluation. The examiner experienced anger upon the impromptu request, and instead of personally evaluating Britt, whom he had seen before, he delegated the examination to a fellow trainee in child psychiatry. After the fellow examined Britt, she concluded that Britt needed to be in an acute psychiatric program. The fellow presented this recommendation to Britt and her mother. Upon hearing this, Britt began to cry and pleaded that she didn't need to be in the hospital. Her mother's demeanor was bland and passive, but she expressed concerns about Britt's fear of hospitalization. Because Britt was so distressed about the possibility of hospitalization, the fellow presented partial hospitalization as an alternative. Britt's mother remained impassive. Britt said that she wanted to see her classmates, hinting that she didn't like the partial hospitalization option either. The examiner asked the fellow to write an appropriate prescription and refer Britt for outpatient therapy. The examiner remained highly aroused with anger toward Britt's mother.

The following night at 3:00 A.M., the examiner was awakened by a call not related to Britt. After the examiner answered the call, Britt's case came to his mind. He began to explore why he was so angry at Britt's mother.

The examiner had evaluated Britt for the first time 6 months earlier for severe depression and a severe obsessive-compulsive disorder. At the time of the evaluation, Britt was experiencing auditory hallucinations commanding her to kill herself. Britt had severe school difficulties centered on profound immaturity and regressive behaviors; her classmates regularly teased and ridiculed her. Britt's mother was skeptical of her suicidal intentions and didn't give any credence to her hallucinations. Britt made allegations of physical abuse by her father and claimed that her father abused alcohol. Her mother denied these complaints.

Britt was a small, unattractive, inhibited, anxious, and immature adolescent. She displayed a regressed demeanor and a somewhat inappropriate affect. She had marked behavior inhibition and endorsed a number of compulsive features, including nail biting and compulsive eating of the skin of the knuckles of both hands. The look of her palms was remarkable: the backs of both hands had large areas of denuded skin. The examiner reflected that Britt's mother had rejected acute care or partial hospitalization options. The examiner had prescribed an antidepressant and a neuroleptic and arranged for Britt to report back a few weeks later.

When the examiner saw Britt the second time, Britt denied suicidal ideation, but she continued complaining of psychotic features and prominent obsessive-compulsive disorder and anxiety symptoms. No significant symptom changes had occurred, partly because Britt had not taken the antidepressant on a consistent basis and because her mother had refused to give her the neuroleptic. The examiner experienced irritation about the lack of compliance.

Britt's school continued to express concerns about her inappropriate behaviors. School officials had also heard Britt's complaints about her father's alcohol abuse and physically abusive behavior. When Britt's mother was presented with these allegations, she explained that these allegations were a thing of the past, that her husband had stopped drinking a number of years earlier, and that he was not physically abusive. She also reported that her husband did not believe that Britt's condition was serious or that she needed psychiatric help. Britt was seen two more times before the latest crisis.

The examiner's introspection in the middle of the night threw light on the intense anger he had felt toward Britt's mother. He was aware that he tended to respond with anger in situations of passivity and helplessness. He came to understand his anger and frustration at the mother as a response to her passivity and helplessness regarding her husband's and daughter's difficulties. The examiner recognized that Britt's mother had been hoping that her husband's alcohol abuse and physically abusive behaviors would go away. She was also hoping that Britt's symptoms were not serious and that they would go away. The examiner realized that Britt's mother had difficulties asserting herself, and this explained her passive and ineffectual behavior with her husband and her daughter.

This insight dissipated the examiner's anger. Armed with these understandings, he approached the mother in a constructive and positive manner. He made her aware of her passive and ineffectual behavior, of her wish that the problems with her husband and her daughter would go away, and of her fears of confronting her husband and her daughter. For some reason, she was afraid of asserting herself with her husband and hesitated to fight for what she felt her daughter needed. She gained an understanding of her difficulties in dealing with her husband's and daughter's problems, changed her attitude, and began to approach these difficulties in a more resolute manner.

The examiner did not direct his raw, "unmetabolized" anger at Britt's mother. Instead, he used private, introspective work to transform the anger into a therapeutic tool. The transformation of a raw feeling (i.e., anger) into a therapeutic insight helped the examiner to help Britt's mother become a more competent parent and a more effective wife.

By using subjective feelings skillfully, the interviewer learned something new and important about the patient's problems. A similar approach may be used when attempting to understand other feelings elicited during the interview (e.g., sadness, anger, sexual feelings). The examiner needs to integrate the subjective responses evoked during the psychiatric examination and make use of the understanding of these responses in configuring the patient's comprehensive diagnostic formulation.

Key Points

- *Countertransference* can be defined as any emotional state or thought process that diverts the examiner from the goal of helping the patient and his or her family in the diagnostic, prognostic and treatment planning process.
- Negative countertransference responses may occur in any psychiatric diagnostic encounter. For the most part, examiners have difficulties identifying emotional responses that have negative influences in the diagnostic evaluation, such as negative prognostications and incoherent treatment planning.
- The examiner can benefit from learning introspective approaches to gain insight and to help avoid intruding and derailing emotional states during the diagnostic and formulating process.

Notes

1. In rereading this chapter, we think now that the evocation of drowsiness by the child could also be connected to the child's father's death. By inducing sleep in the examiner, the child was enacting the father's death and his sense of abandonment. This connected to the examiner's stated responses with drowsiness when he faced situations in which he felt overwhelmed; in short, when the father died, a part of his son died too. This illuminated that the patient did not care anymore—that he was in a progressively deteriorating course, in a path of death.

Sample Format/ Protocol for Documentation of Psychiatric Evaluation of Children and Adolescents

Reprinted with permission from Clarity Child Guidance Center, San Antonio, Texas.

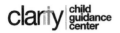

INITIAL PSYCHIATRIC ASSESSMENT

Patient Name _____

Age _____ Date _____ Time _____

B/P_____P_____HT_____WT_____T*_____

I.   **BRIEF PROBLEM FOCUSED HISTORY:**

1. Reason for Referral (Chief Complaint):

_____
_____
_____
_____

2. History of present illness (including time of onset, evolution of major symptoms, contributing medical

problems, if any)

_____
_____
_____
_____
_____
_____
_____
_____
_____
_____
_____
_____
_____
_____
_____
_____
_____
_____

#	Yes	No	Unknown		Comments
1.				Hearing Problems	
2.				Vision Problems	
3.				Headaches	
4.				Head Injury	
5.				Blackouts/Fainting	
6.				Seizures/Convulsions	
7.				EEG/ Brain Wave Test	
8.				Diabetes (Anyone in Family)	
9.				Asthma/ Breathing Problems	
10.				Serious Accident/Injury	
11.				Surgery	
12.				Congenital Defects	
13.				Female Problems/Pregnancy	
14.				Venereal Disease	
15.				Enuresis/Encopresis	
16.				GI Problems	
17.				Urinary Problems	
18.				Cardiovascular	
19.				Respiratory	
Onset Date of Menses:					
Date of last Menses					

3. Psychological Trauma:

	Current Within 2 weeks	Past Over 2 weeks	None
☐ Physical Abuse	☐	☐	☐
☐ Sexual Abuse	☐	☐	☐
☐ Emotional Abuse	☐	☐	☐
☐ Severe Childhood Neglect	☐	☐	☐
☐ Loss of Family Member/Friends	☐	☐	☐
☐ Domestic Violence	☐	☐	☐
☐ Disruption of Living Arrangement and Support	☐	☐	☐
☐ Other	☐	☐	☐

Comments: _____

4. Patient past history (including any significant medical and developmental information):

Past Medical History　　　　　**Development History**　　　　　**Social History**

_____　　　　_____　　　　_____

_____　　　　_____　　　　_____

_____　　　　_____　　　　_____

_____　　　　_____　　　　_____

_____　　　　_____　　　　_____

Legal Issues: _____

Substance Use: _____

Educational: _____

History of allergies and /or medication adverse reactions: _____

_____

5. Family psychiatric history:

_____

_____

_____

_____

_____

_____

_____

_____

6. History of any previous psychiatric/mental health treatment (or past outpatient care):

_____

_____

_____

_____

_____

7. Medications:

Current: _____   **Past:** _____

_____   _____

_____   _____

_____   _____

_____   _____

II. **PATIENT MENTAL STATUS:** **Patient's Age:** _____

A. **APPEARANCE**

    1. **Ethnicity:** ☐ Caucasian ☐ Hispanic ☐ African/American ☐ Other _____

    2. **Dress:** ☐ Casual ☐ Neat ☐ Sloppy ☐ Bizarre

    3. **Grooming:** ☐ Good ☐ Fair ☐ Poor

    4. **Hygiene:** ☐ Good ☐ Fair ☐ Poor

    5. **Age:** ☐ Appears Age ☐ Younger ☐ Older

    6. **Gait:** ☐ Normal ☐ Broad ☐ Narrow ☐ Variable

    7. **Activity level:** ☐ Increased ☐ Decreased ☐ Neither

    8.   **Speech:**

        RATE: ☐ Increased ☐ Decreased ☐ Neither Increased/Decreased ☐ Mute

        VOLUME: ☐ Increased ☐ Decreased ☐ Neither Increased/Decreased

        ARTICULATION: ☐ Good ☐ Fair ☐ Poor

        Errors in Sound Production _____ ☐ Stuttering ☐ Slurring

    9. **Anxious/Tense:** ☐ Yes ☐ No

    10. **Angry:** ☐ Yes ☐ No

B. **RELATEDNESS:**

    1. ☐ Cooperative ☐ Uncooperative ☐ Distant

    2. ☐ Friendly ☐ Unfriendly

    3. Eye contact: ☐ Good ☐ Poor

C. **MOOD AND AFFECT:**

    Mood: Angry: ☐ Mild ☐ Moderate ☐ Severe

            Depressed: ☐ Mild ☐ Moderate ☐ Severe

            Elated: ☐ Mild ☐ Moderate ☐ Severe

            ☐ Euthymic:

    Affect: ☐ Appropriate ☐ Inappropriate

           Range: ☐ Increased ☐ Decreased ☐ Neither Increased/Decreased

           Intensity: ☐ Increased ☐ Decreased ☐ Neither Increased/Decreased

D. **SENSORIUM:**

    1. Orientation: ☐ Person ☐ Place ☐ Time

    2. Memory: Age Appropriate ☐ Yes ☐ No

    3. Concentration: Age Appropriate ☐ Yes ☐ No

E. **INTELLECTUAL FUNCTION:**

    ☐ Average ☐ Above Average ☐ Below Average

    Based on:

    ☐ Vocabulary ☐ Complexity of concepts

F.   THOUGHT:

1. Coherent: ☐ Yes   ☐ No
2. Logical: ☐ Yes   ☐ No
3. Goal Directed: ☐ Yes   ☐ No
4. Responses to Similarities: ☐ Abstract   ☐ Concrete
5. Flight of Ideas: ☐ Yes   ☐ No
6. Looseness of Association ☐ Yes   ☐ No
7. Obsessive Thoughts: ☐ Yes   ☐ No

Content if yes_____

_____

8. Hallucinations: ☐ Yes   ☐ No

Content if yes_____

_____

9. Delusions: ☐ Yes   ☐ No

Content if yes: _____

_____

10. Suicidal thoughts: ☐ Yes   ☐ No

Content if yes: _____

_____

11. Suicidal plans: ☐ Yes   ☐ No

Content if yes: _____

_____

12. Homicidal thoughts: ☐ Yes   ☐ No

Content if yes: _____

_____

13. Judgment: ☐ Good   ☐ Fair ☐ Poor
14. Insight: ☐ Good   ☐ Fair ☐ Poor
15. Superego Functioning: ☐ Good   ☐ Fair   ☐ Poor

III.   SUICIDE RISK ASSESSMENT

Circle each item based on information already assessed. Do ask question of parent/child if factor has already been assessed, but assess any items that you do not have data on.

RISK FACTOR	LOW RISK	MILD RISK	MODERATE RISK	SERIOUS RISK
Score	0	1	2	3
Gender	Female		Male	
Age	1–14 years		15–19 years	
Family History of Suicide	None	Suicide > | 3 years ago	Suicide 1 to 3 years ago	Suicide in past 12 months
History of Attempts	None	Attempt > 3 years ago	Attempt 1 to 3 years ago	Attempt in past 12 months
Lethality of Most Recent Attempt	No attempt or ideation only	Gesture	Non-lethal	Lethal or potentially lethal
Intent	No intent to die	Minimal intent	Moderate intent	Clear intent
Support System	Good	Minimal	Conflicted	None
Loss or Trauma in Last 6 Months	None	Moderate	Serious	Multiple
Impulsiveness/Aggression	None	Mild	Moderate	Severe
Substance Abuse	None	Recreational	Abuse	Dependence
Hopelessness	Hopeful	Some hope	Ambivalent	Hopeless

TOTAL SCORE:_____

If Suicide Risk Assessment score > 12, document precautions in the Admission Orders.

MITIGATING FACTORS FOR SUICIDE RISK

Yes	No	Unknown	Easy access to a variety of clinical interventions and support for help seeking
Yes	No	Unknown	Family and community support (connectedness)
Yes	No	Unknown	Supportive school relationships/involvement
Yes	No	Unknown	Support from ongoing mental health and/or medical care relationships
Yes	No	Unknown	Skills in problem solving, conflict resolution, and nonviolent ways of handling disputes
Yes	No	Unknown	Cultural and/or religious beliefs that discourage suicide and support instincts for self-preservation
Yes	No	Unknown	Other:
Yes	No	Unknown	Other:

IV.   **RISK FACTORS:**

		Current	Past	None
Physical Abuse		☐	☐	☐
Sexual Abuse		☐	☐	☐
Neuropsychiatric Deficits		☐	☐	☐
Runaway		☐	☐	☐
Sexual Behaviors		☐	☐	☐
Suicidal		☐	☐	☐
Violence risk to others	**(Within 6 months)**	☐	☐	☐
Violence risk to self	**(Within 6 months)**	☐	☐	☐
Sexually Transmitted Diseases		☐	☐	☐
Gangs or Arrests		☐	☐	☐
Substance Abuse		☐	☐	☐
History of psychiatric hospitalizations		☐	☐	☐
History of family psychiatric Illness		☐	☐	☐

If yes is indicated in risk factors, please comment if information is not in the history section.

_____

_____

_____

_____

_____

_____

_____

_____

_____

_____

V.   DIAGNOSTIC FORMULATION

	PREDISPOSING	PERPETUATING	PRECIPITATING	PROTECTIVE
BIO				
PSYCHO				
SOCIAL				

TREATMENT FOCUS FOR THIS INPATIENT STAY (Summary of Formulation)

_____
_____
_____
_____
_____
_____
_____
_____

PROGNOSIS_____
_____
_____
_____

VI.   DIAGNOSIS

AXIS I: (Primary)_____; _____;

_____; _____;

_____; _____;

AXIS II: _____; _____;

AXIS III: _____; _____;

AXIS IV:

☐ Problems with primary support groups _____

☐ Problems related to the social environment _____

☐ Educational problem _____

☐ Housing problems _____

☐ Economic problems _____

☐ Problems with access to health care services _____

☐ Problems related to interaction with the legal system/crime _____

☐ Other psychosocial and environmental problems _____

AXIS V. GAF: Present: _____   Highest past Year_____

Plan:
1. Reviewed prior records   ☐ Yes   ☐ No
2. Obtained collateral information   ☐ Yes   ☐ No
3. Labs   ☐ Yes   ☐ No
4. Other: _____
5. Medications:

Name	Dose	Target	Symptom

VII. **REASON FOR ADMISSION** (check all that are applicable):

- ☐ Suicidal risk
- ☐ Self-mutilative risk
- ☐ Hallucinations or delusions directing person to harm themselves
- ☐ Agitation or psychomotor retardation resulting in an inability to care for self
- ☐ Inability to comply with prescribed medical health regimens due to concurrent psychiatric illness and failure to comply is potentially hazardous to the life of the person.
- ☐ Severe eating disorder which requires 24 hours a day medical observation, supervision, and intervention.
- ☐ Severe substance abuse disorder, which requires 24 hours a day medical observation, supervision, and intervention.
- ☐ Evaluation and treatment cannot be carried out safely or effectively in a less restrictive setting because of severely disruptive behaviors and other behaviors which may include runaway behavior, placing the person at risk, and physical, sexual or psychological abuse.
- ☐ Homicidal risk.
- ☐ Risk of assaultive behavior.
- ☐ Hallucinations or delusions directing the person to harm others.
- ☐ Acute onset or psychosis or clinical deterioration in someone with a chronic psychosis rendering the person unmanageable and the person is in need of assessment and treatment in a safe and therapeutic setting.
- ☐ Proposed treatment or therapy requires 24 hours a day medical supervision and treatment.
- ☐ The individual requires medication therapy or complex diagnostic evaluation where the person's level of functioning prevents cooperation with treatment.
- ☐ The person, because of psychiatric symptoms, is ordered by the court to undergo assessment and treatment in a hospital.
- ☐ Other: _____

VIII. **PATIENT and FAMILY EDUCATION:**

The following have been reviewed with the patient and guardian:

	PATIENT			FAMILY		
Reason for Hospitalization	☐Yes	☐No	☐NA	☐Yes	☐No	☐NA
Diagnosis	☐Yes	☐No	☐NA	☐Yes	☐No	☐NA
Risks of Hospitalization	☐Yes	☐No	☐NA	☐Yes	☐No	☐NA
Discharge Goals	☐Yes	☐No	☐NA	☐Yes	☐No	☐NA
Initial Plan of Care	☐Yes	☐No	☐NA	☐Yes	☐No	☐NA

Physician Signature: _____ Date/Time: _____

Printed name: _____ M. D.

Physician Signature: _____ Date/Time: _____

Printed name: _____ M. D

Bibliography

Ablon SL: The therapeutic action of play. J Am Acad Child Adolesc Psychiatry 35(4):545–547, 1996 8919718

Achenbach TM: Clinical data systems: rating scales and interviews, in Psychiatry, Revised Edition, Vol 2. Edited by Michels R, Cooper AM, Guze SB, et al. Philadelphia, PA, Lippincott-Raven, 1995, pp 1–14

Achenbach TM: Assessment, diagnosis, nosology, an taxonomy of child and adolescent psychopathology, in Handbook of Clinical Psychology, Vol 2: Children and Adolescents. Edited by Hersen M, Gross AM. New York, Wiley, 2008, pp 429–457

Aggarwal R, Guanci N, Appareddy VL: Issues in treating patients with intellectual disabilities. Psychiatric Times, August 14, 2013, pp 9–13

Akiskal HS: Developmental pathways to bipolarity: are juvenile-onset depressions pre-bipolar? J Am Acad Child Adolesc Psychiatry 34(6):754–763, 1995 7608049

Akiskal HS, Akiskal K: Mental status examination: the art and science of the clinical interview, in Diagnostic Interviewing, 2nd Edition. Edited by Hersen M, Turner SM. New York, Plenum, 1994, pp 25–51

Akiskal HS, Puzantian VR: Psychotic forms of depression and mania. Psychiatr Clin North Am 2:419–439, 1979

Allen JG: The spectrum of accuracy in memories of childhood trauma. Harv Rev Psychiatry 3(2):84–95, 1995 9384933

American Psychiatric Association: Diagnostic and Statistical Manual of Mental Disorders, 4th Edition. Washington, DC, American Psychiatric Association, 1994

American Psychiatric Association: Diagnostic and Statistical Manual of Mental Disorders, 4th Edition. Washington, DC, American Psychiatric Association, 2000

American Psychiatric Association: Diagnostic and Statistical Manual of Mental Disorders, 5th Edition. Arlington, VA, American Psychiatric Association, 2013

Anderson SC: Effects of confrontation by high- and low-functioning therapists. J Couns Psychol 15:411–416, 1968

Digits at the end of journal articles are PubMed ID numbers.

Angold A: Clinical interviewing with children and adolescents, in Child and Adolescent Psychiatry: Modern Approaches. Edited by Rutter M, Taylor E, Hersov L. Oxford, England, Blackwell Scientific, 1994, pp 51–63

Armando M, Pontillo M, Vicari S: Psychosocial interventions for very early and early onset schizophrenia: a review of treatment efficacy. Curr Opin Psychiatry 28(4):312–323, 2015 26001923

Asarnow JR, Baraff LJ, Berk M, et al: Pediatric emergency department suicidal patients: two-site evaluation of suicide ideators, single attempters, and repeat attempters. J Am Acad Child Adolesc Psychiatry 47(8):958–966, 2008 18596552

Ash P: Children and adolescents, in Textbook of Violence Assessment and Management. Edited by Simon RI, Tardiff K. Washington, DC, American Psychiatric Publishing, 2008, pp 359–380

Asher SR, Erdley C, Gabriel SW: Peer relations, in Development Through Life: A Handbook for Clinicians. Edited by Rutter M, Hay DF. Oxford, England, Blackwell Scientific, 1994, pp 456–487

Axelson D, Goldstein B, Goldstein T, et al: Diagnostic precursors to bipolar disorder in offspring of parents with bipolar disorder: a longitudinal study. Am J Psychiatry 172(7):638–646, 2015 25734353

Bacciagaluppi M: The relevance of attachment research to psychoanalysis and analytic social psychology. J Am Acad Psychoanal 22(3):465–479, 1994 7844022

Bark C, Resch F: Neurobiology of depression in childhood and adolescence, in Biological Child Psychiatry: Recent Trends and Developments. Edited by Banaschewski T, Rohde LA. Basel, Switzerland, S Karger, 2008, pp 53–81

Barker ED, Arseneault L, Brendgen M, et al: Joint development of bullying and victimization in adolescence: relations to delinquency and self-harm. J Am Acad Child Adolesc Psychiatry 47(9):1030–1038, 2008 18665001

Barkley RA: ADHD and the Nature of Self-Control. New York, Guilford, 1997

Barkley RA: Etiologies of ADHD, in Attention-Deficit Hyperactivity Disorder: A Handbook for Diagnosis and Treatment, 4th Edition. Edited by Barkley RA. New York, Guilford, 2015, pp 356–390

BBCnewsbeat: Amanda Todd: memorial for teenage cyberbullying victim. October 17, 2012. Available at http://www.bbc.co.uk/newsbeat/article/19960162/amanda-todd-memorial-for-teenage-cyberbullying-victim. Accessed February 7, 2016.

Beauchaine TP, Hong J, Marsh P: Sex differences in autonomic correlates of conduct problems and aggression. J Am Acad Child Adolesc Psychiatry 47(7):788–796, 2008 18520959

Bedi G, Carrillo F, Cecchi GA, et al: Automated analysis of free speech predicts psychosis onset in high-risk youth. NPJ Schizophrenia, published online August 26, 2015. doi:10.1038/npjschz.2015.30

Belluck P: Panel urges screening for maternal depression. New York Times, Jan 27, 2016, A1, 13

Belsky J, Cassidy J: Attachment theory and evidence, in Development Through Life: A Handbook for Clinicians. Edited by Rutter M, Hay DF. Oxford, England, Blackwell Scientific, 1994, pp 373–402

Belson K: As worries rise and players flee, a Missouri school board cuts football. New York Times, September 28, 2015, B11

Ben Zeev Ghidoni B: Rett syndrome. Child Adolesc Psychiatr Clin N Am 16(3):723–743, 2007 17562589

Benedek EP, Schetky DH: Problems in validating allegations of sexual abuse. Part 1: factors affecting perception and recall of events. J Am Acad Child Adolesc Psychiatry 26(6):912–915, 1987a 3429411

Benedek EP, Schetky DH: Problems in validating allegations of sexual abuse. Part 2: clinical evaluation. J Am Acad Child Adolesc Psychiatry 26(6):916–921, 1987b 3429412

Benjamin S, Lauterbach MD, Stanislawski AL: Congenital and acquired disorders presenting as psychosis in children and young adults. Child Adolesc Psychiatr Clin N Am 22(4):581–608, 2013 24012075

Bennet TL, Dittmar C, Ho MR: The neuropsychology of traumatic brain injury, in The Neuropsychology Handbook, 2nd Edition, Vol 2. Edited by Horton AM, Wedding D, Webster J. New York, Springer, 1997, pp 123–172

Berkelhammer LD: Pediatric neuropsychological evaluation, in Handbook of Clinical Psychology, Vol 2: Children and Adolescents. Edited by Hersen M, Gross AM. New York, Wiley, 2008, pp 497–519

Berman AL, Carroll TA: Adolescent suicide: a critical review. Death Educ 8(1):53–63, 1984

Bernet W: False statements and the differential diagnosis of abuse allegations. J Am Acad Child Adolesc Psychiatry 32(5):903–910, 1993 8407762

Bernstein GA, Borchardt CM, Perwien AR: Anxiety disorders in children and adolescents: a review of the past 10 years. J Am Acad Child Adolesc Psychiatry 35(9):1110–1119, 1996 8824054

Berthelot N, Ensink K, Bernazzani O, et al: Intergenerational transmission of attachment in abused and neglected mothers: the role of trauma-specific reflective functioning. Infant Ment Health J 36(2):200–212, 2015 25694333

Biederman J, Faraone S, Mick E, et al: Attention-deficit hyperactivity disorder and juvenile mania: an overlooked comorbidity? J Am Acad Child Adolesc Psychiatry 35(8):997–1008, 1996 8755796

Biederman J, Ball SW, Monuteaux MC, et al: New insights into the comorbidity between ADHD and major depression in adolescent and young adult females. J Am Acad Child Adolesc Psychiatry 47(4):426–434, 2008 18388760

Birmaher B, Williams DT: Acquired brain disorders, in Child and Adolescent Psychiatry: A Comprehensive Textbook, 2nd Edition. Edited by Lewis M. Baltimore, MD, Williams & Wilkins, 1996, pp 363–374

Bishop DVM: Speech and language difficulties, in Child and Adolescent Psychiatry: Modern Approaches, 4th Edition. Edited by Rutter M, Taylor E. Oxford, England, Blackwell Scientific, 2002, pp 664–681

Black B, Uhde TW: Psychiatric characteristics of children with selective mutism: a pilot study. J Am Acad Child Adolesc Psychiatry 34(7):847–856, 1995 7649954

Blader JC, Pliszka SR, Kafantaris V, et al: Prevalence and treatment outcomes of persistent negative mood among children with attention-deficit/hyperactivity disorder and aggressive behavior. J Child Adolesc Psychopharmacol 26(2):164–173, 2016 26745211

Blair RJR: The neurobiology of aggression, in Neurobiology of Mental Illness, 3rd Edition. Edited by Charney DS, Nestler EJ. New York, Oxford University Press, 2009, pp 1307–1320

Blazei RW, Iacono WG, McGue M: Father-child transmission of antisocial behavior: the moderating role of father's presence in the home. J Am Acad Child Adolesc Psychiatry 47(4):406–415, 2008 18388763

Boomsma DI, van Beijsterveldt CEM, Bartels M, et al: Genetic and environmental influences on anxious/depression: a longitudinal study in 3- to 12-year-old children, in Developmental Psychopathology and Wellness: Genetic and Environmental Influences. Edited by Hudziak JJ, Washington, DC, American Psychiatric Publishing, 2008, pp 161–189

Boothby N: Political violence and development: an ecologic approach to children in war zones. Child Adolesc Psychiatr Clin N Am 17(3):497–514, vii, 2008 18558309

Borelli JL, West JL, Decoste C, et al: Emotionally avoidant language in the parenting interviews of substance-dependent mothers: associations with reflective functioning, recent substance use, and parenting behavior. Infant Ment Health J 33(5):506–519, 2012 23049148

Borum R, Bartel PA, Forth AE (eds): Structured Assessment of Violence Risk in Youth. New York, Guilford, 2005

Bowden CL, Rhodes L: Mania in children and adolescents: recognition and treatment. Psychiatr Ann 26(7):S430–S434, 1996

Bowlby J: Attachment and Loss, Vol 1: Attachment. New York, Basic Books, 1969

Braungart-Rieker JM, Zentall S, Lickenbrock DM, et al: Attachment in the making: mother and father sensitivity and infants' responses during the Still-Face Paradigm. J Exp Child Psychol 125:63–84, 2014 24833270

Brent D, Maalouf F: Depressive disorders in childhood and adolescence, in Rutter's Child and Adolescent Psychiatry, 6th Edition. Edited by Thapar A, Pine DS, Leckman JF, et al. New York, Wiley Blackwell, 2015, pp 874–892

Brent DA, Melhem NM, Oquendo M, et al: Familial pathways to early onset suicide attempt: a 5.6-year prospective study. JAMA Psychiatry 72(2):160–168, 2015 25548996

Bridge JA, Greenhouse JB, Weldon AH, et al: Suicide trends among youths aged 10 to 19 years in the United States, 1996–2005 (editorial). JAMA 300(9):1025–1026, 2008 18768413

Brotman MA, Guyer AE, Lawson ES, et al: Facial emotion labeling deficits in children and adolescents at risk for bipolar disorder. Am J Psychiatry 165(3):385–389, 2008 18245180

Brown GW, Rutter M: The measurements of family activities and relationships: a methodological study. Hum Relat 2(3 suppl):241–263, 1996

Bruck M, Ceci SJ: Children's testimony: a scientific framework for evaluating the reliability of children's statements, in Rutter's Child and Adolescent Psychiatry, 6th Edition. Edited by Thapar A, Pine DS, Leckman JF, et al. New York, Wiley Blackwell, 2015, pp 250–260

Bureau JF, Yurkowski K, Schmiedel S, et al: Making children laugh: parent-child dyadic synchrony and preschool attachment. Infant Ment Health J 35(5):482–494, 2014 25798498

Burns CD, Cortell R, Wagner BM: Treatment compliance in adolescents after attempted suicide: a 2-year follow-up study. J Am Acad Child Adolesc Psychiatry 47(8):948–957, 2008 18596554

Burrous CE, Crockenberg SC, Leerkes EM: Developmental history of care and control, depression and anger: correlates of maternal sensitivity in toddlerhood. Infant Ment Health J 30(2):103–123, 2009

Calof D: Chronic self-injury in adult survivors of childhood abuse: sources, motivations, and functions of self-injury (part I). Treating Abuse Today 5(3):11–17, 1995a

Calof D: Chronic self-injury in adult survivors of childhood abuse: sources, motivations, and functions of self-injury (part II). Treating Abuse Today 5(4/5):31–36, 1995b

Cantwell DP: Attention deficit disorder: a review of the past 10 years. J Am Acad Child Adolesc Psychiatry 35(8):978–987, 1996 8755794

Caplan R: Thought disorder in childhood. J Am Acad Child Adolesc Psychiatry 33(5):605–615, 1994 8056724

Carey B: Scientists home in on cause of schizophrenia: study finds 'pruning' of brain synapses go awry. The New York Times, Jan 28, 2016, pp 1, A18

Carlson GA: Child and adolescent mania—diagnostic considerations. J Child Psychol Psychiatry 31(3):331–341, 1990 2180969

Carlson GA: Affective disorders and psychosis in youth. Child Adolesc Psychiatr Clin N Am 22(4):569–580, 2013 24012074

Carlson GA, Youngstrom EA: Clinical implications of pervasive manic symptoms in children. Biol Psychiatry 53(11):1050–1058, 2003 12788250

Castle DJ: Bipolar mixed states: still mixed up? Curr Opin Psychiatry 27(1):38–42, 2014 24270474

Centers for Disease Control and Prevention, National Center for Injury Prevention and Control: 10 Leading Causes of Death by Age Group, United States—2013. Atlanta, GA, National Center for Injury Prevention and Control, Centers for Disease Control and Prevention, 2016. Available at: http://www.cdc.gov/injury/wisqars/pdf/leading_causes_of_death_by_age_group_2013-a.pdf. Accessed February 7, 2016.

Cepeda C: Psychotic Symptoms in Children and Adolescents: Assessment, Differential Diagnoses and Treatment. New York, Routledge Taylor and Francis, 2007

Cepeda C: Clinical Manual for the Psychiatric Interview of Children and Adolescents: General Principles of Interviewing. Washington, DC, American Psychiatric Publishing, 2010

Charman T, Hood JK, Howlin P: Psychological assessment in the clinical context, in Rutter's Child and Adolescent Psychiatry, 6th Edition. Edited by Thapar A, Pine DS, Leckman JF, et al. New York, Wiley-Blackwell, 2015, pp 436–448

Cicchetti D, Toth SL: A developmental psychopathology perspective on child abuse and neglect. J Am Acad Child Adolesc Psychiatry 34(5):541–565, 1995 7775351

Clegg J, Gillott A, Jones J: Conceptual issues in neurodevelopmental disorders: lives out of synch. Curr Opin Psychiatry 26(3):289–294, 2013 23519204

Cloninger CR: A systematic method for clinical description and classification of personality variants. A proposal. Arch Gen Psychiatry 44(6):573–588, 1987 3579504

Cloninger CR, Adolfsson R, Svrakic NM: Mapping genes for human personality. Nat Genet 12(1):3–4, 1996 8528246

Cohen JA: Helping adolescents affected by war, trauma, and displacement (editorial). J Am Acad Child Adolesc Psychiatry 47(9):981–982, 2008 18714193

Cohen NJ, Horodezky NB: Language impairments and psychopathology (letter). J Am Acad Child Adolesc Psychiatry 37(5):461–462, 1998 9585644

Cohen R: Case formulation and treatment planning, in Basic Handbook of Child Psychiatry, Vol 1. Edited by Noshpitz JD, Berlin IN. New York, Basic Books, 1979, pp 633–640

Coleman L: Medical examination for sexual abuse: have we been misled? The Champion, November 1989, pp 5–12

Confidentiality of alcohol and drug abuse patient records, 2005, 42 CFR 2.14

Cook EH, Leventhal BL: Neuropsychiatric disorders of childhood and adolescence, in Textbook of Neuropsychiatry, 2nd Edition. Edited by Yudofsky SC, Hales RE. Washington, DC, American Psychiatric Press, 1992, pp 639–661

Cornblatt BA, Carrión RE, Auther A, et al: Psychosis prevention: a modified clinical high-risk perspective from the recognition and prevention (RAP) program. Am J Psychiatry 172(10):986–994, 2015 26046336

Costello AJ: Structured interviewing, in Child and Adolescent Psychiatry: A Comprehensive Textbook. Edited by Lewis M. Baltimore, MD, Williams & Wilkins, 1996, pp 457–464

Cox AD: Diagnostic appraisal, in Child and Adolescent Psychiatry: Modern Approaches. Edited by Rutter M, Taylor E, Hersov L. Oxford, England, Blackwell Scientific, 1994, pp 22–33

Cox A, Hopkinson K, Rutter M: Psychiatric interviewing techniques, II. Naturalistic study: eliciting factual information. Br J Psychiatry 138:283–291, 1981a 7272628

Cox A, Rutter M, Holbrook D: Psychiatric interviewing techniques, V. Experimental study: eliciting factual information. Br J Psychiatry 139:29–37, 1981b 7296187

Cox JL, Holden JM, Sagovsky R: Detection of postnatal depression. Development of the 10-item Edinburgh Postnatal Depression Scale. Br J Psychiatry 150:782–786, 1987

Crowley TJ, Sakai JT: Substance related and addictive disorders, in Rutter's Child and Adolescent Psychiatry, 6th Edition. Edited by Thapar A, Pine DS, Leckman JF, et al. New York, Wiley Blackwell, 2015, pp 931–949

Cummings J: Neuropsychiatry, in Manual of Psychiatric Disorders. Edited by Simpson GM. New York, Impact Communications, 1995a, pp 109–136

Cummings J: Neuropsychiatry: clinical assessment and approach to diagnosis, in Comprehensive Textbook of Psychiatry, Vol 1, 6th Edition. Edited by Kaplan HI, Sadock BJ. Baltimore, MD, Williams & Wilkins, 1995b, pp 167–187

Cvejic M: Sleep disorders in infants and children, in Mayo Clinical Neurology Board Review. Clinical Neurology for Initial Certification and MOC. Edited by Flemming KD, Jones LK. Rochester, MN, Mayo Clinic Scientific Press, 2015, pp 819–823

David DH, Gelberg L, Suchman NE: Implications of homelessness for parenting young children: a preliminary review from a developmental attachment perspective. Infant Ment Health J 33(1):1–9, 2012 22685362

Debnath M, Venkatasubramanian G: Recent advances in psychoneuroimmunology relevant to schizophrenia therapeutics. Curr Opin Psychiatry 26(5):433–439, 2013 23867655

Denckla MB: The neurobehavioral examination in children, in Behavioral Neurology and Neuropsychology. Edited by Feinberg TE, Farah MJ. New York, McGraw-Hill, 1997, pp 721–728

Dennis M: Acquired disorders of language in children, in Behavioral Neurology and Neuropsychology. Edited by Feinberg TE, Farah MJ. New York, McGraw-Hill, 1997, pp 737–754

Di Leo JH: Children's Drawings as Diagnostic Aids. New York, Brunner/Mazel, 1973

Dickstein DP: The path to somewhere: moving toward a better biological understanding of irritability (editorial). Am J Psychiatry 172(7):603–605, 2015 26130199

Dickstein DP: Mechanisms distinguishing irritability in children and adolescents (editorial). Am J Psychiatry 173(7):653–654, 2016 27363546

Dolan M: Neurobiological disturbances in callous-unemotional youths (editorial). Am J Psychiatry 165(6):668–670, 2008 18519530

Egger HL: Psychiatric assessment of young children. Child Adolesc Psychiatr Clin N Am 18(3):559–580, 2009 19486838

Espelage DL, Holt MK: Suicidal ideation and school bullying experiences after controlling for depression and delinquency. J Adolesc Health 53(1 suppl):S27–S31, 2013 23790197

Famularo R, Stone K, Popper C: Preadolescent alcohol abuse and dependency. Am J Psychiatry 142:1187–1189, 1985

Faraone SV, Biederman J, Weber W, et al: Psychiatric, neuropsychological, and psychosocial features of DSM-IV subtypes of attention-deficit/hyperactivity disorder: results from a clinically referred sample. J Am Acad Child Adolesc Psychiatry 37(2):185–193, 1998 9473915

Feinstein C, Singh S: Social phenotypes in neurogenetic syndromes. Child Adolesc Psychiatr Clin N Am 16(3):631–647, 2007 17562583

Fenichel GM: Clinical Pediatric Neurology: A Signs and Symptoms Approach, 5th Edition. Philadelphia, PA, Elsevier Saunders, 2005

Fisher PW, Chin EM, Vidair HB: Use of structured interviews, rating scales, and observational methods in clinical settings, in Rutter's Child and Adolescent Psychiatry, 6th Edition. Edited by Thapar A, Pine DS, Leckman JF et al. New York, Wiley-Blackwell, 2015, pp 419–435

Fitzgerald PA: Endocrine disorders, in Current Medical Diagnosis and Treatment, 54th Edition. Edited by Papadakis MA, McPhee SJ. McGraw Hill Education, 2015, pp 1081–1183

Flanagan EP: Nondegenerative dementias and encephalopathies, in Mayo Clinic Neurology Board Review. Clinical Neurology for Initial Certification and MOC. Edited by Flemming K, Jones L. Rochester, MN, Mayo Clinic Scientific Press, 2015, pp 299–310

Fleitlich-Bilyk B, Lock J: Eating disorders, in Biological Child Psychiatry: Recent Trends and Developments. Edited by Banaschewski T, Rohde LA. Basel, Switzerland, S Karger, 2008, pp 138–152

Flouri E, Kallis C: Adverse life events and psychopathology and prosocial behavior in late adolescence: testing the timing, specificity, accumulation, gradient, and moderation of contextual risk. J Am Acad Child Adolesc Psychiatry 46(12):1651–1659, 2007 18030087

Flykt M, Punamäki R, Belt R, et al: Maternal representations and emotional availability among drug-abusing and nonusing mothers and their infants. Infant Ment Health J 33(2):123–138, 2012

Forth AE, Kosson D, Hare RD: The Hare PCL: Youth Version. Toronto, ON, Multi-Health Systems, 2003

Frankel FH: Dissociation: the clinical realities. Am J Psychiatry 153(7 suppl):64–70, 1996

Foss-Feig J, MacPartland JC: Autism spectrum disorders and psychiatry: update on diagnosis and treatment considerations. Psychiatr Times 33(6):41–44, 2016

Frazier Norbury C, Paul R: Disorders of speech, language, and communication (Chapter 52), in Rutter's Child and Adolescent Psychiatry, 6th Edition. Edited by Thapar A, Pine DS, Leckman JF, et al. London, Wiley Blackwell, 2015, pp 683–699

Freeman AJ, Youngstrom EA, Youngstrom JK, et al: Disruptive mood dysregulation disorder in a community mental health clinic: prevalence, comorbidity and correlates. J Child Adolesc Psychopharmacol 26(2):123–130, 2016 26745325

Freud A: The concept of developmental lines (1965), in An Anthology of the Psychoanalytic Study of the Child. Edited by Eissler RS, Freud A, Kris M, et al. New Haven, CT, Yale University, 1977, pp 11–30

Freud A: Child analysis as the study of mental growth (normal and abnormal) (1979), in The Course of Life: Psychoanalytic Contributions Towards Understanding Personality Development, Vol 1: Infancy and Early Childhood. Edited by Greenspan SI, Pollock GH. Bethesda, MD, Mental Health Study Center, National Institute of Mental Health, 1980, pp 1–10

Freud S: The Ego and the Id (1923), in The Standard Edition of the Complete Psychological Works of Sigmund Freud, Vol 19. Translated and edited by Strachey J. London, Hogarth, 1962, pp 3–66

Fuller D: The AMSIT (student handout). San Antonio, TX, University of Texas Health Science Center at San Antonio, Department of Psychiatry, 1998

Galanter CA, Leibenluft E: Frontiers between attention deficit hyperactivity disorder and bipolar disorder. Child Adolesc Psychiatr Clin N Am 17(2):325–346, viii–ix, 2008 18295149

Galdiolo S, Roskam I: From me to us: the construction of family alliance. Infant Ment Health J 37(1):29–44, 2016 26715070

Garralda ME: Hallucinations in children with conduct and emotional disorders: I. The clinical phenomena. Psychol Med 14(3):589–596, 1984a 6494367

Garralda ME: Hallucinations in children with conduct and emotional disorders: II. The follow-up study. Psychol Med 14(3):597–604, 1984b 6494368

Geller B, Luby J: Child and adolescent bipolar disorder: a review of the past 10 years. J Am Acad Child Adolesc Psychiatry 36(9):1168–1176, 1997 9291717

Geller B, Luby J: Mania in young children (letter). J Am Acad Child Adolesc Psychiatry 37(10):1005, 1998

Ghuman JK, Arnold LE, Anthony BJ: Psychopharmacological and other treatments in preschool children with attention-deficit/hyperactivity disorder: current evidence and practice, in Advances in Preschool Psychopharmacology. Edited by Luby JL, Riddle MA. New Rochelle, NY, Mary Ann Liebert, 2009, pp 221–261

Gillberg C: Epidemiology of early onset schizophrenia, in Schizophrenia in Children and Adolescents. Edited by Remschmidt H. Cambridge, United Kingdom, Cambridge University Press, 2001, pp 43–59

Glaser D: Child sexual abuse (Chapter 30), in Rutter's Child and Adolescent Psychiatry, 6th Edition. Edited by Thapar A, Pine DS, Leckman JF, et al. London, Wiley Blackwell, 2015, pp 376–388

Gold AP: Evaluation and diagnosis by inspection, in Child and Adolescent Neurology for Psychiatrists. Edited by Kaufman DM, Solomon GE, Pfeffer CR. Baltimore, MD, Williams & Wilkins, 1992, pp 1–12

Goodman GS, Saywitz KJ: Memories of abuse: interviewing children when sexual victimization is suspected. Child Adolesc Psychiatr Clin N Am 4:645–661, 1994

Goodman R: Brain disorders, in Child and Adolescent Psychiatry: Modern Approaches. Edited by Rutter M, Taylor E, Hersov L. Oxford, England, Blackwell Scientific, 1994, pp 172–190

Goodwin FK, Jamison KR: Childhood and adolescence, in Manic-Depressive Illness. Edited by Goodwin FK, Jamison KR. New York, Oxford University Press, 1990, pp 186–209

Goodwin FK, Jamison KR: Manic-Depressive Illness: Bipolar Disorders and Recurrent Depression, 2nd Edition. New York, Oxford University Press, 2007

Goodyer IM: Depression in childhood and adolescence, in Handbook of Affective Disorders, 2nd Edition. Edited by Paykel ES. New York, Guilford, 1992, pp 585–600

Gothelf D: Preface: neuropsychiatric genetic syndromes. Child Adolesc Psychiatr Clin N Am 16(special issue):xvii–xx, 2007

Gottschalk MG, Domschke K: Novel developments in genetic and epigenetic mechanisms of anxiety. Curr Opin Psychiatry 29(1):32–38, 2016 26575296

Grados MA: The neurobiological basis of anxiety in children and adolescents, in Biological Child Psychiatry: Recent Trends and Developments. Edited by Banaschewski T, Rohde LA. Basel, Switzerland, S Karger, 2008, pp 67–81

Grados MA, Riddle MA: Two times four is four: OCD dimensions, classes, and categories. J Am Acad Child Adolesc Psychiatry 47(7):731–733, 2008 18574396

Grafman J, Rickard T: Acalculia, in Behavioral Neurology and Neuropsychology. Edited by Feinberg TE, Farah MJ. New York, McGraw-Hill, 1997, pp 219–225

Green AH: Child sexual abuse: immediate and long-term effects and intervention. J Am Acad Child Adolesc Psychiatry 32(5):890–902, 1993 8407761

Grills-Taquechel A, Ollendick TH: Diagnostic interviewing, in Handbook of Clinical Psychology, Vol 2: Children and Adolescents. Edited by Hersen M, Gross AM. New York, Wiley, 2008, pp 458–479

Groopman J: How Doctors Think. Boston, Houghton Mifflin, 2007

Gunlicks ML, Weissman MM: Change in child psychopathology with improvement in parental depression: a systematic review. J Am Acad Child Adolesc Psychiatry 47(4):379–389, 2008 18388766

Guy W: Physical and Neurological Examination for Soft Signs, in ECDEU Assessment Manual for Psychopharmacology (Revised). DHEW Publ No ADM-76-338. Rockville, MD, U.S. Department of Health, Education, and Welfare, Public Health Service, Alcohol, Drug Abuse, and Mental Health Administration, 1976, pp 383–406

Hagerman RJ, Narcisa V, Hagerman PJ: Fragil X: a molecular and treatment model for autism spectrum disorder, in Autism Spectrum Disorder. Edited by Amaral DG, Dawson G, and Geschwind DH. New York, Oxford University Press, 2011, pp 801–824

Hajek T, McIntyre R, Alda M: Bipolar disorders, type 2 diabetes mellitus, and the brain. Curr Opin Psychiatry 29(1):1–6, 2016 26575297

Harris JC: Developmental Neuropsychiatry: Assessment, Diagnosis, and Treatment of Developmental Disorders, Vol 2. New York, Oxford University Press, 1995a

Harris JC: Memory, in Developmental Neuropsychiatry Fundamentals, Vol 1. New York, Oxford University Press, 1995b, pp 138–153

Hartlage LC, Williams BL: Pediatric neuropsychology, in The Neuropsychology Handbook, Vol 2, 2nd Edition. Edited by Horton AM, Wedding D, Webster J. New York, Springer, 1997, pp 211–235

Health Insurance Portability and Accountability Act of 1996 (HIPAA; Pub.L. 104–191, 110 Stat. 1936, enacted August 21, 1996)

Hechtman L: ADHD and bipolar disorder. ADHD Rep 7(2):1–4, 1999

Heim C, Shugart M, Graighead WE, et al: Neurobiological and psychiatric consequences of child abuse and neglect. Dev Psychobiol 52(7):671–690, 2010 20882586

Heindel WC, Salloway S: Memory systems in the human brain. Psychiatr Times 16:19–21, 1999

Henderson SW, Martin A: Formulation and integration, in Lewis's Child and Adolescent Psychiatry: A Comprehensive Textbook, 4th Edition. Edited by Martin A, Volkmar FR, Lewis M. Philadelphia, PA, Lippincott Williams & Wilkins, 2007, pp 377–382

Henrich CC, Shahar G: Social support buffers the effects of terrorism on adolescent depression: findings from Sderot, Israel. J Am Acad Child Adolesc Psychiatry 47(9):1073–1076, 2008 18664998

Heyman I, Skuse D, Goodman R: Brain disorders and psychopathology (Chapter 31), in Rutter's Child and Adolescent Psychiatry, 6th Edition. Edited by Thapar A, Pine DS, Leckman JF, et al. London, Wiley Blackwell, 2015, pp 389–401

Hickok G: The Myth of Mirror Neurons: The Real Neuroscience of Communication and Cognition. New York, WW Norton, 2014

Hinshaw SP: Lessons from research on the developmental psychopathology of girls and women. J Am Acad Child Adolesc Psychiatry 47(4):359–361, 2008 18356701

Hollander E, Benzaquen SD: Is there a distinct OCD spectrum? CNS Spectrums 1:17–26, 1996

Holz NE, Laucht M, Meyer-Lindenberg A: Recent advances in understanding the neurobiology of childhood socioeconomic disadvantage. Curr Opin Psychiatry 28(5):365–370, 2015 26147616

Hopkinson K, Cox A, Rutter M: Psychiatric interviewing techniques, III. Naturalistic study: eliciting feelings. Br J Psychiatry 138:406–415, 1981 7284707

Hornstein NL, Putnam FW: Clinical phenomenology of child and adolescent dissociative disorders. J Am Acad Child Adolesc Psychiatry 31(6):1077–1085, 1992 1429408

Hsiao EY, Bregere C, Malkova N, et al: Modeling features of autism in rodents, in Autism Spectrum Disorders. Edited by Amaral DG, Dawson G, Geschwind DH. New York, Oxford University Press, 2011, pp 935–959

Huth-Bocks AC, Muzik M, Beeghly M, et al: Secure base scripts are associated with maternal parenting behavior across contexts and reflective functioning among trauma-exposed mothers. Attach Hum Dev 16(6):535–556, 2014 25319230

Huz I, Nyer M, Dickson C, et al: Obsessive-compulsive symptoms as a risk factor for suicidality in U.S. college students. J Adolesc Health 58(4):481–484, 2016

Hymel S, Swearer SM: Four decades of research on school bullying: An introduction. Am Psychol 70(4):293–299, 2015 25961310

Jankovic J, Fahn S: Choreas, in Merritt's Neurology, 12th Edition. Edited by Rowland LP, Pedley TA. Philadelphia, PA, Lippincott Williams & Wilkins, 2010, pp 727–734

Jansen DE, Veenstra R, Ormel J, et al: Early risk factors for being a bully, victim, or bully/victim in late elementary and early secondary education: the longitudinal TRAILS study. BMC Public Health 11:440, 2011 21645403 Available at: http://bmcpublichealth.biomedcentral.com/articles/10.1186/1471-2458-11-440. Accessed February 7, 2016.

Jenkins JM, Curwen T: Change in adolescents' internalizing symptomatology as a function of sex and the timing of maternal depressive symptomatology. J Am Acad Child Adolesc Psychiatry 47(4):399–405, 2008 18388768

Judd FK, Burrows GD: Anxiety disorders and their relationship to depression, in Handbook of Affective Disorders, 2nd Edition. Edited by Paykel ES. New York, Guilford, 1992, pp 77–87

Kagan J: Galen's Prophesy: Temperament in Human Nature. New York, Basic Books, 1994

Kaminer Y: Adolescent substance abuse, in Textbook of Substance Abuse Treatment, 4th Edition. Edited by Galanter M, Kleber HD. Washington, DC, American Psychiatric Publishing, 2008, pp 525–535

Kandel ER: A new intellectual framework for psychiatry. Am J Psychiatry 155(4):457–469, 1998 9545989

Kapczinski F, Vieta E, Andreazza AC, et al: Allostatic load in bipolar disorder: implications for pathophysiology and treatment. Neurosci Biobehav Rev 32(4):675–692, 2008 18199480

Kariuki-Nyuthe C, Gomez-Mancilla B, Stein DJ: Obsessive compulsive disorder and the glutamatergic system. Curr Opin Psychiatry 27(1):32–37, 2014 24270485

Katz P: The first few minutes: the engagement of the difficult adolescent. Adolesc Psychiatry 17:69–81, 1990 2240435

Keitner GI, Miller IW: Family functioning and major depression, in The Transmission of Depression in Families and Children: Assessment and Intervention. Edited by Sholevar GP, Schwoeri L. Northvale, NJ, Jason Aronson, 1994, pp 7–30

Keller J, Shen L, Gomez RG, et al: Hippocampal and amygdalar volumes in psychotic and nonpsychotic unipolar depression. Am J Psychiatry 165(7):872–880, 2008 18450931

Kendall PC, Peterman JS, Cummings CM: Cognitive-behavioral therapy, behavioral therapy, and related treatments in children, in Rutter's Child and Adolescent Psychiatry. Edited by Thapar A, Pine DS, Leckman JF, et al. New York, Wiley Blackwell, 2015, pp 496–509

Kennard BD, Hughes JL, Stewart SM, et al: Maternal depressive symptoms in pediatric major depressive disorder: relationship to acute treatment outcome. J Am Acad Child Adolesc Psychiatry 47(6):694–699, 2008 18434919

Kim HF, Schultz PE, Wilde EA, et al: Laboratory testing and imaging studies in psychiatry, in American Psychiatric Publishing Textbook of Psychiatry, 5th Edition. Edited by Hales RE, Yudofsky SC, Gabbard GO. Washington, DC, American Psychiatric Publishing, 2008, pp 19–72

King BH, State MW, Shah B, et al: Mental retardation: a review of the past 10 years. Part I. J Am Acad Child Adolesc Psychiatry 36(12):1656–1663, 1997 9401326

Kinsbourne M, Wood FB: Disorders of mental development, in Child Neurology, 7th Edition. Edited by Menkes JH, Sarnat HB, Maria BL. Philadelphia, PA, Lippincott Williams & Wilkins, 2006, pp 1097–1156

Kleinman A: Foreword, in DSM-5® Handbook on the Cultural Formulation Interview. Edited by Lewis-Fernández R, Aggarwal NK, Hinton L, et al. Arlington, VA, American Psychiatric Publishing, 2016, pp xvii–xix

Klimes-Dougan B, Ronsaville D, Wiggs EA, et al: Neuropsychological functioning in adolescent children of mothers with a history of bipolar or major depressive disorders. Biol Psychiatry 60(9):957–965, 2006 16934765

Kratochwill TR, Morris RJ, Robinson J: Historical perspectives, in Handbook of Clinical Psychology, Vol 2: Children and Adolescents. Edited by Hersen M, Gross AM. New York, Wiley, 2008, pp 3–38

Kovacs M, Pollock M: Bipolar disorder and comorbid conduct disorder in childhood and adolescence. J Am Acad Child Adolesc Psychiatry 34(6):715–723, 1995 7608044

Lajiness-O'Neill R, Beaulieu I: Neuropsychological and psychoeducational testing, in Pediatric Neuropsychiatry. Edited by Coffey CE, Brumback RA. Philadelphia, PA, Lippincott Williams & Wilkins, 2006, pp 75–95

Lampe L: Avoidant personality disorder as a social anxiety phenotype: risk factors, associations and treatment. Curr Opin Psychiatry 29(1):64–69, 2016 26651009

Laplante DP, Brunet A, Schmitz N, et al: Project Ice Storm: prenatal maternal stress affects cognitive and linguistic functioning in 5 1/2-year-old children. J Am Acad Child Adolesc Psychiatry 47(9):1063–1072, 2008 18665002

Larsen PD: Clinical neuropsychiatric assessment of children and adolescents (Chapter 3), in Pediatric Neuropsychiatry. Edited by Coffey CE, Brumback RA. Baltimore, MD, Lippincott Williams & Wilkins, 2006, pp 49–73

Lask B, Britten C, Kroll L, et al: Children with pervasive refusal. Arch Dis Child 66(7):866–869, 1991 1863102

Latas M, Milovanovic S: Personality disorders and anxiety disorders: what is the relationship? Curr Opin Psychiatry 27(1):57–61, 2014 24270478

Lefkovics E, Baji I, Rigó J: Impact of maternal depression on pregnancies and on early attachment. Infant Ment Health J 35(4):354–365, 2014 25798487

Leon RL: Psychiatric Interviewing: A Primer. New York, Elsevier North-Holland, 1982

Lewis M: Borderline disorders in childhood. Child Adolesc Psychiatr Clin N Am 3:31–42, 1994

Lewis M: Memory and psychoanalysis: a new look at infantile amnesia and transference. J Am Acad Child Adolesc Psychiatry 34(4):405–417, 1995 7751254

Lewis M: Psychiatric assessment of infants, children and adolescents, in Child and Adolescent Psychiatry: A Comprehensive Textbook, 2nd Edition. Edited by Lewis M. Baltimore, MD, Williams & Wilkins, 1996, pp 440–453

Lewis-Fernández R, Aggarwal NK, Kirmayer LJ: Cultural formulation before DSM-5, in DSM-5 Handbook on the Cultural Formulation Interview. Edited by Lewis-Fernandez R, Aggarwal NK, Hinton L, et al. Arlington, VA, American Psychiatric Publishing, 2016, pp 1–26

Lieberman AF, Padron E, Van Horn P, et al: Angels in the nursery: the intergenerational transmission of benevolent parental influences. Infant Ment Health J 26(6):504–520, 2005

Lion JR: Clinical assessment of violent patients, in Clinical Treatment of the Violent Person. Edited by Roth LH. New York, Guilford, 1987, pp 1–19

Loeber R, Hay DF: Developmental approaches to aggression and conduct problems, in Development Through Life: A Handbook for Clinicians. Edited by Rutter M, Hay DF. Oxford, England, Blackwell Scientific, 1994, pp 488–515

Lovegrove PJ, Henry KL, Slater MD: Examination of the predictors of latent class typologies of bullying involvement among middle school students. J Sch Violence 11(1):75–93, 2012 22606069

Mah L, Szabuniewicz C, Fiocco AJ: Can anxiety damage the brain? Curr Opin Psychiatry 29(1):56–63, 2016 26651008

Mahler MS, Pine F, Bergman A: The Psychological Birth of the Human Infant. New York, Basic Books, 1974

Malmquist CP: School violence, in Textbook of Violence Assessment and Management. Edited by Simon RI, Tardiff K. Washington, DC, American Psychiatric Publishing, 2008, pp 537–553

Malone JC, Levendosky AA, Dayton CJ, et al: Understanding the "ghosts in the nursery" of pregnant women experiencing domestic violence: prenatal maternal representations and histories of childhood maltreatment. Infant Ment Health J 31(4):432–454, 2010

Mantell DM: Ethical and Legal Issues, in Handbook of Clinical Psychology, Vol 2: Children and Adolescents. Edited by Hersen M, Gross AM. New York, Wiley, 2008, pp 94–137

Marcus MD, Wildes JE: Disordered eating in obese individuals. Curr Opin Psychiatry 27(6):443–447, 2014 25247456

Marmot M: Better parenting skills may break the poverty–disease connection. Sci Am 314(3):23–24, 2016

Marvin RS, Britner PA: Normative development: the ontogeny of attachment, in Handbook of Attachment: Theory, Research, and Clinical Applications, 2nd Edition. New York, Guilford, 2008, pp 269–294

Mash EJ: Treatment of child and family disturbance: a behavioral-systems perspective, in Treatment of Childhood Disorders. Edited by Mash EJ, Barkley RA. New York, Guilford, 1989, pp 3–36

Mash EJ, Dozois DJA: Child psychopathology: a developmental systems perspective, in Child Psychopathology. Edited by Mash EJ, Barkley RA. New York, Guilford, 1996, pp 3–60

Mataix-Cols D, Nakatani E, Micali N, et al: Structure of obsessive-compulsive symptoms in pediatric OCD. J Am Acad Child Adolesc Psychiatry 47(7):773–778, 2008 18344900

Maughan B, Collishaw S: Development and psychopathology: a life course perspective, in Rutter's Child and Adolescent Psychiatry, 6th Edition. Edited by Thapar A, Pine DS, Leckman JF, et al. New York, Wiley Blackwell, 2015, pp 5–16

Mayes SD, Waxmonsky JD, Calhoun SL, et al: Disruptive mood dysregulation disorder symptoms and association with oppositional defiant and other disorders in a general population child sample. J Child Adolesc Psychopharmacol 26(2):101–106, 2016 26745442

McDonnell MA, Glod C: Prevalence of psychopathology in preschool-age children. J Child Adolesc Psychiatr Nurs 16(4):141–152, 2003 14748450

McHale JP, Sullivan MJ: Family systems, in Handbook of Clinical Psychology, Vol 2: Children and Adolescents. Edited by Hersen M, Gross AM. New York, Wiley, 2008, pp 192–226

Meier MH, Caspi A, Reichenberg A, et al: Neuropsychological decline in schizophrenia from the premorbid to the postonset period: evidence from a population-representative longitudinal study. Am J Psychiatry 171(1):91–101, 2014 24030246

Menkes JH, Falk RF: Chromosomal anomalies and contiguous-gene syndromes, in Child Neurology, 7th Edition. Edited by Menkes JH, Sarnat HB, Maria BL. Philadelphia, PA, Lippincott William & Wilkins, 2006, pp 227–257

Miller M, Hemenway D: Guns and suicide in the United States (editorial). N Engl J Med 359(10):989–991, 2008 18768940

Mills-Koonce WR, Appleyard K, Barnett M, et al: Adult attachment style and stress as risk factors for early maternal sensitivity and negativity. Infant Ment Health J 32(3):277–285, 2011 24855326

Miranda R, Scott M, Hicks R, et al: Suicide attempt characteristics, diagnoses, and future attempts: comparing multiple attempters to single attempters and ideators. J Am Acad Child Adolesc Psychiatry 47(1):32–40, 2008 18174823

Moffitt TE, Houts R, Asherson P, et al: Is adult ADHD a childhood-onset neurodevelopmental disorder? Evidence from a four-decade longitudinal cohort study. Am J Psychiatry 172(10):967–977, 2015 25998281

Mohl P: Brief psychotherapy, in Comprehensive Textbook of Psychiatry, 6th Edition. Edited by Kaplan HI, Sadock BJ. Baltimore, MD, Williams & Wilkins, 1995, pp 1879–1880

Monahan J: Structured risk assessment of violence, in Textbook of Violence Assessment and Management. Edited by Simon RI, Tardiff K. Washington, DC, American Psychiatric Publishing, 2008, pp 17–33

Monahan J, Steadman H, Appelbaum P: Classification of Violence Risk. Lutz, FL, Psychological Assessment Resources, 2005

Moncreiff J: New evidence from clinical study reports reveals misclassification, misrepresentation, and underreporting of serious harm. BMJ 352:i217, 2016 26823531

Mongelli L, Celona L, Schram J, et al: Why the 'bully killing' teen finally snapped. New York Post, June 19, 2014. Available at: http://nypost.com/2014/06/19/bully-killing-teen-was-afraid-for-his-life/. Accessed February 7, 2016.

Monk CS, Pine DS: Childhood anxiety disorders: a cognitive neurobiological perspective, in Neurobiology of Mental Illness, 3rd Edition. Edited by Charley DS, Nestler EJ. New York, Oxford University Press, 2009, pp 1153–1172

Moore BE, Fine BD: Psychoanalytic Terms and Concepts. New Haven, CT, Yale University Press, 1990

Mossman D, Weston CG: Divorce, custody, and parental consent for psychiatric treatment. Curr Psychiatr 7(8):63–67, 2008

Moura PJ, Lombroso PJ, Mercadante MT: Autism, in Biological Child Psychiatry: Recent Trends and Developments. Edited by Banaschewski T, Rohde LA. Basel, Switzerland, S Karger, 2008, pp 21–38

Muller RJ: Doing Psychiatry Wrong: A Critical and Prescriptive Look at a Faltering Profession. New York, Analytic Press, 2008

Munir KM: The co-occurrence of mental disorders in children and adolescents with intellectual disability/intellectual developmental disorder. Curr Opin Psychiatry 29(2):95–102, 2016 26779862

Nagera H: Early Childhood Disturbances, the Infantile Neuroses, and the Adulthood Disturbances. New York, International Universities Press, 1966

Nehring WM: Down syndrome, in Primary Care of the Child with a Chronic Condition, 5th Edition. Edited by Allen PJ, Vessey JA, Schapiro NA. Mosby Elsevier, 2010, pp 447–469

Neul JL: Rett syndrome and MECP2-related disorders, in Autism Spectrum Disorders. Edited by Amaral DG, Dawson G, Geschwind DH. New York, Oxford University Press, 2011, pp 776–800

Newman LK, Steel Z: The child asylum seeker: psychological and developmental impact of immigration detention. Child Adolesc Psychiatr Clin N Am 17(3):665–683, 2008 18558318

Ngo V, Langley A, Kataoka SH, et al: Providing evidence-based practice to ethnically diverse youths: examples from the Cognitive Behavioral Intervention for Trauma in Schools (CBITS) program. J Am Acad Child Adolesc Psychiatry 47(8):858–862, 2008 18645419

Nickels KC: Neurological development and developmental disabilities, in Mayo Clinic Neurology Board Review: Clinical Neurology for Initial Certification and MOC. Edited by Flemming KD, Jones LK. Rochester, MN, Mayo Clinic Scientific Press, 2015, pp 675–680

Nurcombe B: Malpractice, in Child and Adolescent Psychiatry: A Comprehensive Textbook. Edited by Lewis M. Baltimore, MD, Williams & Wilkins, 1996, pp 1134–1145

Nurcombe B: Clinical decision making in psychiatry, in Current Diagnosis and Treatment: Psychiatry, 2nd Edition. Edited by Ebert MH, Loosen PT, Nurcombe B, et al. New York, McGraw Hill Medical, 2008a, pp 1–6

Nurcombe B: Psychological reactions to acute and chronic systemic illness in pediatric patients, in Current Diagnosis and Treatment: Psychiatry, 2nd Edition. Edited by Ebert M, Loosen PT, Nurcombe B, et al. New York, McGraw-Hill Medical, 2008b, pp 675–678

O'Brien JD: Children with attention-deficit hyperactivity disorder and their parents, in Psychotherapies with Children and Adolescents. Edited by O'Brien JD, Pilowsky DJ, Lewis OW. Washington, DC, American Psychiatric Press, 1992, pp 109–124

O'Connor TG, Bredenkamp D, Rutter M: Attachment disturbances and disorders in children exposed to early severe deprivation. Infant Ment Health J 20(1):10–29, 1999

Olino TM, Pettit JW, Klein DN, et al: Influence of parental and grandparental major depressive disorder on behavior problems in early childhood: a three-generation study. J Am Acad Child Adolesc Psychiatry 47(1):53–60, 2008 18174825

Oliveira PS, Soares I, Martins C, et al: Indiscriminate behavior observed in the strange situation among institutionalized toddlers: relations to caregiver report and to early family risk. Infant Ment Health J 33(2):187–196, 2012 25552781

Otnow Lewis D: Conduct disorder, in Child and Adolescent Psychiatry: A Comprehensive Textbook. Edited by Lewis M. Baltimore, MD, Williams & Wilkins, 1991, pp 561–573

Otnow Lewis D: Diagnostic evaluation of the child with dissociative identity disorder/multiple personality disorder. Child Adolesc Psychiatr Clin N Am 5(2):303–331, 1996

Owens J: Epidemiology of sleep disorders during childhood, in Principles and Practice of Pediatric Sleep Medicine. Edited by Sheldon SH, Ferber R, Kryger MH. Philadelphia, PA, Elsevier/Saunders, 2005, pp 27–33

Parfitt Y, Ayers S: Postnatal mental health and parenting: the importance of parental anger. Infant Ment Health J 33(4):400–410, 2012

Parker G, Paterson A: Melancholia: definition and management. Curr Opin Psychiatry 27(1):1–6, 2014 24270479

Patankar VC, Sangle JP, Shah HR, et al: Neurological soft signs in children with attention deficit hyperactivity disorder. Indian J Psychiatry 54(2):159–165, 2012 22988324

Pavuluri MN, Bogarapu S: Brain model for pediatric bipolar disorder, in Biological Child Psychiatry: Recent Trends and Developments. Edited by Banaschewski T, Rohde LA. Basel, Switzerland, S Karger, 2008, pp 39–52

Pavuluri MN, Herbener ES, Sweeney JA: Psychotic symptoms in pediatric bipolar disorder. J Affect Disord 80(1):19–28, 2004 15094254

Pendleton Jones B, Butters N: Neuropsychological assessment, in The Clinical Psychology Handbook, 2nd Edition. Edited by Hersen M, Kazdin AE, Bellack AS. New York, Pergamon, 1991, pp 406–429

Pennington B: The Development of Psychopathology: Nature and Nurture. New York, Guilford, 2002

Perkins DO, Jeffries CD, Cornblatt BA, et al: Severity of thought disorder predicts psychosis in persons at clinical high-risk. Schizophr Res 169(1–3):169–177, 2015 26441004

Perlman SB, Fournier JC, Bebko G, et al: Emotional face processing in pediatric bipolar disorder: evidence for functional impairments in the fusiform gyrus. J Am Acad Child Adolesc Psychiatry 52(12):1314–1325.e3, 2013 24290464

Perry JC: Maternal defense mechanisms influence infant development. Am J Psychiatry 173(2):99–100, 2016 26844788

Pfeffer C: The suicidal child, in The Evaluation of Childhood Suicidal Risk by Clinical Interview. Edited by Pfeffer C. New York, Guilford, 1986, pp 173–192

Pfeffer C: Attempted suicide in children and adolescents: causes and management, in Child and Adolescent Psychiatry: A Comprehensive Textbook. Edited by Lewis M. Baltimore, MD, Williams & Wilkins, 1991, pp 664–672

Phillips D: Concussions in a required class: boxing at military academies. The New York Times, September 29, 2015, A1, A15

Phillips KA, Stein DJ: Handbook on Obsessive-Compulsive and Related Disorders. Washington, DC, American Psychiatric Publishing, 2015

Pies RW: Must we now consider SRIs neuroleptics? J Clin Psychopharmacol 17(6):443–445, 1997 9408805

Pike A, Plomin R: Importance of nonshared environmental factors for childhood and adolescent psychopathology. J Am Acad Child Adolesc Psychiatry 35(5):560–570, 1996 8935202

Pilowsky DJ, Wickramaratne P, Talati A, et al: Children of depressed mothers 1 year after the initiation of maternal treatment: findings from the STAR*D-Child Study. Am J Psychiatry 165(9):1136–1147, 2008 18558646

Pliszka S: Bipolar disorder and ADHD: comments on current controversy. ADHD Rep 7:9–11, 1999

Popma A, Vermeiren R: Conduct disorder, in Biological Child Psychiatry: Recent Trends and Developments. Edited by Banaschewski T, Rohde LA. Basel, Switzerland, S Karger, 2008, pp 153–165

Porter E: Push marriage? Not for the sake of the children. The New York Times, March 23, 2016, pp B1–B3

Posey DJ, McDougle CJ: Treating autism spectrum disorders. Preface. Child Adolesc Psychiatr Clin N Am 17(4):xv–xviii, 2008 18775365

Post RM, Leverich GS, Fergus E, et al: Parental attitudes towards early intervention in children at high risk for affective disorders. J Affect Disord 70(2):117–124, 2002 12117623

Pruett KD: The art of the science: a child, family, and systems-centered approach, in Lewis's Child and Adolescent Psychiatry: A Comprehensive Textbook, 4th Edition. Edited by Martin A, Volkmar FR, Lewis M. Philadelphia, PA, Lippincott Williams & Wilkins, 2007, pp 2–11

Pryse-Phillips W: Companion to Clinical Neurology, 2nd Edition. New York, Oxford University Press, 2003

Puig-Antich J, Gittelman R: Depression in childhood, in Handbook of Affective Disorders. Edited by Paykel ES. New York, Guilford, 1982, pp 379–392

Puig-Antich J, Blau S, Marx N, et al: Prepubertal major depressive disorder: a pilot study. J Am Acad Child Psychiatry 17(4):695–707, 1978 744852

Purves D, Augustine GJ, Fitzpatrick D, et al (eds): Neuroscience, 5th Edition. Sunderland, MA, Sinauer Associates, 2012

Putnam FW: Dissociative disorders in children and adolescents. A developmental perspective. Psychiatr Clin North Am 14(3):519–531, 1991 1946022

Quinsey G, Harris G, Rice M, et al: Violent Offenders: Appraising and Managing Risk, 2nd Edition. Washington, DC, American Psychological Association, 1996

Racker H: Transference and Countertransference. London, Hogarth, 1968

Raine A, Brennan P, Mednick SA: Birth complications combined with early maternal rejection at age 1 year predispose to violent crime at age 18 years. Arch Gen Psychiatry 51(12):984–988, 1994 7979887

Ramchandani PG, Stein A, O'Connor TG, et al: Depression in men in the postnatal period and later child psychopathology: a population cohort study. J Am Acad Child Adolesc Psychiatry 47(4):390–398, 2008 18388761

Ramos MC, Bennett DC: Cyberbullyng: who hurts, and why. Psychiatric Times, January 29, 2016

Rapin I: Introduction. Autism turns 65: a neurologist's bird's eye view, in Autism Spectrum Disorders. Edited by Amaral DG, Dawson G, Geschwind DH. New York, Oxford University Press, 2011, pp 3–14

Remschmidt H: Schizophrenia in children and adolescents, in Biological Child Psychiatry: Recent Trends and Developments. Edited by Banaschewski T, Rohde LA. Basel, Switzerland, S Karger, 2008, pp 118–137

Rhebergen D, Graham R: The re-labelling of dysthymic disorder to persistent depressive disorder in DSM-5: old wine in new bottles? Curr Opin Psychiatry 27(1):27–31, 2014 24270481

Riddle MA, Yershova K, Lazzaretto D, et al: The preschool attention-deficit/hyperactivity disorder treatment study (PATS) 6-year follow-up. J Am Acad Child Adolesc Psychiatry 52(3):264–278, 2013

Roessner V, Rothenberger A: Neurobiological background of tic disorders, in Biological Child Psychiatry: Recent Trends and Developments. Edited by Banaschewski T, Rohde LA. Basel, Switzerland, S Karger, 2008, pp 95–117

Rosário MC, Alvarenga P, Mathis MA, et al: Obsessive-compulsive disorder in childhood, in Biological Child Psychiatry: Recent Trends and Developments. Edited by Banaschewski T, Rohde LA. Basel, Switzerland, S Karger, 2008, pp 82–94

Rosenblum O, Mazet P, Benony H: Mother and infant affective involvement states and maternal depression. Infant Ment Health J 18(4):350–363, 1997

Rotella F, Fioravanti G, Ricca V: Temperament and personality in eating disorders. Curr Opin Psychiatry 29(1):77–83, 2016 26575294

Rumsey JM: Brain imaging of reading disorders (letter). J Am Acad Child Adolesc Psychiatry 37(1):12, 1998 9444890

Rush AJ, First MD, Blacker D: Handbook of Psychiatric Measures, 2nd Edition. Washington, DC, American Psychiatric Publishing, 2007

Russ SW: Psychodynamic, in Handbook of Clinical Psychology, Vol 2: Children and Adolescents. Edited by Herson M, Gross AM. New York, Wiley, 2008, pp 173–191

Rutter M, Brown GW: The reliability and validity of measures of family life and relationships in families containing a psychiatric patient. Soc Psychiatry 1(1):38–53, 1966

Sankar R, Koh S, Wu J, et al: Paroxysmal disorders, in Child Neurology, 7th Edition. Edited by Menkes JH, Sarnat HB, Maria BL. Philadelphia, PA, Lippincott, Williams & Wilkins, 2006, pp 857–942

Santos A, Meyer-Lindenberg A: Neuroimaging of Williams-Beuren syndrome, in Understanding Neuropsychiatric Disorders: Insights From Neuroimaging. Edited by Shelton ME, Turetsky BI. Cambridge, England, Cambridge University Press, 2011, pp 537–554

Sarver DE, Rapport MD, Kofler MJ, et al: Hyperactivity in attention-deficit/hyperactivity disorder (ADHD): impairing deficit or compensatory behavior? J Abnorm Child Psychol 43(7):1219–1232, 2015 25863472

Saxe GN, Stoddard F, Hall E, et al: Pathways to PTSD, part I: children with burns. Am J Psychiatry 162(7):1299–1304, 2005 15994712

Sbordone RJ: The ecological validity of neuropsychological testing, in The Neuropsychology Handbook, Vol 1, 2nd Edition. Edited by Horton AM, Wedding D, Webster J. New York, Springer, 1997, pp 365–392

Scheid JM: Children in foster care: issues and concerns. Psychiatric Times 33(6):16, 21–22, 2016

Schildkrout B: Distinguishing between medical and psychiatric conditions. The Carlat Report: Psychiatry 13(11–12):1, 6–7, 8, 2015

Schneider M, Kay J: Rebecca Ann Sedwick suicide: two girls arrested for 'terrorizing' bullied victim. The Huffington Post (online), October 15, 2013. Available at: http://m.huffpost.com/us/entry/rebecca-ann-sedwick_n_4100350.html. Accessed February 7, 2016

Schneiderman G, Winders P, Tallett S, et al: Update on bereavement risk (letter). J Am Acad Child Adolesc Psychiatry 35(2):132–133, 1996 8720621

Schore N: Affect Regulation and the Origin of the Self: The Neurobiology of Emotional Development. Hillsdale, NJ, Erlbaum, 1994

Schreier HA: Hallucinations in nonpsychotic children: more common than we think? J Am Acad Child Adolesc Psychiatry 38(5):623–625, 1999 10230196

Schulenberg SE, Kaster JT, Nassif C, et al: Assessment of psychopathology, in Handbook of Clinical Psychology, Vol 2: Children and Adolescents. Edited by Hersen M, Gross AM. Hoboken, NJ, Wiley, 2008, pp 520–550

Scott S: Oppositional and conduct disorders, in Rutter's Child and Adolescent Psychiatry, 6th Edition. Edited by Thapar A, Pine DS, Leckman JF, et al. New York, Wiley Blackwell, 2015, pp 913–930

Sekar A, Bialas AR, de Rivera H, et al: Schizophrenia risk from complex variation of complement component 4. Nature 530(7589):177–183, 2016 26814963

Senay EC: Diagnostic interview and mental status examination, in Substance Abuse: A Comprehensive Textbook, 3rd Edition. Edited by Lowinson JH, Ruiz P, Millman RB, et al. Baltimore, MD, Williams & Wilkins, 1997, pp 365–367

Shaffer D: Discussion of "Predictive validity of the suicide scale among adolescents in Group home treatment." J Am Acad Child Adolesc Psychiatry 35(2):172–174, 1996

Shapiro T: The psychodynamic formulation in child and adolescent psychiatry. J Am Acad Child Adolesc Psychiatry 28(5):675–680, 1989 2793795

Sharma T, Guski LS, Freund N, et al: Suicidality and aggression during antidepressant treatment: systematic review and meta-analysis based on clinical study reports. BMJ 352:i65, 2016 26819231

Shea SC: Psychiatric Interviewing: The Art of Understanding, 2nd Edition. Philadelphia, PA, WB Saunders, 1998

Sheldon SH: Introduction to pediatric sleep medicine, in Principles and Practice of Pediatric Sleep Medicine. Edited by Sheldon SH, Ferber R, Kryger MH. Philadelphia, PA, Elsevier/Saunders, 2005a, pp 1–16

Sheldon SH: Preface, in Principles and Practice of Pediatric Sleep Medicine. Edited by Sheldon SH, Ferber R, Kryger MH. Philadelphia, PA, Elsevier/Saunders, 2005b, p vii

Shenton ME, Turetsky BI (eds): Preface, in Understanding Neuropsychiatric Disorders: Insights From Neuroimaging. Cambridge, UK, Cambridge University Press, 2011, pp xiii–xiv

Sher Y, Garcia R, Maldonado JR: Neuropsychiatric masquerades: diagnosis and treatment. Psychiatr Times February 19, 2016

Sheridan MD: From Birth to Five Years: Children's Developmental Progress, 2nd Edition. Revised and updated by Frost M, Sharma A. London, Routledge, 1997

Singh MK: In this issue/abstract thinking: update your socioeconomic status. J Am Acad Child Adolesc Psychiatry 51(9):853–854, 2012

Singh T: Pediatric bipolar disorder: diagnostic challenges in identifying symptoms and course of illness. Psychiatry (Edgmont) 5(6):34–42, 2008 19727283

Shlafer RJ, Raby KL, Lawler JM, et al: Longitudinal associations between adult attachment states of mind and parenting quality. Attach Hum Dev 17(1):83–95, 2015 25316283

Smith BH, Barkley RA, Shapiro CJ: Attention-deficit/hyperactivity disorder, in Assessment of Childhood Disorders, 4th Edition. Edited by Mash EJ, Barkley RA. New York, Guilford, 2007, pp 53–123

Soczynska JK, Zhang L, Kennedy SH, et al: Are psychiatric disorders inflammatory-based conditions? Psychiatric Times, October 8, 2012

Solanto M: Executive function deficits in adults with ADHD, in Attention-Deficit/Hyperactivity Disorder: A Handbook for Diagnosis and Treatment, 4th Edition. Edited by Barkley RA. New York, Guilford, 2015, pp 256–266

Solomon J, George C: The measurements of attachment security and related constructs in infancy and early childhood, in Handbook of Attachment: Theory, Research and Clinical Applications, 2nd Edition. New York, Guilford, 2008, pp 383–416

Sperner-Unterweger B, Fuchs D: Schizophrenia and psychoneuroimmunology: an integrative view. Curr Opin Psychiatry 28(3):201–206, 2015 25768084

Spirito A, Brown L, Overholser J, et al: Attempted suicide in adolescence: a review and critique of the literature. Clin Psychol Rev 9(3):335–363, 1989

Spreen O, Risser AH, Edgell D: Developmental Neuropsychology. New York, Oxford University Press, 1995

Stacks AM, Muzik M, Wong K, et al: Maternal reflective functioning among mothers with childhood maltreatment histories: links to sensitive parenting and infant attachment security. Attach Hum Dev 16(5):515–533, 2014 25028251

Starcevic V, Brakoulias V: New diagnostic perspectives on obsessive-compulsive personality disorder and its links with other conditions. Curr Opin Psychiatry 27(1):62–67, 2014 24257122

Stein MB, Sareen J: Generalized anxiety disorder: clinical practice. N Engl J Med 373(21):2059–2068, 2015

Steinhauer J: Verdict in MySpace suicide case. New York Times, November 26. 2008. Available at: http://www.nytimes.com/2008/11/27/us/27myspace.html?_r=0, 2008. Accessed June 30, 2016.

Stewart SE, Rosario MC, Baer L, et al: Four-factor structure of obsessive-compulsive disorder symptoms in children, adolescents, and adults. J Am Acad Child Adolesc Psychiatry 47(7):763–772, 2008 18520961

Stoddard FJ, Saxe G, Ronfeldt H, et al: Acute stress symptoms in young children with burns. J Am Acad Child Adolesc Psychiatry 45(1):87–93, 2006 16327585

Strakowski SM: Managing bipolar disorder: practical tips. The Carlat Report: Psychiatry 14(1):1, 4–5, 7, 2016

Sullivan EM, Annest JL, Simon TR, et al: Suicide trends among persons aged 10–24 years—United States, 1994–2012. MMWR Morb Mortal Wkly Rep 64(8):201–205, 2015 25742379

Sundheim ST, Myers RM, Voeller KK: Intellectual disability, in Pediatric Neuropsychiatry. Edited by Coffey CE, Brumback RA. Philadelphia, PA, Lippincott Williams & Wilkins, 2006, pp 151–186

Swaiman KF: Neurological examination of the older child, in Pediatric Neurology Principles and Practice, Vol 1, 4th Edition. Edited by Swaiman KF, Ashwal S, Ferriero DM. Maryland Heights, MO, Mosby Elsevier, 2006, pp 17–35

Swaiman KF, Wu I: Cerebral palsy, in Pediatric Neurology: Principles and Practice, Vol 1, 4th Edition. Edited by Swaiman KF, Ashwal S, Ferriero DM. Philadelphia, PA, Maryland Heights, MO, Mosby Elsevier, 2006, pp 491–504

Swartz HA, Frank E, Zuckoff A, et al: Brief interpersonal psychotherapy for depressed mothers whose children are receiving psychiatric treatment. Am J Psychiatry 165(9):1155–1162, 2008 18558645

Swedo SE, Rapoport JL, Leonard H, et al: Obsessive-compulsive disorder in children and adolescents: clinical phenomenology of 70 consecutive cases. Arch Gen Psychiatry 46(4):335–341, 1989 2930330

Swedo SE, Leckman JF, Rose NR: From research subgroup to clinical syndrome: modifying the PANDAS criteria to describe PANS (pediatric acute-onset neuropsychiatric syndrome). Pediatrics & Therapeutics 2(2):1–8, 2012

Swillen A: The importance of understanding cognitive trajectories: the case of 22q11.2 deletion syndrome. Curr Opin Psychiatry 29(2):133–137, 2016 26779858

Szobot CM, Bukstein O: Substance use disorders in adolescence, in Biological Child Psychiatry: Recent Trends and Developments. Edited by Banaschewski T, Rohde LA. Basel, Switzerland, S Karger, 2008, pp 166–180

Takizawa R, Maughan B, Arseneault L: Adult health outcomes of childhood bullying victimization: evidence from a five-decade longitudinal British birth cohort. Am J Psychiatry 171(7):777–784, 2014 24743774

Taliaferro LA, Oberstar JV, Borowsky IW: Prevention of youth suicide: the role of the primary care physician. J Clin Outcomes Manag 19(6):270–285, 2012

Tarasoff v Regents of the University of California, 131 Cal Rptr 14,551 P2d 334 (1976)

Tardiff K: Clinical risk assessment of violence, in Textbook of Violence Assessment and Management. Edited by Simon RI, Tardiff K. Washington, DC, American Psychiatric Publishing, 2008, pp 3–16

Tarrier N, Johnson J: Introduction: case formulation, in Cognitive Behavior Therapy, 2nd Edition. Edited by Tarrier N, Johnson J. New York, Routledge, Taylor & Francis Group, 2016, pp 1–13

Taylor GJ: Why publish a special issue on psychoanalysis and psychosomatics? J Am Acad Psychoanal Dyn Psychiatry 36(1):1–10, 2008 18399743

Taylor MA, Sierls FS, Abrams R: The neuropsychiatric evaluation, in Textbook of Neuropsychiatry. Edited by Hales RE, Yudofsky SC. Washington, DC, American Psychiatric Press, 1987, pp 3–6

Terr LC, Bloch DA, Michel BA, et al: Children's memories in the wake of Challenger. Am J Psychiatry 153(5):618–625, 1996 8615406

Thompson RA, Goodwin R, Meyer S: Social development: psychological understanding, self-understanding, and relationships, in Handbook of Preschool Mental Health: Development, Disorders, and Treatment. Edited by Luby JL. New York, Guilford, 2006, pp 3–22

Tillman R, Geller B: Diagnosis, prognosis and personalized medicine, in Treatment of Bipolar Disorder in Children and Adolescents. Edited by Geller B, DelBello MP. New York, Guilford, 2008, pp 9–23

Towbin KE: Paying attention to stimulants: height, weight, and cardiovascular monitoring in clinical practice (editorial). J Am Acad Child Adolesc Psychiatry 47(9):977–980, 2008 18580503

Towbin KE: Physical examination and medical investigation, in Rutter's Child and Adolescent Psychiatry, 6th Edition. Edited by Thapar A, Pine DS, Leckman JF, et al. New York, Wiley Blackwell, 2015, pp 449–459

Towbin KE, Riddle MA: Obsessive-compulsive disorder in children and adolescents, in Child and Adolescent Psychiatry: A Comprehensive Textbook, 2nd Edition. Edited by Lewis M. Baltimore, MD, Williams & Wilkins, 1996, pp 684–692

Tranel D: Neuropsychological assessment Psychiatr Clin North Am 15(2):283–299, 1992 1603724

Tully EC, Iacono WG, McGue M: An adoption study of parental depression as an environmental liability for adolescent depression and childhood disruptive disorders. Am J Psychiatry 165(9):1148–1154, 2008 18558644

Turnbull HR, Stowe MJ, Turnbull AP, et al: Public policy and developmental disabilities, in Handbook of Developmental Disabilities. Edited by Odom SL, Horner RH, Snell ME, et al. New York, Guilford, 2007, pp 15–34

Turner SM, Hersen M: The interviewing process, in Diagnostic Interviewing, 2nd Edition. Edited by Hersen M, Turner SM. New York, Plenum, 1994, pp 3–24

Twemlow SW, Sacco FC: Preventing Bullying and School Violence. Washington, DC, American Psychiatric Publishing, 2012

U.S. Customs and Border Protection: United States Border Patrol Southwest Family Unit Subject and Unaccompanied Alien Children Apprehensions Fiscal Year 2016. Available at: www.cbp.gov/newsroom/stats/southwest-border-unaccompanied-children/fy-2016. Accessed February 7, 2016.

van der Kolk BA, Pelcovitz D, Roth S, et al: Dissociation, somatization, and affect dysregulation: the complexity of adaptation to trauma. Am J Psychiatry 153(7 suppl):83–93, 1996 8659645

van der Ploeg R, Steglich C, Salmivalli C, et al: The intensity of victimization: associations with children's psychosocial well-being and social standing in the classroom. PLoS One 10(10):e0141490, 2015 26513576

Van Meter AR, Burke C, Kowatch RA, et al: Ten-year updated meta-analysis of the clinical characteristics of pediatric mania and hypomania. Bipolar Disord 18(1):19–32, 2016 26748678

van Os J: 'Schizophrenia' does not exist. BMJ 352:i375, 2016; doi: 10.1136/bmj.i375

Viding E, McCrory E: Developmental risk for psychopathy, in Rutter's Child and Adolescent Psychiatry. Edited by Thapar A, Pine DS, Leckman JF, et al. New York, Wiley Blackwell, 2015, pp 966–980

Vitiello B: Ethical and regulatory aspects in the treatment of children and adolescents with bipolar disorder, in Treatment of Bipolar Disorder in Children and Adolescents. Edited by Geller B, DelBello MP. New York, Guilford, 2008, pp 392–404

Voeller KKS: Social and emotional learning disabilities, in Behavioral Neurology and Neuropsychology. Edited by Feinberg TE, Farah MJ. New York, McGraw-Hill, 1997, pp 795–801

Volkmar FR: Reactive attachment disorders of infancy or early childhood, in Comprehensive Textbook of Psychiatry, 6th Edition. Edited by Kaplan HI, Sadock BJ. Baltimore, MD, Williams & Wilkins, 1995, pp 2354–2359

Volkmar FR: Childhood and adolescent psychosis: a review of the past 10 years. J Am Acad Child Adolesc Psychiatry 35(7):843–851, 1996 8768343

Wagner KD: New findings about youth suicide. Psychiatric Times, June 16, 2015

Wagner KD: Bullying and depression in youths. Psychiatric Times, February 8, 2016

Walsh J, Hepper EG, Marshall BJ: Investigating attachment, caregiving, and mental health: a model of maternal-fetal relationships. BMC Pregnancy Childbirth 14:383, 2014 25406583

Wang S: How to think about the risk of autism. The New York Times, Sunday, March 30, 2014, Sunday Review, p. 7

Warren SL, Oppenheim D, Emde RN: Can emotions and themes in children's play predict behavior problems? J Am Acad Child Adolesc Psychiatry 35(10):1331–1337, 1996 8885587

Webster C, Douglas K, Eaves D, et al: HCR-20 Assessing Risk for Violence, Version II. Burnaby, BC, Simon Frazier University, Mental Health, Law and Policy Institute, 1997

Wechsler D: Wechsler Intelligence Scale for Children, 4th Edition. San Antonio, TX, Pearson Assessment, 2003

Weiner MF, Moll P: Theories of personality and psychopathology: other dynamic schools, in Comprehensive Textbook of Psychiatry, 6th Edition. Edited by Kaplan HI, Sadock BJ. Baltimore, MD, Williams & Wilkins, 1995, pp 500–550

Weinshel EM, Renik O: Psychoanalytic technique, in Textbook of Psychoanalysis. Edited by Nersessian E, Kopff Jr RG. Washington, DC, American Psychiatric Press, 1996, pp 423–454

Weisbrot DM: Prelude to a school shooting? Assessing threatening behaviors in childhood and adolescence. J Am Acad Child Adolesc Psychiatry 47(8):847–852, 2008 18645417

Williams DT: Delirium and catatonia, in Lewis's Child and Adolescent Psychiatry: A Comprehensive Textbook. Edited by Martin A, Volkmar FR. Philadelphia, PA, Lippincott Williams & Wilkins, 2007, pp 647–655

Williams DT, Pleak R, Hanesian H: Neuropsychiatric disorders of childhood and adolescence, in Textbook of Neuropsychiatry. Edited by Hales RE, Yudofsky SC. Washington, DC, American Psychiatric Press, 1987, pp 365–386

Wolitzky-Taylor KB, Ruggiero KJ, Danielson CK, et al: Prevalence and correlates of dating violence in a national sample of adolescents. J Am Acad Child Adolesc Psychiatry 47(7):755–762, 2008 18520962

Wozniak J, Biederman J, Mundy E, et al: A pilot family study of childhood-onset mania. J Am Acad Child Adolesc Psychiatry 34(12):1577–1583, 1995 8543528

Young JG, Leven L, Ludman W, et al: Interviewing children and adolescents, in Psychiatric Disorders in Children and Adolescents. Edited by Garfinkel BD, Carlson GA, Weller E. Philadelphia, PA, WB Saunders, 1990, pp 443–468

Youngstrom EA, Freeman AJ, Jenkins MM: The assessment of children and adolescents with bipolar disorder. Child Adolesc Psychiatr Clin N Am 18(2):353–390, viii–ix, 2009 19264268

Zeanah CH, Smyke AT: Disorders of attachment and social engagement, in Rutter's Child and Adolescent Psychiatry, 6th Edition. Edited by Thapar A, Pine DS, Leckman JF, et al. New York, Wiley Blackwell, 2015, pp 795–805

Zhang W, Deng W, Yao L, et al: Brain structural abnormalities in a group of never-medicated patients with long-term schizophrenia. Am J Psychiatry 172(10):995–1003, 2015 26085040

Zimmerman M, Chelminski I, Young D: The frequency of personality disorders in psychiatric patients. Psychiatr Clin North Am 31(3):405–420, 2008 18638643

Zola S: Amnesia: neuroanatomic and clinical aspects, in Behavioral Neurology and neuropsychology. Edited by Feinberg TE, Farah MJ. New York, McGraw-Hill, 1997, pp 447–461

Zuckerman ML, Vaughan BL, Whitney J, et al: Tolerability of selective serotonin reuptake inhibitors in thirty-nine children under age seven: a retrospective chart review, in Advances in Preschool Psychopharmacology. Edited by Luby JL, Riddle MA. New Rochelle, NY, Mary Ann Liebert, 2009, pp 7–16

Index

Page numbers printed in **boldface** *type refer to tables or figures. Page numbers followed by* n *indicate note numbers.*